The Adolescent Athlete

The Adolescent Athlete

A Practical Approach

Edited by

Lyle J. Micheli, MD

Clinical Professor, Department of Orthopaedic Surgery, Harvard Medical School; Director, Division of Sports Medicine, Children's Hospital Boston; O'Donnell Family Professor of Orthopaedic Sports Medicine, Children's Hospital Boston, Boston Massachusetts, USA

Laura Purcell, MSc, MD, FRCPC, FAAP, Dip Sport Med

Assistant Professor, Departments of Internal Medicine, Pediatrics, and Family Medicine, Schulich School of Medicine at the University of Western Ontario; Pediatric Emergency Consultant, Children's Hospital of Western Ontario; Pediatric Sport Medicine Physician, Fowler Kennedy Sport Medicine Clinic, London, Ontario, Canada

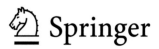 Springer

Lyle J. Micheli, MD
Clinical Professor
Department of Orthopaedic Surgery
Harvard Medical School
Director
Division of Sports Medicine
Children's Hospital Boston
O'Donnell Family Professor of
  Orthopaedic Sports Medicine
Children's Hospital Boston
Boston, MA, USA

Laura Purcell, MSc, MD, FRCPC,
  FAAP, Dip Sport Med
Assistant Professor
Departments of Internal Medicine,
  Pediatrics, and Family Medicine
Schulich School of Medicine at the
  University of Western Ontario
Pediatric Emergency Consultant
Children's Hospital of Western Ontario
Pediatric Sport Medicine Physician
Fowler Kennedy Sport Medicine Clinic
London, ON, Canada

Alice Y. Chen, Medical Illustrator, is responsible for Figures 3.1A, 3.1B, 3.3A, 3.4A, 3.5A, 4.5, 6.2, 7.1, 10.1, 11.1A, 11.1B, and 13.1A

Library of Congress Control Number: 2007925042

ISBN: 978-0-387-35964-9   e-ISBN: 978-0-387-49825-6

Printed on acid-free paper.

9 8 7 6 5 4 3 2 1

springer.com

Preface

Good health should be a goal of all children and adolescents, as well as the parents and guardians who care for them. Regular physical activity is part of achieving this goal. Sports can provide manifold benefits, including fitness, motor skill development, teamwork, and of course, *fun*. As with any pursuit that provides such benefits, however, there are risks involved, particularly for growing athletes. Physicians and other health professionals caring for active children should be able to provide appropriate care and advice for sport and fitness-related medical issues.

This book is written as a practical guide for those of us who provide care for young athletes. The focus is on musculoskeletal injuries that occur in this unique population, as well as conditions that may present as a musculoskeletal injury, but may have more serious consequences. The first section of the book focuses on rehabilitation and diagnostic imaging of musculoskeletal conditions in adolescents. The second section—organized according to anatomical region—addresses specific injuries that adolescents may sustain as a result of sport/activity participation. Each of these body part–specific chapters begins with a review of the relevant anatomy, followed by details of clinical evaluation. Specific injuries, such as acute and chronic injuries, are described in detail, including the management/treatment of each condition. Prevention of injuries and return to play guidelines are given full shrift. Each chapter concludes with "clinical pearls" that provide an insight into the way each of our expert authors practice their craft. Given the distinguished group of authors who graciously agreed to contribute to this resource, just these pearls themselves are worth the "price of admission"!

This prompts us to thank all those who generously donated their time and expertise to this project, particularly the chapter authors and our editors at Springer. Without their contributions, this project would not have come to fruition.

Lyle J. Micheli, MD
Laura Purcell, MSc, MD, FRCPC, FAAP, Dip Sport Med

Contents

Contributors

Donald S. Bae, MD
Instructor, Department of Orthopaedic Surgery, Harvard Medical School; Associate in Orthopaedic Surgery, Harvard Medical School, Children's Hospital Boston, Boston, MA, USA

John P. Batson, MD, FAAP
Clinical Associate Professor, Department of Pediatrics, University of South Carolina School of Medicine; Youth Sports Medicine, The Moore Orthopaedic Clinic, Columbia, SC, USA

Treg Brown, MD
Attending Physician, Southern Orthopedic Associates; Assistant Clinical Professor, Department of Orthopaedic Surgery, Tulane University, Herron, IL USA

Michelina C. Cassella, PT
Director, Department of Physical Therapy and Occupational Therapy, Children's Hospital Boston, Boston, MA, USA

Vernon M. Chapman, MD
Assistant Clinical Professor, Department of Radiology, The Children's Hospital/Radiology Imaging Associates, Denver, CO, USA

Christine Curtis, BS
Research Coordinator, Department of Orthopedics, Division of Sports Medicine, Harvard Medical School, Children's Hospital Boston, Boston, MA, USA

Jessica Flynn Deede, MD
Fellow, Department of Orthopedics, Division of Sports Medicine, Harvard University, Children's Hospital Boston, Boston, MA, USA

Pierre d'Hemecourt, MD, FACSM
Director of Primary Care/Sports Medicine, Division of Sports Medicine, Children's Hospital Boston, Boston, MA, USA

John A. Guido, Jr., MHS, PT, ATC, SCS, CSCS
Director, Sports Therapy and Director, Sports Performance, Texas Metroplex Institute for Sports Medicine and Orthopedics, Grand Prairie, TX 75050, USA

Diego Jaramillo, MD, MPH
Radiologist-in-Chief and Professor, Department of Radiology, Children's Hospital of Philadelphia, University of Pennsylvania, Philadelphia, PA, USA

Hamish Kerr, MBChB, MSc
Assistant Professor, Department of Medicine, Albany Medical Center, Latham, MA, USA

Margaret Lee, MD
Family Practice Resident, Department of Family and Community Medicine, University of California, San Francisco, CA, USA

Mark D. Locke, MD, FAAP
Pediatric Orthopaedic Surgeon, The Moore Orthopaedic Clinic, Columbia, SC, USA

Anthony Luke MD, MPH
Assistant Professor and Director, Primary Care Sports Medicine, Departments of Orthopedics and Family and Community Medicine, University of California, San Francisco, San Francisco, CA, USA

Angus M. McBryde, Jr., MD, FACS
Foot and Ankle Orthopaedic Surgeon, Alabama Sports Medicine and Orthopaedic Center, St. Vincent's Hospital, Birmingham, AL, USA

Michelle McTimoney, MD, FRCPC, Dip Sport Med
Pediatrician, Department of Emergency Medicine, IWK Health Center, Dalhousie University, Halifax, Nova Scotia, Canada

Lyle J. Micheli, MD
Clinical Professor, Department of Orthopaedic Surgery, Harvard Medical School; Director, Division of Sports Medicine, Children's Hospital Boston; O'Donnell Family Professor of Orthopaedic Sports Medicine, Children's Hospital Boston, Boston, MA, USA

Jason H. Nielson, MD
Attending, Department of Orthopedics, Sunrise Children's Hospital, Henderson, NV, USA

Laura Purcell, MSc, MD, FRCPC, FAAP, Dip Sport Med
Assistant Professor, Departments of Internal Medicine, Pediatrics, and Family Medicine, Schulich School of Medicine at the University of Western Ontario; Pediatric Emergency Consultant, Children's Hospital of Western Ontario; Pediatric Sport Medicine Physician, Fowler Kennedy Sport Medicine Clinic, London, ON, Canada

Kathleen Richards, BS
Clinical Manager, Department of Physical Therapy, Children's Hospital Boston, Boston, MA, USA

Marc Safran, MD
Associate Professor, Director, UCSF Sports Medicine, Departments of Orthopedics and Family and Community Medicine, University of California, San Francisco, San Francisco CA, USA

Angela D. Smith, MD
Department of Orthopaedics, The Sports Medicine and Performance Center at the Children's Hospital of Philadelphia, King of Prussia, PA, USA

Merrilee Zetaruk, MD, FRCPC
Associate Professor, Faculty of Medicine, Department of Pediatrics and Child Health, University of Manitoba, Winnipeg, Manitoba, Canada

Introduction

Sports participation by children and adolescents has exploded in recent years. In the United States, more than 35 million children participate in organized sport, with millions of others participating at a recreational level (1). Children are becoming involved at younger and younger ages, and are often participating in sports year-round. They are also participating at more and more competitive levels, necessitating training with increased intensity.

Injuries related to sports participation occur frequently (2), accounting for more than one third of all injuries (3). The majority of injuries occur in young athletes, with an estimated 2.6 million emergency visits per year related to sport injury for those aged 5–24 years (4). Childhood injuries are a frequent reason for visits to primary care offices as well, accounting for 1 of every 10 visits, with >25% of adolescent visits attributable to sports (5). Musculoskeletal injuries are the third most common reason for adolescents to seek medical attention, with knee pain being the most frequent complaint (6).

With the increasing participation of today's youth in sports, it is imperative that health care providers taking care of these children and adolescents are prepared to address their unique needs. Young athletes have specific needs that set them apart from adult athletes. Understanding the developmental changes that occur during childhood and adolescence, which result in different injury patterns and psychological issues, is essential to provide exceptional care for young athletes. Knowledge of the physical and emotional development, as well as the level of skill and motivation, of adolescents will help prevent injuries and promote healthy participation and enjoyment of sport.

Benefits of Sports

The benefits of sports include psychosocial, physical, and health-related benefits. Sports provide an enjoyable opportunity for children and adolescents to be active. Being active helps youths to achieve a healthy weight

1

and increase physical fitness. Sports may provide youth the opportunity to develop independence, identify with a peer group, and increase social interaction. Youths can achieve success by improving and mastering new skills and participating in a common goal. This success can improve their sense of self-esteem and can help build confidence (7).

Older children who participate in sports are less likely to adopt risky behaviors, such as smoking, doing drugs, and breaking the law. Sports participation is associated with elevated social status among peer groups, and it may provide opportunities for traveling with a team, as well as the possibility of athletic scholarships (7).

Positive sport experiences may go a long way to maintaining exercise and sport during the adult years. By adopting a healthy active lifestyle, adolescents may reduce the risk of chronic health problems in adulthood, such as cardiovascular disease, obesity, and Type II diabetes (7).

Adults play an important role in providing positive sports experiences for children. They teach children motor skills, the rules of the sport, and sportsmanship. Adults can act as role models for youth, and are instrumental in organizing sporting opportunities for children. However, organized sports should be developmentally appropriate for children so that they have fun being physically active (8–11). Children should be encouraged to participate in a variety of activities and avoid early specialization (12).

Sport Readiness

"Sport readiness" implies a certain level of physical, cognitive, and emotional development that allows the acquisition of the necessary skills to meet the demands of sports (8–11). Although there are many benefits to sport, sporting activities must be developmentally appropriate to ensure that children enjoy the activity. Placing children in sports that are beyond their developmental ability can cause frustration and loss of enjoyment, and ultimately lead to the decision not to participate (8–11).

One aspect of sport readiness is motor development. Learning and mastering fundamental motor skills such as throwing, running, and jumping, is an innate process, independent of gender or physical maturity. Each fundamental skill is composed of a sequence of developmental stages that all children progress through, but at variable rates. Most children have acquired some fundamental skills by preschool age. However, it is not until children reach 6 yr of age that sufficient combinations of fundamental skills are attained to allow them to begin organized sports (8–11).

Choosing appropriate sport activities can be guided by knowledge of the developmental capabilities of children of various ages (Table I.1). Sports activities can be modified to match children's developmental levels by simple modifications, such as shorter games, smaller equipment, and frequent changing of positions (8–11).

TABLE I.1. Developmental skills and sport recommendations during childhood and adolescence.

	Middle childhood 6–9yr	Late childhood 10–12yr	Early adolescence 13–15yr	Late adolescence 16–18yr
Motor skills	• Mature fundamental sport skills • Posture, balance improving • Beginning transitional skills (e.g., throwing for accuracy)	• Improving transitional skills • Mastering complex motor skills (e.g., layup in basketball)	• Tremendous growth • Loss of flexibility • Differences with timing of puberty	• Continued growth into adulthood • Mature sport skills
Learning	• Short attention span • Limited memory and rapid decision-making	• Attention span improving but remains selective • Improving memory	• Improved attention span • Good memory skills, able to memorize plays and strategize	• Good attention span, memory skills
Skill emphasis	• Emphasize fundamental skills • Encourage beginning transitional skills	• Emphasize skill development • Increasing emphasis on tactics and strategy	• Promote individual strengths	• Promote individual strengths
Suggested activities	Entry level soccer and baseball; swimming; running; gymnastics; skating; dance; racquet sports	Entry-level football, basketball, ice hockey	Early-maturing boys: track and field, basketball, ice hockey Late-maturing girls: gymnastics, skating	All sports depending on interest

Source: Purcell, 2005. Adapted with permission from Paediatrics and Child Health.

By middle childhood, most children achieve mature patterns of fundamental motor skills and are beginning to learn transitional skills (Table I.1). Transitional skills are fundamental abilities performed in combination or with variation, for example, throwing for distance or accuracy. Improvement of transitional skills progresses through late childhood, and by the time they reach adolescence, most youths are able to master complex motor skills, such as a lay-up in basketball. Motor skills continue to improve throughout adolescence (8–11).

Cognitive development is another aspect of determining sport readiness. Young children have short attention spans, limited memory, and an inability to make rapid decisions. Sports activities for young children should therefore concentrate on mastering fundamental skills and the development of transitional skills. Instruction should be short, rules should be flexible, and the emphasis should be on fun, not competition. As children grow older, their memory improves and their attention spans increase, but may remain selective. Older children are capable of learning strategy and tactics, and can begin to master more complex play combinations (8–11).

Children are unique from adults in that they are growing, which predisposes them to unique injuries. Growth during adolescence is particularly marked. There are dramatic increases in muscle mass, muscle strength, and cardiopulmonary endurance during this period. Adolescents continue to increase both fat mass and fat-free mass, although during puberty, girls tend to accumulate fat mass at a greater rate. Muscle strength increases in both sexes, but is greater in boys. Loss of flexibility and a temporary decrease in coordination and balance is common during adolescence (13).

Growth, Maturation, and Development

As children progress through adolescence to adulthood, they are subject to three interacting processes: growth, maturation, and development (14,15). As they grow, children increase in height and weight, in lean and fat tissues, and in the size of their organs. Maturation is the state of maturity, in which growth has been completed. Development is the process of learning appropriate behaviors in society. Children develop behaviorally in the acquisition of motor skills, as well as cognitively, emotionally, socially, and morally. It is important to be aware of these interactions in children and adolescents, and how they may potentially affect a youth's ability to participate in sports (14,15).

Sexual Maturity

Adolescence is marked by sexual growth and maturity, i.e., the process of puberty. Secondary sexual characteristics, including pubic hair in both sexes, breast development and menarche in girls, and penis and testes development in boys, forms the basis of assessment of sexual maturity (14). Tanner developed a sexual maturation scale based on the development of secondary sexual characteristics (Table I.2) (16).

Puberty can affect sports performance (14,15). The onset of puberty can be quite variable and can result in differences in physical attributes important to sport. Boys who mature early are taller, stronger, and have greater muscle mass than those who enter puberty later, and are therefore usually better suited to sports requiring physical strength, such as American football. Girls who mature late have narrower shoulders and hips, and are well-suited to esthetic sports, such as figure skating and dance (8–15).

TABLE I.2. Tanner staging.

A. Girls

Tanner stage	Stage of development	Pubic hair	Breasts
Stage 1	Preadolescence	No pubic hair	Juvenile breasts with elevated papilla and small flat areola
Stage 2	Early adolescence (10–13 yrs)	Sparse, long, and straight, slightly pigmented	Buds form papilla, and areola form small mound
Stage 3	Middle adolescence (12–14 yrs)	Dark and curly	Continued enlargement of breast bud and areola, with no separation of breast contour
Stage 4	Middle adolescence	Coarse in texture; number of hairs continue to curl and increase	Papilla and areola separate to form a secondary mound
Stage 5	Late adolescence 14–16 yrs	Adult triangle pattern with spread to surface of medial thigh	Mature areola mound recedes into contour of the breast, nipples project

B. Boys

Tanner stage	Stage of development	Pubic hair	Penis/testes
Stage 1	Preadolescence	No pubic hair	Identical to early childhood
Stage 2	Early adolescence (10.5–14 yrs)	Sparse, long, and straight, slightly pigmented at base of penis	Enlargement of testes and scrotum; reddish color and enlargement of penis
Stage 3	Middle adolescence (12.5–15 yrs)	Increase curl and pigmentation, spreading laterally	Continued growth, penis increases in length
Stage 4	Middle adolescence	Coarse in texture, more adult in distribution	Continued growth of testes and scrotum skin darkens, penis grows in width, glans penis develops
Stage 5	Late adolescence (14–16 yrs)	Mature distribution with spreading to medial thigh	Mature adult size and shape of testes, scrotum, and penis

Source: Adapted by permission from Tanner JM. Growth at Adolescence. 2nd ed. Osney Mead, Oxford: Blackwell Scientific Ltd.; 1962. © Blackwell Scientific Publications.

Skeletal Maturity

Children's bones are different from those in adults in that they are still growing. The reaction of growing bones to trauma is therefore different. Growing bones are not as dense, are more porous, and possess a striated cortex with loosely attached periosteum. Bones in children have a growth plate complex, which includes the epiphysis, physis, and diaphysis. The developing physis or growth plate is especially vulnerable to injury, and if growth plate injuries are not managed properly, can lead to permanent disability (17).

The physis is located between the epiphysis and metaphysis (Figure I.1). It is a cartilaginous plate where endochondral growth occurs, resulting in bone lengthening. It is the weakest link in the bone–ligament complex, which results in different injury patterns in children. Injuries in adults are more likely to be ligament ruptures, whereas in children, because the ligament is stronger than the physis, a child is more likely to sustain a growth plate injury, particularly in the knee and ankle (17).

As skeletal maturity approaches, the physis narrows and is replaced by bone until it closes. This results in unique injuries at this age, particularly in ankle injuries. Fractures in young children usually occur parallel to the physis, whereas in adolescents, fractures occur through the physis and into the articular surface (Figure I.1) (17,18).

Another unique feature of children's bones is the presence of apophyses. An apophysis is a prominence of bone that is also a center of growth of the bone. It acts as an attachment for muscle groups. Apophyses are found around the pelvis, the patella, the tibial tubercle, the calcaneus, and the base of the fifth metatarsal, and are sites of avulsion injuries in growing athletes. During growth spurts, muscles and tendons get stretched out and can result in increased tension at the sites of attachment, causing inflammation and pain (apophysitis). Some examples of apophysities include

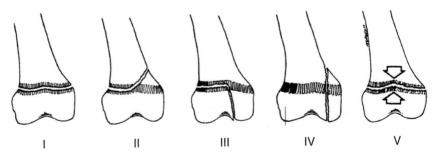

| I | II | III | IV | V |

FIGURE I.1. Salter–Harris classification of growth plate injuries. From Micheli LJ, Musculoskeletal trauma in children. In: Green M, Haggerty RJ, eds. Ambulatory Peds. 1984; 3(1):195–196. Reprinted with permission from The Ambulatory Pediatric Association.

Osgood–Schlatter and Sever's diseases. With sufficient force, the muscles attached to apophyses can pull off a piece of bone, resulting in an avulsion fracture. These injuries are commonly seen in adolescents who are going through growth spurts (18).

Risk of Injury

Injuries are an inevitable part of participating in sports. Certain injuries are associated with particular sports, such as patellar tendonitis and ankle injuries in basketball (19). Certain sports are associated with more injuries. Girls' cross-country, football, wrestling, and girls' soccer have been associated with the greatest number of injuries, based on injury rate/1,000 athletic exposures (19). Ankle and knee injuries are among the most common injuries as a result of sports (6,19).

Various methods of preventing injuries can be employed. Preparticipation physicals can help identify medical problems, previous injuries, or risk factors for further injury in young athletes. By assessing an athlete's general health, level of fitness, flexibility, strength and joint stability, treatment or preconditioning recommendations can be made to reduce injury risk before sports participation. Appropriate sport-specific conditioning programs can prepare athletes for the demands of their particular sport (20).

Ensuring a proper diet and conditioning in all adolescent athletes is key to maintaining general health. Rest is also important for growing athletes to recuperate from sport, particularly during times of growth when injury risk is higher. Avoidance of overtraining will help ensure athletes are not developing overuse injuries or burning out. Participating in a variety of activities will help ensure children develop a variety of skills and help prevent overuse injuries (12). Making sure that injuries are properly rehabilitated will help prevent further injury (20).

Parents, coaches, and trainers can reduce the incidence of injuries by ensuring the proper use of protective equipment, ensuring safe play conditions, enforcing rules, and providing appropriate supervision. Ensuring the proper selection of sporting events can also minimize injuries. Sports should be matched to the child's interest and abilities (8–11,20).

Conclusion

Sports are a great way for youth to be physically active. There are many benefits to sports participation, including physical health, skill development, and social interaction. Children and adolescents can get the most out of sports when the activities are geared towards their interests and developmental level.

The risk of injury is inherent to sports participation. Children and adolescents are subject to unique injuries because they are still growing.

Injuries can be prevented by ensuring children are in good physical condition, by the use of proper equipment and by ensuring that playing conditions are safe. Participating in a variety of activities will also help minimize injuries.

References

1. Stirling JM, Landry GL. Sports medicine training during pediatric residency. Arch Pediatr Adolesc Med 1996;150:211–215.
2. Metzl JD. Sports medicine in pediatric practice: keeping pace with the changing times. Pediatr Ann 2000;29:146–148.
3. Bijur PE, Trumble A, Harel Y, Overpeck MD, Jones D, Scheidt PC. Sports and recreation injuries in US children and adolescents. Arch Pediatr Adolesc Med 1995;149:1009–1016.
4. Burt CW, Overpeck MD. Emergency visits for sports-related injuries. Ann Emerg Med 2001;37:301–308.
5. Hambidge SJ, Davidson AJ, Gonzales R, Steiner JF. Epidemiology of pediatric injury-related primary care office visits in the United States. Pediatrics 2002; 109:559–565.
6. Ziv A, Boulet JR, Slap GB. Utilization of physician offices by adolescents in the United States. Pediatrics 1999;104:35–41.
7. Landry GL. Benefits of sports participation. In: Sullivan JA and Anderson SJ, eds. Care of the Young Athlete. Rosemont, Illinois: American Academy of Orthopaedic Surgeons and American Academy of Pediatrics; 2000:1–8.
8. Purcell L. Sport readiness in children and youth. Paediatr Child Health 2005; 10:343–344.
9. Patel DR, Pratt HD, Greydanus DE. Pediatric neurodevelopment and sports participation: When are children ready to play sports? Pediatr Clin N Am 2002;49:505–531.
10. Nelson MA. Developmental skills and children's sports. Physician Sportsmed 1991;19:67–79.
11. Harris S. Readiness to participate in sports. In: Sullivan JA, Anderson SJ, eds. Care of the Young Athlete. Rosemont, Illinois: American Academy of Orthopaedic Surgeons and American Academy of Pediatrics; 2000:19–24.
12. International Federation of Sports Medicine. Position statement on excessive physical training in children and adolescents. Clin J Sport Med 1991;1:262–264.
13. Gomez JE. Growth and maturation. In: Sullivan JA, Anderson SJ, eds. Care of the Young Athlete. Rosemont, Illinois: American Academy of Orthopaedic Surgeons and American Academy of Pediatrics; 2000:25–32.
14. Malina RM. Growth and maturation: applications to children and adolescents in sports. In: Birrer RB, Griesemer BA, Cataleto MB, eds. Philadelphia: Lippincott, Williams and Wilkins; 2002:39–58.
15. Baxter-Jones ADG and Malina RM. Growth and maturation issues in elite young athletes: normal variation and training. In: Maffuli N, Chan KM, Macdonald R, Malina RM and Parker AW, eds. Sport Medicine for Specific Ages and Abilities. London: Churchill Livingstone; 2001:95–108.

16. Tanner JM. Growth at adolscence, 2nd ed. Osney Mead, Oxford: Blackwell Scientific Ltd; 1962.
17. Thornton A and Gyll C. Children's fractures. London: WB Saunders 1999:2.
18. Martin TJ and Martin JS. Special issues and concerns for the high school- and college-aged athletes. Pediatr Clin N Am 2002;49:533–552.
19. Rice SG. Risks of injury during sports participation. In: Sullivan JA, Anderson SJ, eds. Care of the Young Athlete. Rosemont, Illinois: American Academy of Orthopaedic Surgeons and American Academy of Pediatrics; 2000:9–18.
20. Barfield WR and Gross RH. Injury prevention. In: Sullivan JA, Anderson SJ, eds. Care of the Young Athlete. Rosemont, Illinois: American Academy of Orthopaedic Surgeons and American Academy of Pediatrics; 2000:121–136.

Section I
Rehabilitation and Diagnosis

1
Principles of Rehabilitation

Michelina C. Cassella and Kathleen Richards

The number of adolescent athletes competing in organized sports has significantly increased over the past several years, thus causing a rise in sport-related injuries. Adolescents are specializing in sports at an earlier age and, in some cases, performing excessive and repetitive training that often leads to overuse injuries. Sport is the number one cause of injuries in 5–17-yr-old children (1). Many sports-related injuries do not receive proper rehabilitation. Adolescents may return to sports training and/or competition too quickly after an injury. This often causes a recurrence of the injury and/or the development of a new injury. Therefore, a comprehensive rehabilitation program to successfully manage an injury is extremely important to ensure the safe return to sport and/or competition. Appropriate rehabilitation and education of athletes, parents, and coaches are essential components in assisting the young athlete's recovery. In addition, the rehabilitation program should include the athlete's personal goals.

The evidence for rehabilitation practice in the field of adolescent sports medicine is often lacking proper research studies, particularly clinical trials. Many of the recommended rehabilitation programs are based on clinical experience, mainly with an adult population.

Before establishing a rehabilitation program, consideration must be given to the adolescent athlete's stage of maturation, which is more important than chronological age. Adolescence is a difficult period to define because of the wide variation in time of onset and termination. Age ranges of 8–19 yr in girls and 10–22 yr in boys are often listed as limits for the adolescent period. During this period, bodily systems become adult both structurally and functionally. Structurally, the rate of growth in stature marks the onset of the adolescent growth spurt. The rate of the statural growth reaches a peak, decelerates, and finally terminates with the attainment of adult stature (2).

Functionally, adolescence is defined by sexual maturation. Tanner and associates developed a sexual maturation scale that correlates with peak height velocity (*see* Table I.1 in the Introduction) (2). Tanner stage 1 is determined by growth hormone production, whereas stages 2–5 are related to sex hormones (3). Therefore, children are described as prepubertal

(Tanner stage 1), pubertal (Tanner stage 3), and postpubertal (Tanner stage 5). Postpubertal individuals are physically adults. Tanner staging is useful in determining the appropriate treatment and rehabilitative interventions. This chapter discusses the principles of rehabilitation, with emphasis on the evidence supporting these principles.

Principles of Rehabilitation

The major principle of rehabilitation is to safely maximize the athlete's abilities, despite an existing and/or a developing impairment. The goals of a rehabilitation program are to control inflammation and pain, promote healing, restore function, safely return to sports training and/or competition, and prevent future injury. In addition, maintaining the athlete's level of physical fitness while recovering from an injury is an essential component of the rehabilitation program.

The rehabilitation program includes assessments of posture, joint range of motion, muscle strength, endurance, balance, coordination, and function (4–8). Posture deviations and muscle weakness and/or tightness often lead to serious imbalances that can cause malalignment, an increase in pain, a decrease in function, and a predisposition to future injury.

Rehabilitation Program

A comprehensive rehabilitation program includes a detailed patient history, a review, an examination of all systems, and the establishment of a plan of care.

Patient History

Information is gathered from both the patient and parent (Table 1.1).

TABLE 1.1. Patient history.

Patient history

- Demographics and developmental history
- Current medical diagnoses
- Previous diagnoses
- Past injuries with dates
- Surgical history with dates and complications (if any)
- Medications
- Chronological age; bone age
- Review of clinical tests (MRI, bone scan, radiograph)
- Past and present activity level
- Recreational versus competitive activity
- Pain assessment at rest, night, with activity (age appropriate pain scale) patient's current concerns and goals[1]

Source: Cassella M, Richards K. Physical therapy/rehabilitation. In: The Pediatric and Adolescent Knee. Micheli L, Kocher, eds. 2006. By permission of Elsevier.

TABLE 1.2. Resting adolescent heart rate by sex and age.

Age	12	13	14	15	16	17
White males	76	76	74	73	70	73
White females	86	83	84	83	84	81
Afro-american males	75	71	73	71	69	66
Afro-american females	81	80	80	80	78	77

Source: Rabbia et al., 2002.

Systems Review

Gathering baseline information before treatment intervention is necessary to establish goals, monitor the effects of both therapeutic and conditioning exercises, and identify risks factors that may contribute to future injury. Systems to review include:

1. Cardiovascular/Pulmonary: Knowledge of normal respiratory rates, heart rates, and blood pressure for adolescents is necessary to monitor their response to treatment (Tables 1.2 and 1.3) (9,10).

2. Integumentary: Assessment of the integumentary system includes skin integrity, color, trophic changes, and scar formation. Blistering, skin temperature, scar tissue pliability, texture, and sensation should be observed. Activities or movements that aggravate the incisional site should be documented in adolescents who have had surgery. Scar types include contracture, hypertrophic, and keloid. A contracture scar is a tightening of surrounding tissues. These scars tend to cause impaired movement. Hypertrophic scar tissue can be caused by the overproduction of connective tissue. They are raised above the skin, thick, red, and itchy. Keloid formations are highly thickened areas of scar tissue. They are larger and more raised than the hypertrophic scars. This type of scarring is often genetic (11).

3. Musculoskeletal: Tightness in the muscle–tendon units seems to occur in the absence of injury as the athlete enters puberty. Adolescent athletes,

TABLE 1.3. Blood pressure for girls and boys by age and height percentile of 50%.

Age	Girls systolic/diastolic	Boys systolic/diastolic
11	103/61	104/61
12	105/62	106/62
13	107/63	108/62
14	109/64	111/63
15	110/65	113/64
16	111/66	116/65
17	111/66	118/67

Source: Staley and Richard, 2001.

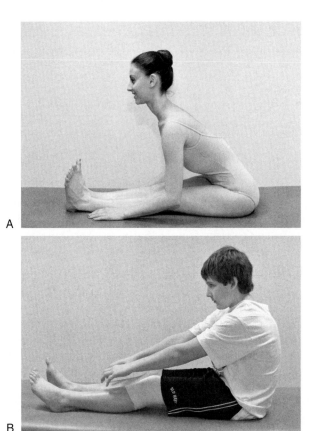

FIGURE 1.1. Hamstring length. **(A)** Normal and better than normal hamstring length. The dancer is able to exceed a 90-degree hip angle keeping her knee straight. **(B)** Tightness in the hamstring. The athlete has had an increase in linear growth; therefore, he is unable to attain a 90-degree hip angle with his knees straight.

particularly males, demonstrate a generalized loss of flexibility, especially in larger muscle groups, such as the hip flexors, hamstring, quadriceps, and triceps surae. Linear growth in the long bones and spine exceeds the rate of growth of the muscle–tendon unit. Therefore, during the adolescent growth spurt, a loss of both strength and flexibility can often occur (Figure 1.1) (12). The loss of strength and flexibility not only impacts the athlete's athletic ability, but also often leads to serious injuries. Therefore, detailed posture, joint range, muscle strength, and functional assessments should be performed at regular intervals to determine the athlete's fitness for sports activities. Specific tests and measurements will enable the professional to establish a baseline for appropriate treatment interventions for an existing injury and to prevent future injuries.

4. Posture: A detailed posture assessment helps the examiner identify deviations and/or malalignment (Table 1.4). Both can have a serious, nega-

Table 1.4. Posture assessment.

Posture Evaluation Form				

Name: _____ Medical Record
NO. _____ D.O.B. _____ Sex ____
Diagnosis _____ Surgical Procedure/Date _____
          Precautions _____

Posterior view			Left	Right
Head	Centered	Tilt		
Shoulders	Level	Elevated		
Scapulae	Level	Elevated		
Spine	Aligned	Shifted		
Waist folds	Symmetrical	Increased		
Pelvis	Level	Elevated		
Knees	Aligned	Varus		
		Valgus		
Heels	Aligned	Varus		
		Valgus		

Anterior view			Left	Right
Head	Centered	Tilt		
Neck folds	Symmetrical	Increased		
Breasts	Symmetrical	Prominent		
Arm length	Equal	Longer		
Pelvis	Level	Elevated		
Knees	Aligned	Varus		
		Valgus		
Forefoot	Aligned			
	Pronated			
	Supinated			

Lateral view		Left	Right
Head	Aligned	Forward	Backward
Cervical (anterior) curve	Normal	Increased	Decreased
Shoulders	Level	Forward	Backward
Scapulae	Aligned	Protracted	Retracted
Thoracic (posterior) curve	Normal	Increased	Decreased
Lumbar (anterior) curve	Normal	Increased	Decreased
Pelvis	Aligned	Anterior Tilt	Posterior Tilt

Adams forward bend test		Left	Right
Thoracic	Negative	Rib hump	Rib hump
Lumbar	Negative	Increased m. bulk	Increased m. bulk
Knees	Aligned	Hyperextension	Hyperextension
Ankles	Aligned	Increased DF	Increased DF
		Increased PF	Increased PF

Source: Cassella M, Richards K. Physical therapy/rehabilitation. In: The Pediatric and Adolescent Knee. Micheli L, Kocher, eds. 2006. By permission of Elsevier.

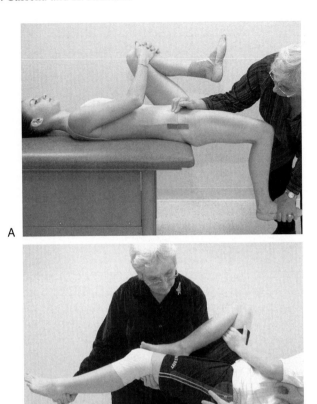

FIGURE 1.2. Thomas test. **(A) Negative** Thomas test. The lumbar spine remains flat on the table, the pelvis is in a neutral position, and the thigh is in contact with the table, indicating appropriate length of the iliopsoas muscle. **(B) Positive** Thomas test. The lumbar spine loses contact with the table, and the pelvis moves anteriorly at 30 degrees of hip flexion, indicating tightness in the iliopsoas muscle.

tive impact on body mechanics and sport-specific techniques. In addition, identifying postural deviations leads the examiner to further investigate specific joint and/or muscle impairments.

  5. Joint range of motion: Standardized testing includes measuring each joint, especially those that impact the athlete's performance. A few examples of tests that measure tightness in muscle groups that are generally affected during the adolescent growth spurt are as follows:

a. Thomas test: The Thomas test measures tightness in the iliopsoas muscle (Figure 1.2). Restricted flexibility in this muscle can cause increased lumbar hyperlordosis, decreased hip extension, and an increase in knee hyperextension. The test is performed passively. The patient is positioned supine with both hips and knees flexed to the chest, with the lower back flat on the table. The patient holds one leg flexed to the chest. The examiner cradles the other leg and has one hand around the pelvis. The examiner's thumb is positioned on the anterior superior iliac spine (ASIS) to determine when the pelvis begins to move anteriorly. The examiner passively lowers the leg. When the ASIS begins to move anteriorly, the test is stopped and the angle of hip flexion is measured (13).

  b. Straight leg raise: The straight leg raise measures hamstring tightness (Figure 1.3). Restricted flexibility in the hamstrings will negatively affect

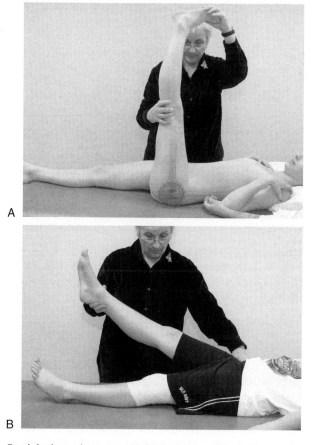

FIGURE 1.3. Straight leg raise test. **(A) Negative** straight leg raise test. The pelvis remains in a neutral position as the straight leg is passively flexed to 90 degrees, indicating appropriate length of the hamstrings muscles. **(B) Positive** straight leg raise test. The pelvis begins to move anteriorly at 40 degrees of hip flexion, indicating tightness in the hamstrings muscles.

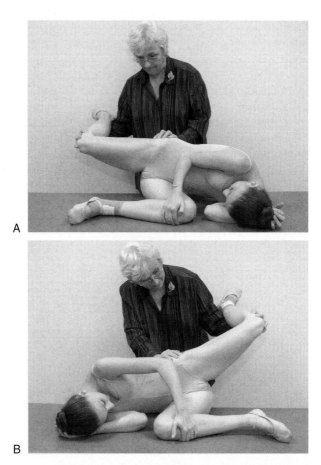

FIGURE 1.4. Ober test. **(A) Negative** Ober test. The thigh and knee are horizontal in relation to the hip joint, indicating normal length of the ITB. **(B) Positive** Ober test. The thigh and knee are above the horizontal in relation to the hip joint indicating a tight ITB.

low back, pelvis, hip, and knee alignment. The straight leg raise test focuses on proximal hamstring tightness. The test is performed passively. The patient is positioned supine with hips and knees extended and the pelvis in a neutral position. The examiner cradles the leg with one arm and has the other hand around the pelvis. The examiner's thumb is positioned on the ASIS. The examiner passively raises the leg, keeping the knee straight. As soon as the ASIS begins to move posteriorly, the test is stopped and the angle of hip flexion is measured (14,15).

c. Ober test: The Ober test measures tightness in the iliotibial band (ITB) (Figure 1.4). Restricted flexibility of the ITB often promotes lateral tracking of the patella. This malalignment of the patella can disrupt knee joint mechanics. Tightness of the ITB not only contributes to knee pain but can also interfere with function. The test is performed passively. The patient is positioned sidelying, with the lumbar spine in flexion. The hips and knees are flexed to the chest. The patient's neck and trunk are also flexed. The patient holds the bottom leg to the chest while the examiner cradles the top leg, keeping the knee flexed. The examiner flexes the hip and then widely abducts and extends the hip to allow the tensor fasciae latae muscle to move over the greater trochanter. The examiner attempts to passively lower the leg to the horizontal position (14).

d. Ely Test: The Ely test measures tightness in the rectus femoris muscle (Figure 1.5). Restricted flexibility in this muscle can also have a negative

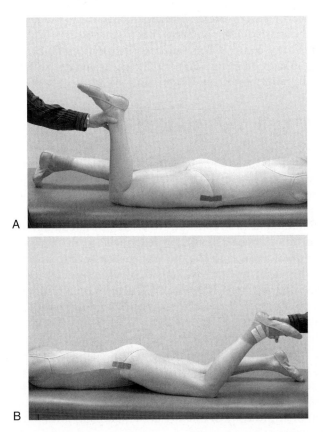

FIGURE 1.5. Ely test. **(A) Negative** Ely test. The anterior hip remains in contact with the table when the knee is flexed to 90 degrees, indicating appropriate length of the rectus femoris muscle. **(B) Positive** Ely test. The anterior hip loses contact with the table and the buttock begins to rise when the knee is flexed to 60 degrees, indicating tightness in the rectus femoris muscle.

effect on patellar alignment. The test is performed passively. The patient is positioned prone, with the hips and knees extended. The examiner grasps the lower leg and slowly flexes the knee. The test is stopped when the hip begins to flex and the buttock begins to rise. The angle of knee flexion is measured (14).

6. Neuromuscular system: The neuromuscular system includes assessment of strength, coordination, balance, proprioception, agility, and gait. Coordination and agility are the ability to perform movements with appropriate speed, distance, direction, rhythm, and muscle tension. When assessing adolescents, normal development of skill acquisition must be taken into consideration so that testing is age appropriate. By age five, the child can hop 10 hops, but a skillful hop that requires flight and distance continues to develop into early adolescence (15). Neuromuscular training describes a progressive exercise regimen that restores synergy and synchrony of the muscle-firing patterns that are necessary for dynamic stability and fine motor control. This is accomplished by enhancing the dynamic muscular stabilization of the joint and by increasing the athlete's cognitive awareness of both joint position and motion.

Establishment of A Plan of Care

A successful rehabilitation program depends not only on physiological factors but also on the emotional and psychosocial attitudes of the adolescent athlete (16). These factors have a significant influence on compliance, performance, and the expectations of both the athlete and the health professional.

Positive communication is the key to a successful rehabilitation program. Communication between health professionals, team members managing the athlete's condition, and the parents is necessary to achieve a positive outcome. The adolescent understands the consequences of compliance, but often focuses on the here and now (17). Education and detailed explanations with the rationale for each activity will help to promote the athlete's compliance.

The rehabilitation program is based on the diagnosis, the goals of treatment, the athlete's expectations, and the anticipated course of healing (Table 1.5). Acute injuries require early medical attention, especially if the injury affects mechanics and performance. An accurate diagnosis is necessary so that the appropriate management can be planned. The goals of rehabilitation are to control inflammation and pain, promote healing, and restore function. Once the athlete has recovered sufficiently, return to sports and/or competition can be considered. Maintaining the athlete's physical fitness during recovery, education on preventing future injuries, and specialized training to increase performance are essential components of the rehabilitation program.

TABLE 1.5. Guidelines for a rehabilitation program based on the stages of healing.

Time	Stages of Healing	Rehabilitation program	Therapeutic goals
Phase 1 Days 1–3	Acute Inflammation	Modified activities, Ice, Compression, Elevation (MICE); crutches, braces, supportive devices PRN	**1. Control Inflammation and Pain** Acute care management Protect affected area (protective weight bearing in lower extremity injuries) Reduce swelling and inflammation Minimize hypoxic damage to tissue
Days 4–7	Repair/Substrate/ Inflammation	Isometric exercises Gentle "pain free" active range of motion	Limit further tissue damage Gradually increase "pain free" range of motion
Phase 2 Days 7–21	Proliferation	Restore active full range of motion Gentle progressive resistive exercises	**2. Promote Healing** Decrease protected status if indicated (i.e partial weight bearing status) Reduce muscle atrophy Improve: range of motion, flexibility, strength
Phase 3 Week 3 to 6	Healing and Maturation	Functional activities as tolerated More complex movements Progress loading (i.e. cycling, light weights)	**3. Restore Function** Continue to restore range of motion and strength Restore proper muscle activation and biomechanics Improve: proprioception, endurance
Phase 4 Week 6–6 mo	Tissue Remodeling	Sport specific training Simulate the demands of the sport/activity Coordination and balance exercises Eccentric loading exercises	**4. Return to Activities and Sports** Restore anatomic form, physiologic function Improve conditioning Return to play/sport Consider training modifications and return to play/sports
plans			**5. Prevent Future Injury** Protective equipment Injury prevention exercises/ programs

Source: Jarvinen TAH, Jarvinen TLN, Kaariainen M, et al. Muscle injuries: biology and treatment. Am J Sports Med, 2005;33(5);745–764. Reprinted by permission of Sage Publications, Inc.

Rehabilitation Plan of Care

The aims of a rehabilitation plan of care are to:

- provide immediate injury care (RICE)
- promote healing
- restore function
- return to sports and/or competition
- prevent future injury.

Immediate Care

The acronym **RICE** (**R**est/modified activity depending on the severity of the injury, **I**ce, **C**ompression, and **E**levation) is applied in acute injuries. Self-treatment or treatment by the coach or trainer on the field should begin immediately after an injury (18,19). A recent article by Bleakley et al. reviewed the evidence for cryotherapy in the acute management of soft tissue injuries and noted the following:

- Applying ice immediately after an acute injury reduced tissue temperature by 10–15°C.
- Ice applied intermittently at 10-min intervals was shown to be more effective at cooling in animal and human tissues.
- Simultaneous ice and compression did not prove to be any more efficient than compression alone. However, the studies did not look at the thickness of the various dressings that may have impeded the cooling effect.
- Cryotherapy or ice application may be most effective when combined with exercises. The cooling effect reduces pain, spasm, and neural inhibition, which allows exercises to begin earlier.

According to Bleakely et al., because of the variables of the studies reviewed, future studies are required to evaluate the effects of cryotherapy at each phase of an injury (20).

Promote Healing

Controlling pain and reducing inflammation facilitates the healing process.

Currently, there are reliable and valid tools to assess pain in neonates, infants, toddlers, school age children, adolescents, and adults. Adolescents are able to accurately report their pain level because they have developed a more complex pain vocabulary. The Visual Analog Scales can be used with the adolescent athlete. It consists of a horizontal or a vertical line exactly 10 cm long, with anchors (0 no pain, 10 extreme pain) at either end. The athlete marks a point through the line that best describes the pain level, which can be read as a percentage or a number (21).

The athlete needs to be able to differentiate between the pain associated with an injury and the discomfort that can be expected from therapeutic exercise. The athlete also needs to understand that pain is the body's sign that there is a problem. However, the athlete should also be informed that delayed muscle soreness might be expected after stretching or strengthening exercises. If recurrent swelling, increased stiffness, loss of motion or severe discomfort occurs at any time during the rehabilitation program, the exercise should be discontinued and the athlete's physician notified. Treatment is only resumed with physician approval.

The application of the following treatment modalities may not only reduce pain and inflammation but may also enhance the healing process (Table 1.6):

Medications are sometimes prescribed in addition to RICE. However, medications should be used judiciously because the athlete's natural healing potential is good. The most commonly prescribed medications for sports-related injuries are nonsteroidal antiinflammatory drugs (NSAIDs). These medications are sometimes used to control inflammation and pain. However, studies in animal models have suggested that some of these medications may interfere with the normal tissue healing process. This issue requires further study in humans. Long-term use of NSAIDs is not indicated for children or adolescents. Pain should not be masked with the use of NSAIDs, or any other type of medication, to allow the athlete to compete. Most NSAIDs, other than ibuprofen and Naprosyn, are not approved for use in children.

Superficial heat and cold increases or decreases tissue temperature at a depth up to 5 cm, depending on the method of delivery (22). The physiological response to heat causes vasodilatation and erythema, whereas the application of cold causes vasoconstriction followed by vasodilatation. Ice can help reduce metabolism and secondary hypoxic injury (20). Both heat and cold can reduce fast and slow nerve fiber sensation (23). The initial goal is to decrease pain and promote relaxation of the tissues. In addition, applying pressure with cold reduces posttraumatic swelling. It is essential to have a

TABLE 1.6. Treatment modalities.

Rice	Massage
Medication	Orthotics and assistive devices
Superficial heat and cold	Therapeutic Ultrasound (deep heat)
Hydrotherapy	Neuromuscular Electrical Nerve Stimulation (NMES)
Acupuncture	Iontophoresis
Transcutaneous Electrical Nerve Stimulation (TENS)	

Source: Rennie and Michlovitz, 1996; Cassella M, Richards K. Physical therapy/rehabilitation. In: Micheli L, Kocher, eds. The Pediatric and Adolescent Knee. Elsevier; 2006. By permission of Elsevier.

proper barrier between the skin and the hot or cold pack to prevent skin irritation and/or damage. There is no clear evidence to demonstrate the effectiveness, indications, duration, and optimal mode of cryotherapy for closed soft-tissue injuries, particularly in children (20). There is no clear evidence that heat has a long-term effect on pain (24).

Hydrotherapy is the immersion of body segments in water, for example in a whirlpool. Water immersion promotes an increase or decrease in superficial tissue temperature in a large body part. The main goal of hydrotherapy is to decrease swelling, relieve joint pain and stiffness, and promote relaxation (25).

Acupuncture describes a family of procedures involving stimulation of anatomical points on the body by a variety of techniques. Acupuncture originated in China over 2,000 yrs ago, and it has been used in the treatment of many health problems, including musculoskeletal injuries, headaches, gastrointestinal problems, and pain (26). An example is the insertion of fine needles into selected acupuncture points to bring the body's systems into "balance."

Transcutaneous electrical nerve stimulation (TENS) is the procedure of applying controlled, low-voltage electrical impulses to the nervous system by passing electricity through the skin. It is effective for the symptomatic treatment of acute and chronic pain. TENS is based on the theory that the peripheral stimulation of large-diameter cutaneous afferent nerve fibers blocks sensation at the spinal cord through the gate control mechanisms (27).

Massage is the manipulation of soft tissues by the hands. Pressure and stretching compresses soft tissue, causing an increase in arterial blood and lymphatic circulation, thus promoting better muscle nutrition and relaxation (28). Massage before performing a series of exercises can promote better mobility, pain reduction, and cardiovascular and neuromuscular relaxation, and it also has psychological benefits (29).

Orthotic and assistive devices are prescribed to support or immobilize a body part, correct or prevent deformity, and/or to assist function. Devices include braces, foot orthotics, shoulder slings, splints, prosthetics, crutches, and many others. Devices such as braces restrict, control, or eliminate joint movement, whereas others, such as prosthetics, assist movement (30). Some orthotic devices can help to reduce pain, decrease swelling, control and enhance movement, and improve proprioception. Proper selection, evaluation, and fit of the orthoses are critical to ensure both safety and patient compliance. Instruction in proper orthotic application and care is a key component to a successful outcome. External supports have been shown to reduce ankle sprains in high-risk recreational activities in adolescents with previous ankle sprains (31).

Therapeutic ultrasound is produced by a transducer, which converts electrical energy into sound energy. Ultrasound produces a thermal effect by increasing tissue temperature 1–2°C at a depth of 5 cm. Nonthermal effects include cavitation and mechanical and chemical alterations (32). The main goal is to increase tissue extensibility and decrease inflammation, swelling, pain, and muscle spasm. In addition, ultrasound can help to reduce joint contractures and scar tissue. Ultrasound should never be applied over open epiphyses (33,34). Although ultrasound is widely used, there is minimal evidence that ultrasound has long-term effects on the outcome of musculoskeletal injuries (35).

Neuromuscular electrical nerve stimulation (NMES) is electrical current applied to the skin that activates motor units, causing an involuntary skeletal muscle contraction (36). The main goal is to provide biofeedback and muscle reeducation to the involved muscles. Neuromuscular electrical nerve stimulation has been shown to enhance muscle function postoperatively (37,38).

Iontophoresis is the transfer of topical medications in the form of applied active ions into the epidermis and mucous membranes of the body by direct current (39). Topical steroids are commonly administered using iontophoresis. The goals of iontophoresis include the reduction of inflammation and edema and the softening of scar tissue.

Restore Function

The goal of restoring function is to achieve independence in all activities with maximum efficiency and effectiveness. Exercises to increase and maintain flexibility, muscle strength, proprioception, speed, power, neuromuscular training, and cardiovascular endurance are the major components for full restoration of function. The rate of exercise progression is based on the athlete's abilities and the nature of the injury. An experienced therapist is helpful in determining the appropriate program.

Early mobilization may be limited because of pain, swelling, internal joint derangement, scar tissue formation, and prolonged immobilization. Prolonged immobilization can often lead to muscle shortening, loss of sarcomeres, atrophy, and weakening of the muscle. After some injuries, tightening of surrounding tissues from scarring may cause impaired movement. The period of muscle–tendon immobilization should be short, usually less than 1 wk, to limit the extent of connective tissue proliferation at the site of injury (40).

Muscle Length (Flexibility)

Limited muscle flexibility can have a detrimental effect on the overall rehabilitation program. Stretching exercises may have to be discontinued while the athlete is recovering from a specific injury. The injured area must be fully healed before resuming a stretching program. However, maintaining the athlete's overall flexibility is essential to ensure fitness when the athlete is ready to return to sports and/or competition. A safe stretching program before activities is best done after a series of "warm-up" exercises. Warm-up exercises increase tissue elasticity, thus protecting the muscle–tendon units from further stretch injury (41). A suggestion for warming-up is to start with global, gentle movements ranging in time from 3–5 min. This will help to increase the muscle and body core temperature (42).

The optimal length of time, frequency, and the type of exercises to improve long-term flexibility needs to be clearly established. Static stretching when the muscle is elongated to tolerance and sustained for a length of time appears to be the safest and most effective method (43). Static hamstring stretches performed once a day, holding each stretch for 30 s, resulted in a significant improvement over a 6-wk period (44). Teaching the athlete how and when to safely stretch is the key to a successful outcome.

Joint Range of Motion

After an injury, restoring joint range of motion may need to begin very slowly with active, assistive exercises done with gravity eliminated. For example, the athlete with an acute knee injury is positioned side lying on his involved side, with the uninvolved leg over a pillow. The side-lying position not only eliminates gravity, but also helps to facilitate active, assistive knee flexion and extension (Figure 1.6). Non–weight-bearing active or passive exercises in the side-lying position can be very comfortable and is less painful. Gentle "contract/relax" exercise techniques can help to quickly regain full, pain-free range of motion (45).

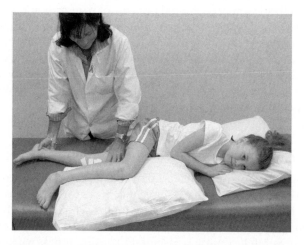

FIGURE 1.6. Active-assisted knee flexion and extension. Side lying on the involved side to facilitate pain-free knee flexion and extension with gravity eliminated.

Joint range of motion can also be increased with manual therapies, including both manipulation and mobilizations. Manipulation is defined as a small-amplitude, high-velocity thrust technique involving a rapid movement beyond a joint's available range of motion. Mobilizations are low-velocity techniques that can be performed in various parts of the available joint range based on the desired effect (46). Mobilization techniques have been shown to produce concurrent effects on pain, sympathetic nervous system activity, and motor activity. Joint mobilizations are considered far safer than manipulations because the patient participates in the technique.

Restore and Improve Strength

Regaining neuromuscular strength and the control to perform functional activities requires a safe, well-designed, age-appropriate, resistive exercise program. Optimal loading of the muscles during strength training exercises includes varying the amount of resistance, repetitions, frequency, speed, and rest intervals (Table 1.7) (47). Appropriate exercise programs are designed to apply controlled, sufficient, but not excessive, stress to healing structures. After an injury, there can often be persistent weakness, muscle atrophy, and painful inhibition. A well-designed exercise program helps to alleviate the sequelae of an injury.

Eccentric loading involves the development of tension while the muscle is contracting and being lengthened, e.g., the downward movement (eccentric) of a biceps curl using a dumbbell. The high forces produced in muscles eccentrically can cause damage and/or injury, particularly in muscle and tendon tears, as well as in overuse injuries (48). However, if the eccentric contractions are applied progressively and repeatedly, the muscle–tendon unit is capable of adapting to these high forces. Eccentric loading exercises have been demonstrated to help in rehabilitation of chronic tendinopathies, such as Achilles and patellar tendinosis, using incline drop squats (49,50).

TABLE 1.7. Guide to strength training in the young athlete.

Number of Exercises	8–12 address all major muscle groups
Frequency	2 nonconsecutive strength training sessions per week
Resistance	60–75% maximal weight load
Repetitions	10–15 repetitions of each exercise
Sets	1 challenging set
Speed	Controlled 3–5 s each rep
Range	Full range of pain-free motion
Technique	Proper posture, biomechanics, and smooth movement
Progression	Increase resistance 5–10% when 15 reps can be completed

Source: Adapted by permission from Faigenbaum and Westcott, 2004.

The term "kinetic chain" refers to the coordinated activities of body segments and the forces generated from proximal to distal. Open kinetic chain (OKC) exercises are performed with the distal lower extremity segment free (Figure 1.7 A). A short arc knee extension, quadriceps-strengthening exercise is an example of an OKC. Closed kinetic chain (CKC) exercises are performed with the distal segment fixed (Figure 1.7 B) (51). An example of a CKC exercise is a leg press. CKC exercises tend to be more functional and safer.

Core stability is the recruitment of the trunk musculature while controlling the position of the lumbar spine during dynamic movements. The stabilization of the central core (trunk) in sports has benefits for preventing injuries, as well as improving performance. The core muscles include the abdominals, extensors, and rotators of the spine. The core muscles act as a bridge between the upper and lower extremities providing stability to the limbs. The strength of the abdominal muscles is critical in maintaining optimal alignment of the trunk and pelvis (7). Figure 1.8 illustrates normal abdominal muscle strength.

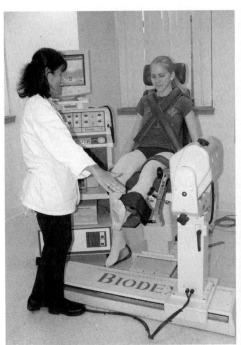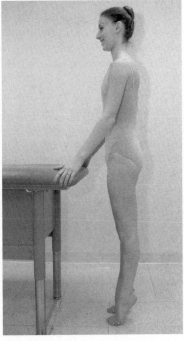

A

B

FIGURE 1.7. OKC and CKC. **(A) OKC** exercise using BIODEX equipment. The distal segment is free as the athlete performs a long-arc quadriceps strengthening exercise. **(B) CKC** exercise. The distal segment is fixed as the dancer performs a gastrocnemius-strengthening exercise.

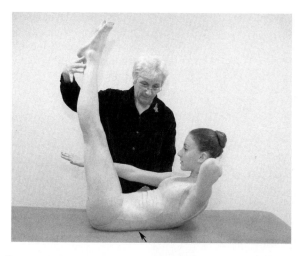

FIGURE 1.8. Core stability. The dancer is able to the keep lumbar spine in contact with the table, while strengthening both the upper and lower abdominal muscles.

Proprioception allows the body to maintain stability and orientation during static and dynamic activities at both the conscious and unconscious level. Mechanoreceptors are the neurosensory cells that are responsible for monitoring joint position and movement. After an injury, proprioception can be diminished from damage of the mechanoreceptors. In addition, loss of tensile properties of static structures such as ligaments or the joint capsule, and the latent response of muscles to provide reflex stabilization of a joint, can also have a negative effect on proprioception (52). A rehabilitation program designed to improve proprioception stimulates the mechanoreceptors that encourage joint stabilization, balance, and postural activities at both the conscious and unconscious level.

Neuromuscular training describes a progressive exercise program that restores synergy and synchrony of the muscle firing patterns required for dynamic stability and fine motor control. This is accomplished by enhancing the dynamic muscular stabilization of the joint and by increasing the cognitive awareness of both joint position and motion. Activities are designed to restore both functional stability around the joint and enhance motor control skills. Use of balance equipment, such as a wobble board and therapeutic exercise balls, can challenge the proprioceptive and balance systems (Figure 1.9). This helps to restore dynamic stability and allow the control of abnormal joint translation during functional activities (53).

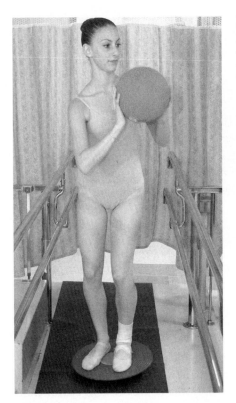

FIGURE 1.9. Dynamic stability (proprioception training). The dancer is catching a medicine ball (weighted), while maintaining her balance on a wobble disc.

Safe Return to Sport/Competition

Athletes are able to safely return to their sport/competition when their injuries are healed and their physical attributes are sufficient to withstand the demands of their activity. A comprehensive rehabilitation program must include progressive exercises to ensure the athlete's readiness for these demands. A program designed for sport-specific activities is implemented when the athlete has achieved full, pain-free, passive and active joint range of motion. In addition, adequate muscle strength and cardiovascular and muscle endurance are essential components in restoring normal movement patterns.

The athlete must have medical clearance before returning to full activity. Functional testing helps to determine the athlete's readiness to return to a specific sport (Table 1.8). Functional tests emphasize skill-related activities and often include assessments of agility, balance, coordination, speed, power, and reaction time (Figure 1.10).

Plyometrics is a natural event that occurs in jumping, hopping, skipping, and even walking. Sport-specific plyometric exercises can be incorporated

TABLE 1.8. Example of functional test for lower extremity.

Test	Goal	Directions	Measure	Normative data (NV)
SLS for Distance	To hop as far forward as possible on one leg	Stand on test leg heel on zero mark. Hop as far forward as possible, landing on test leg.	Horizontal distance hopped from heel at start position to heel on landing position.	Age 14.5 NV = 119.9–155.1 cm
SLS Triple Jump for Distance	To hop as far forward 3 consecutive times	Start position as above. Hops 3 consecutive times on the test leg. On the final hop, hop for maximal distance. Hold landing foot stationary for 1 s.	Horizontal distance hopped from heel at starting positon to heel on landing position.	Unknown
SLS Vertical Jump	To jump as high as possible and land on one leg	Record standing reach. Jump on test leg touching wall with chalked hand. Landing on same leg. Record reach.	Maximal height jumped minus patient's standing reach height.	Age 14.3–15.8 NV = 46.9–49.0 cm
SLS 6 m Hop for Distance	To hop 6 m as quickly as possible	Stand on test leg. Hop forward for 6 m as quickly as possible.	Time to nearest 0.01 s.	Unknown

Source: Manske R, Smith B, Wyatt F. Test-retest reliability of lower extremity functional tests after a closed kinetic chain isokinetic testing bout. J Sport Rehab 2003;12(2):119–132. Reprinted with permission from Human Kinetics.

into the athlete's functional programs (Figure 1.11). The principle of plyometric training is the stretch-shortening cycle, which is when the muscle is stretched eccentrically and immediately contracted, leading to an increase in the force of the contraction. Plyometric training increases the athlete's power and speed. An example of a plyometric program consists of 1 set of 5–10 repetitions of low-intensity drills, such as squat jumps and medicine ball chest passes, performed 2 times per week. Depending on the athlete's ability, the program may progress to multiple hops, jumps, and throws (54). A recent study demonstrated that jumping power and running velocities were improved in prepubescent boys that performed plyometric exercises; the improvements were maintained after a brief period of reduced training compared with matched controls (55). Another study of female athletes ages 15.3 ± 0.9 yr who underwent 6 wk of training, which included

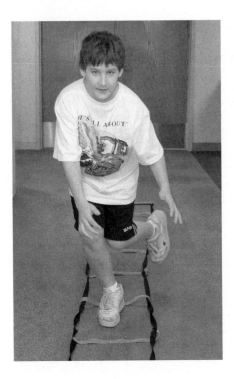

FIGURE 1.10. Agility and balance. The athlete is instructed to jump within the rungs of a ladder to promote agility, balance, and coordination.

plyometric training, core strengthening, and balance and speed training, showed improved measures of performance and movement biomechanics (56).

Prevention of Future Injuries

Prevention is the ideal management for all sports injuries. However, because the nature of sport activities involves risk-taking and, in some cases, pushing individuals to the limits of performance, injuries are bound to occur. The risk factor that is associated most with future injury is a previous history of a similar injury (57).

Preseason conditioning and "warm-up" exercises can often help to reduce injuries. Preseason conditioning, such as treadmill running on a 40-degree incline twice a week and plyometric sessions, reduced injuries in adolescent competitive female soccer players (58). A structured program of "warm-up" exercises was shown to prevent knee and ankle injuries in young female handball players by approximately 50% (59).

Proprioception and neuromuscular training continue to be areas of injury-prevention research. A recent study showed that a 6-mo home-based weekly balance-training program using a wobble board improved static and dynamic balance (60). Balance training has been particularly important in the reduction of anterior cruciate ligament (ACL) injuries, especially for female athletes (61). Another study (PEP: Preventative Injury and Enhance-

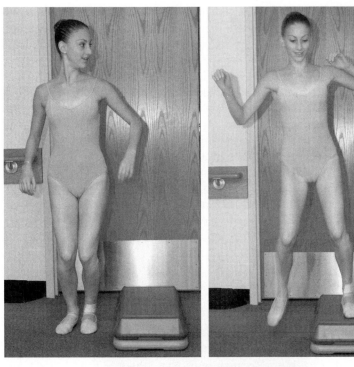
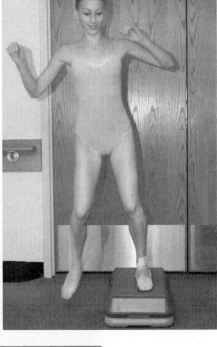

A   B

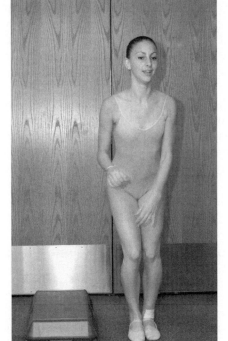

C

FIGURE 1.11. Plyometrics. The jump sequence is an example of a plyometric exercise. The dancer (A) jumps up to (B) a high step and (C) back down to the floor.

ment Program) of female soccer players aged 14–18 participating in a neuromuscular training program consisting of basic "warm-up" activities, stretching techniques for the trunk and lower extremity, strengthening exercises, plyometric activities, and specific agility drills, had 88% less ACL injuries in the first year and 74% less in the second year (62).

To reduce the risk of reinjury when returning to an intensive training schedule, the athlete must maintain a high level of fitness during the rehabilitation phase. Selection of an appropriate aerobic conditioning program must take into account the athlete's injury, physical ability, and condition. The athlete should begin slowly and not be overexerted with the aerobic activity. Activities such as swimming, low impact exercises, and strengthening of the uninjured area will help to maintain this high level of fitness. Suggested increases for frequency, intensity, and duration are approximately 5–10 % per week, depending on the athlete's level of fitness (64). Adequate periods of recovery should be planned between training sessions.

Summary

An athlete can often lose confidence after a serious injury, even if the injury is healed. A well-designed rehabilitation program that not only focuses on the injured area but also maintains the athlete's fitness level and incorporates sport-specific functional exercises, will help to alleviate the athlete's fear. The skill and movement of the sport are broken down into individual parts and are progressed slowly to build the athlete's confidence. Placing appropriate demands on the recovered injured area will not only help the athlete safely return to sports but also to decrease fear and apprehension.

A successful rehabilitation program includes a comprehensive team approach. Communication between the physician, physiotherapist, athletic trainer, coach, and athlete is essential to determine the athlete's readiness to return to sport. A successful program returns the athlete to his or her preinjury level without putting the athlete or others at risk for injury.

References

1. Damore DT, Metzl JD, Ramundo M, et al. Patterns in childhood sports injury. Pediatr Emerg Care 2003;4:19(2):65–67.
2. Malina R, Bouchard C, Bar-Or O. Biological maturation: concepts and assessment. In: Malina R, Bouchard C, Bar-Or O, eds. Growth, Maturation and Physical Activity. Champaign, Ill: Human Kinetics; 2004:277–305.
3. Bass SL. The prepubertal years: a uniquely opportune stage of growth when the skeleton is most responsive to exercise. Sports Med 2000;2:73–78.

4. Kendall HO, Kendall FP. Posture and Pain. Baltimore: Williams and Wilkins; 1952.
5. Green WB. The Clinical Measurement of Joint Motion. Rosemont, Chicago: American Academy of Orthopaedic Surgeons; 1993.
6. Norkin C, White DJ. Measurement of Joint Range of Motion: A Guide to Goniometry. 2nd edition. Philadelphia: F.A. Davis; 1985.
7. Kendall FP, McCreary KE. Muscles: Testing and Function. 4th ed. Baltimore: Williams & Wilkins; 1993.
8. Hislop HJ, Montgomery J. Daniels and Worthingham's Muscle Testing. Philadelphia: W. B. Saunders; 1995.
9. Rabbia F, Grosso T, Cat Genova G, et al. Assessing resting heart rate in adolescent: determinants and correlates. J Hum Hypertens 2002; 16(5):327–332.
10. National Institutes of Health. Blood Pressure Tables for Children and Adolescent. In: Fourth Report on the Diagnosis, Evaluation, and Treatment of High Blood Pressure in Children and Adolescents. Department of Health and Human Services, National Heart Lung and Blood Institute. May 2004. http://www.nhlbi.nih.gov/guidelines/hypertension/child_tbl.htm. Accessed December 22, 2006.
11. Staley MJ, Richard PL. Burns. In: Schmitz TJ, O'Sullivan SB, eds. Physical rehabilitation: assessment and treatment. 3rd ed. Philadelphia: F.A. Davis; 2001:845–872.
12. Micheli LJ. Overuse syndromes in children in sport: the growth factor. Ortho Clinic North AM 1983;14:337–360.
13. Thomas HO. Diseases of the Hip, Knee and Ankle Joints with Their Deformities: Treated by a New and Efficient Method. Liverpool, England: T Dorr & Co; 1876.
14. Ober F. Backache. American Lecture Series No. 243. Springfield, Ill: Charles Thomas Publisher, 1955.
15. Bradley NS. Motor control: developmental aspects of motor control in skill acquisition. In: Campbell SK, ed. Physical Therapy for Children. 3rd ed. Philadelphia: W.B. Saunders C; 2000:45–87.
16. Feltz DL, Ewing ME. Psychological characteristics of the elite young athlete. Med Sci Sports Exerc. 2002; 19:98–105.
17. Patel DR. Pediatrics neurodevelopment and sports participation: when are children ready to play sports. Pediatr Clin North Am 2002;49:505–531.
18. Micheli LJ. Diagnosing and treating your sports injury. In: The Sports Medicine Bible. Micheli LJ, Jenkins M, eds. New York: Harper Perennial; 1995:42–59.
19. MacAuley D. What is the role of ice in soft tissue injury? In: MacAuley D, Best T, eds. Evidence-based sports medicine. London: BMJ Publishing Group; 2002: 45–62.
20. Bleakley GA, McDonough S, MacAuley D. The use of ice in the treatment of acute soft tissue injury: a systematic review of randomized trials. Am J Sports 2004; 32:251–261.
21. Gaffney A, McGrath PJ, Dick B. Measuring pain in children: developmental and instrument issues. In: Pain in infants, children and adolescents. Schechter NL, Berde CB, Yaster M, eds. Philadelphia: Lippincott, Williams and Wilkins; 2003:128–141.
22. Starkey C. Thermal agents. In: Starkey C, ed. Therapeutic Modalities. 3rd ed. Philadelphia: F.A. Davis; 2004:110–169.

23. Rennie GA, Michlovitz S. Biophysical principles of heat and superficial heating agents. In: Michlovitz S, ed. Thermal Agents in Rehabilitation. 3rd ed. Philadelphia: F.A. Davis; 1996:107–139.
24. Curkovic B, Vitulic V, Babic-Naglic D, et al. The influence of heat and cold on the pain threshold in rheumatoid arthritis. Z Rheumatol 1993;52: 289–291.
25. Walsh MT. Hydrotherapy: the use of water as a therapeutic agent. In: Michlovitz S, ed. Thermal Agents in Rehabilitation. 3rd ed. Philadelphia: F.A. Davis; 1996:138–168.
26. Vickers A, Zollman C. ABC of complimentary medicine. Acupuncture BMJ 1999 Oct; 319(7215):973–976.
27. Smith JL, Madsen JR. Neurosurgical procedures for the treatment of pain. In: Schechter ML, Berde CV, Yaster M, eds. Pain in infants, Children, and Adolescents. Philadelphia: Lippincott, Williams & Wilkins; 2003:329–338.
28. Beard G, Wood E. Massage Principles and Techniques. Philadelphia: W.B. Saunders; 1964.
29. Starkey C. Mechanical modalities. In: Starkey C, ed. Therapeutic Modalities. 2nd ed. Philadelphia: F.A. Davis; 2004:305–344.
30. Cordova ML, Scott BD, Ingersol CD, Leblanc MG. Effects of ankle support on lower extremity functional performance: meta-analysis. Med Sci Sports Exerc 2005;37:635–641.
31. Handoll H, Rowe BH, Quinn KM, et al. Interventions for preventing ankle injuries. Cochrane Database System Rev. 2001;(3):CD000018.
32. Mcdiarmid T, Ziskin M, Michlovitz S. Therapeutic ultrasound. In: Michlovitz S, ed. Thermal Agents in Rehabilitation. 3rd ed. Philadelphia: F.A. Davis; 1996: 168–207.
33. Gann, N. Ultrasound: current concepts. Clin Manage 1991; 11:64–69.
34. Deforest RE, Herrick JF, Janes JM, Kursen FH. Effects of ultrasound on growing bones: experimental study. Arch Phys Med Rehabil 1953;34: 21–31.
35. Baker KG, Robertson VJ, Duck FA. A review of therapeutic ultrasound: biophysical effects. Phys Ther 2001;74:845–850.
36. Nelson R, Currier D. Clinical Electrotherapy. Connecticut: Appleton & Lange; 1991.
37. Robertson VJ, Ward AR. Vastus medialis electrical stimulation to improve lower extremity function following a lateral release. J Ortho Sports Phys Ther 2002;32:437–446.
38. Fitzgerald GK, Piva SR, Irrgang JJ. A modified neuromuscular electrical stimulation protocol for quadriceps strengthening following anterior cruciate ligament reconstruction. J Orthop Sports Phys Ther 2003;33:492–501.
39. Kahn KM, Cook JL, Bonar F, et al. Histopathology of common tendinopathies: update and implications for clinical management. Sports Med 1999;27:393–408.
40. Jarvinen TAH, Jarvinen TLN, Kaariainen M, et al. Muscle injuries. The American Journal of Sports Med 2005; 33:745–764.
41. Safran MR, Garrett Jr WE, Seaber AV, et al. The role of warmup in muscular injury prevention. Am J Med 1998;6:123–129.

42. Alter J. Stretch and Strengthening. Boston: Houghton Mifflin Company; 1986.
43. Bandy WD, Irion JM, Briggler M. The effect of static stretch and dynamic range of motion training on the flexibility of the hamstring muscles. J Ortho Sports Phys Ther 1998;27:295–300.
44. Bandy WD, Irion JM. The effect of time on static stretch on the flexibility of the hamstring muscles. Phys Ther 1994;74:845–850.
45. Knott M. Voss D. Proprioceptive Neuromuscular Facilitation. New York: Harper Brothers; 1956.
46. Sran M, Kahn K. Spinal manipulation versus mobilization. CMAJ 2002;7(9): 1–30.
47. Faigenbaum A, Westcott W. Strength training guidelines. In: Youth Strength Training: A Guide for Fitness Professionals from The American Council on Exercise. Monterey, CA: Healthy Learning Books & Videos; 2004:17–26.
48. Archambault JM, Wiley JP, Bray RC. Exercise loading of tendons and the development of overuse injuries: a review of current literature. Sports Med 1995;20:77–89.
49. Alfredson LC, Pietila T, Jonsson P, et al. Heavy-load eccentric calf muscle training for the treatment of chronic Achilles tendonosis. Am J Sports Med 1998;26:360–366.
50. Young MA, Cook JL, Purdam CR, et al. Eccentric decline squat protocol offers superior results at 12 months compared with traditional eccentric protocol for patellar tendinopathy in volleyball players. Br J Sports Med 2005;39:102–105.
51. Kibler WB. Closed kinetic chain rehabilitation for sports injuries. Phys Med Rehabil Clin North Am 2000;11:369–696.
52. Borsa PA, Lephart SM, Irrang JJ, et al. The effects of joint position and direction of motion on proprioceptive sensibility in anterior cruciate ligament deficient athletes. Am J Sports Med 1997;25:336–340.
53. Bahr R, Lian O. A two-fold reduction in the incidence of ankle sprains in volleyball. Scand J Med Sci Sports 1997;7:172–177.
54. Faigenbaum AD, Yap CW. Are plyometrics safe for children? J Strength Cond Rex 2000;22:45–46.
55. Dialli O, Dore E, Duche P, Van Praagh E. Effects of plyometric training followed by reduced training program on physical performance of prepubescent soccer players. J Sports Med Phys Fitness 2001; 41:341–348.
56. Myer GD, Ford KR, Palumbo JB, Hewett TE. Neuromuscular training improves performance in lower extremity biomechanics in female athletes. Sports Med 2000;30:309–325.
57. Lysens R, Steverlynck A, Van den Auweele Y. The predictability of sports injuries. Sports Med 1984;1:6–10.
58. Heidt RS, Sweeterman LM, Carlonas RL, et al. Avoidance for soccer injuries with preseason conditioning. Am J Sports Med 2000;28:659–662.
59. Olsen OE, Myklebust G, Engebresten L, et al. Exercises to prevent lower extremity injuries in youth sports: cluster randomized control trial. BMJ 2005;330:449–455.
60. Emery CA, Cassidy JD, Klassen TP, et al. Development of a clinical static and dynamic standing balance measurement tool appropriate for use in adolescents. CMAJ 2005;172:749–754.

61. Hewett TE, Myer GD, Ford KR, et al. Biomechanics measure of neuromuscular control and valgus loading of the knee predict anterior cruciate ligament injury risk in female athletes: a prospective study. Am J Sports Med 2005;33: 492–501.
62. Mandelbaum BR, Silvers HJ, Watanabe DS, et al. Effectiveness of neuromuscular training and proprioceptive training in preventing anterior cruciate ligament injuries in female athletes: two year follow-up. Am J Sport Med 2005;33: 1003–1011.
63. Micheli LJ. The Sports Medicine Bible. New York: Harper Collins; 1995.

2
Diagnostic Imaging

Vernon M. Chapman and Diego Jaramillo

Diagnostic imaging is frequently performed in the evaluation of adolescent sports-related injuries. Imaging often helps determine the nature and severity of injuries and is important for deciding appropriate management. There are several diagnostic imaging techniques available for examining the musculoskeletal system. An understanding of the principles, advantages, and disadvantages of these techniques and their clinical application in adolescent patients is important for optimal imaging evaluation.

Imaging Techniques

Radiography

Radiography is the oldest diagnostic imaging technology, dating back to the discovery of x-rays by physicist Wilhelm Roentgen in 1895. Radiography continues to be the most fundamental and frequently utilized technique in diagnostic radiology departments. Radiographs are created by placing the body part of interest between an x-ray source and a film. The body part absorbs the x-rays depending on the density of its various tissues, and the x-rays that pass through are used to generate the image (1). A typical radiograph examination is performed in less than 10 min. Radiographic images, as well as images from all other modalities, are recorded on film ("hard copy") or, increasingly often, kept in a digital format on a picture archive and communication system (PACS).

   Five basic tissue densities are evaluated in radiographs: bone, soft tissue, fat, air, and metal. The first three are most important in the evaluation of radiographs obtained for orthopedic injuries before any surgical intervention. Though bone is the most basic structure evaluated on radiographs, close inspection of the surrounding soft tissues and fat is often useful for assessing the presence or severity of an injury. This is particularly important in disorders such as Osgood–Schlatter's disease, where detection of edema of the prepatellar soft tissues and of Hoffa's fat pad is more diagnostic than detection of osseous irregularity of the tibial tubercle.

The advantages of radiography are high spatial resolution, widespread availability, low cost, and brief exam time. High spatial resolution allows the identification of very subtle injuries, such as nondisplaced fractures. The availability, low cost, and rapid acquisition of radiographs means that radiography may be performed almost anywhere, in nearly any patient.

The disadvantages of radiography are its limited soft tissue contrast, two-dimensional imaging, and radiation exposure. Though excellent for assessing bone pathology, radiography is extremely limited in evaluating soft tissue pathology, including injury to ligaments, tendons, and muscles. Furthermore, radiographs are two-dimensional depictions of three-dimensional structures; although it is common to obtain multiple views, true three-dimensional images cannot be reconstructed from radiographic data. Though radiography has associated radiation exposure, it is substantially less than that associated with computed tomography or nuclear medicine bone scan.

Computed Tomography

In computed tomography (CT), an x-ray source and detector rotate around a patient as the patient moves through the center of rotation. The data acquired are then computer reconstructed into a series of two-dimensional slices of the area of interest. Whereas older CT scanners consisted of a single x-ray source and a single detector, modern scanners use one or two x-ray sources and 64 or more detectors, acquiring data continuously in a helical fashion as the patient moves through the scanner. The result is faster examinations with thinner slices and improved postprocessing capability.

In CT, tissues are depicted based on their x-ray attenuation relative to the reference value of water, which is assigned a value of zero (expressed in Hounsfield units [HU]). The resulting images can be viewed in the axial plane or reformatted to sagittal, coronal, or oblique planes (2). The soft tissue contrast on CT can be accentuated with the use of iodinated intravenous contrast, which is commonly performed for evaluation of the chest, abdomen, and pelvis. Evaluation of the musculoskeletal system, on the other hand, rarely requires intravenous contrast, unless vascular injury is suspected.

The advantages of CT are rapid scan time and three-dimensional imaging. On a modern multidetector CT scanner, imaging of the head, spine, chest, abdomen, pelvis, and/or extremities can be performed in less than 1 min. The scan data can then be used to construct three-dimensional images, which are frequently useful in the preoperative assessment of orthopedic injuries.

The disadvantages of CT are radiation exposure, cost, and availability. The radiation exposure varies, depending on the type of examination, but is several orders of magnitude greater than radiographs. In general, a CT examination delivers a radiation dose that is equivalent to that of 100–250 conventional radiographs. This is an important consideration in regard to risk of radiation-induced malignancies, particularly in young patients whose tissues are more susceptible to radiation carcinogenesis and who have to carry the burden of the radiation damage for many years. It has been estimated that one CT examination carries a risk of malignancy of 1 in 1,000, but with the exposure factors used currently in most pediatric institutions, the risk may be only a fraction of this (3). The cost is substantially greater than that of radiography, which, coupled with its limited availability (depending on location), may limit patient access to CT.

Magnetic Resonance Imaging

Magnetic resonance imaging (MRI) utilizes differences in the frequency of spinning protons in various tissues to create images. Images are obtained using a complex array of gradients and delivered radio frequency pulses, with the patient lying in a strong magnetic field (approximately 10,000 times as strong as the earth's magnetic field) (4). Over the past several decades, MRI has become a powerful technique for evaluating many organ systems, particularly the musculoskeletal system. It is the imaging method of choice for the spine, joints, and soft tissues.

The advantages of MRI are excellent soft tissue contrast, three-dimensional imaging, and lack of radiation exposure. The tissue contrast achieved with MRI far surpasses that of radiography, CT, or any other modality, making it the best modality for evaluating both osseous and nonosseous musculoskeletal trauma. Although the mineralized portions of bone are poorly visualized, the marrow and surrounding tissues are seen well and serve as indicators of injury. Like CT, MRI allows multiplanar imaging, and image data may be used to create three-dimensional images. Furthermore, MRI is associated with no radiation exposure, which is a particularly appealing attribute in the pediatric population.

The disadvantages of MRI are long examination time, cost, limited availability, and contraindications. Most musculoskeletal MRI exams require between 30 min and 1 h, depending on the site being imaged. Sedation is rarely required for older children and younger adolescents suffering sports-related injuries, but patients with injuries may become "fidgety," leading to motion-degraded images. The cost of an MRI examination is greater than any other musculoskeletal imaging modality, with the possible exception of a nuclear medicine bone scan and positron emission tomography (PET). As with CT, the high cost, coupled with the limited availability of MRI (depending on location), limits access of some patients to this modality. Furthermore, some patients are unable to have an MRI examination because of certain indwelling metallic objects (aneurysm clips, cardiac pacer/defibrillator devices, etc.).

Nuclear Medicine

The most commonly performed nuclear medicine study for musculoskeletal pathology is a bone scan. For a bone scan, imaging is performed after intravenous injection of a radiopharmaceutical. Depending on the indication, imaging may be performed at multiple time points (three-phase; most commonly used for infection) or at a single, delayed time point (most commonly for fracture or metastatic disease).

Bone scans may be viewed as planar (two-dimensional) images or as a series of three-dimensional multiplanar images, using single-photon emission computed tomography (SPECT). Using SPECT improves the sensitivity of the bone scan for detecting lesions, particularly in the spine (5). Recently, PET imaging using phosphate compounds has been used to provide high-resolution images of the bone. The role of PET, or PET combined with CT, for the evaluation of sports medicine injuries is not yet defined.

The advantages of the nuclear medicine bone scan are whole-body imaging and the ability to detect subtle bone injuries. Whereas other modalities require focused exams, a bone scan includes whole body planar images with additional focused images, as needed. This, coupled with its sensitivity for bone pathology, makes the bone scan an excellent tool for evaluating injuries with little or no radiographic abnormality, such as stress fractures.

The disadvantages of the bone scan are radiation exposure, low resolution and specificity, and very limited depiction of soft tissue pathology. The radiation exposure is between that of radiography and CT, with the highest dose to the bladder. The resolution of the images obtained is less than CT or MRI, resulting in the grainy appearance of the images. Though abnormal radiotracer uptake on a bone scan indicates pathology, the exact cause can frequently not be determined without additional imaging.

Ultrasound

Ultrasound uses sound waves of frequencies greater than those of audible sound to penetrate tissues and create images that may be viewed in real-time. An ultrasound examination involves a technologist and/or physician placing a probe over the area of interest with gel, and possibly a spacer, between the probe and the skin to maximize image quality (6). Ultrasound examinations take approximately 15–30 min to perform, depending on the size and complexity of the area being imaged. As discussed later in this chapter, there is increasing enthusiasm for using ultrasonography for the evaluation of musculotendinous injuries.

The advantages of ultrasound are lack of radiation exposure, relative low cost, dynamic imaging, and portability. Because ultrasound utilizes percussion waves rather than electromagnetic radiation, there is no risk of induced malignancy. In addition, the examination is relatively inexpensive, between that of radiography and CT. Unlike any other modality, ultrasound allows the user to view the area of interest in real time.

The major disadvantage of ultrasound is user variability and nonvisualization of bone. The quality and success of an ultrasound examination is highly dependant on the experience and skill of the person scanning, whether it is a technologist or physician. This is particularly true with musculoskeletal ultrasound, as these exams are rarely performed in most radiology departments, limiting user familiarity with the examinations. Although ultrasound nicely depicts muscle and other soft tissues, the interface of soft tissue with bone reflects all sound, preventing evaluation of osseous structures.

Arthrography

Arthrography involves the intraarticular injection of contrast and subsequent imaging with fluoroscopy, CT, or MRI. Nearly all injections are performed with fluoroscopic or sonographic guidance and include iodinated and/or gadolinium-based contrast material. The injection takes approximately 10min, with variable time involved thereafter, depending on the wait and time to perform subsequent imaging.

The major advantage of arthrography is improved visualization of the joint space, articular surfaces, and cartilage (particularly with MR arthrography) because of joint distention and increased image contrast. In addition, radiation exposure is low (except with CT arthrography) and limited to the joint.

The disadvantages of arthrography are its cost and invasiveness. Though much of the former results from the cost of the subsequent imaging (frequently MRI), the examination does require a procedure. Accordingly, the procedure portion of the examination carries a small risk of bleeding and infection. Indirect arthrography, in which contrast material injected intravenously diffuses into the synovial space, is possible with MRI. Indirect MR arthrography is useful in joints in which joint distention is not crucial, such as the wrist and hip, but is of limited value in the shoulder.

Sites of Injury

Head and Face

Injuries associated with participation in sports and recreational activities account for approximately 21% of all traumatic brain injuries in children. Though death in children participating in sports activities is rare, the most common cause of death is brain injury. As with all sport injuries in children and adolescents, the majority of head and face injuries are the result of falls, collisions, or being struck by an object (7).

The imaging evaluation of a patient with suspected intracranial trauma begins with an unenhanced head CT. CT is a rapid means of assessing for intracranial hemorrhage, parenchymal contusion, and fracture (Figure 2.1) and may be performed in conjunction with CT of the chest, abdomen, pelvis, or extremities in a patient with multisystem trauma. Prompt diagnosis of intracranial injury is important for timely neurosurgical evaluation and possible intervention. Furthermore, the head CT may be repeated serially to evaluate for change in intracranial hemorrhage.

If the initial head CT is negative and the patient's clinical exam remains concerning for intracranial injury, MRI of the brain may be performed. MRI is excellent for demonstrating subtle parenchymal injuries, such as acute and chronic blood products, diffuse axonal injury, and changes of ischemia or infarction (8).

Similar to the assessment of intracranial injury, CT is the primary modality for evaluating patients with suspected facial fractures (9). The pattern and extent of these fractures is clearly depicted, and the data may be reformatted in any plane or used to create three-dimensional images for surgical planning (Figure 2.2). In addition, associated hematomas, sinus hemorrhage, optic canal involvement, and intracranial injury are well demonstrated.

Spine

Sports-related injuries of the spine in adolescents include acute fracture/subluxation, disc herniation, and spondylolysis. Fracture or subluxation of the spine during participation in sports is extremely rare and most commonly affects the cervical spine. Whereas in younger children injuries tend to occur in the upper cervical spine, older children and adolescents tend to injure the lower cervical spine. Given that the incidence of injury is extremely low and the risk of radiation exposure in young patients is significant, it is prudent to begin the imaging evaluation with conventional radiographs. However, with a history of severe trauma or focal neurologic deficit, CT or MRI may be necessary (10). The former is most useful for assessing for fracture or subluxation (Figure 2.3) and the latter is best for determining ligamentous or cord injury.

Disc herniations are best imaged by MRI, as radiographs and CT provide little useful information. MRI clearly depicts the herniations, as well as the mass effect on surrounding structures, such as the spinal cord and descending and exiting nerve roots. In addition, findings on MRI can distinguish between a disc herniation and slipped ring apophysis, a rare condition that is most common in the lower lumbar spine and may mimic a disc herniation clinically.

Patients with suspected spondylolysis may be imaged with radiographs, nuclear medicine bone scan, or CT. Oblique radiographs demonstrate the bony disruption through the pars interarticularis and are performed

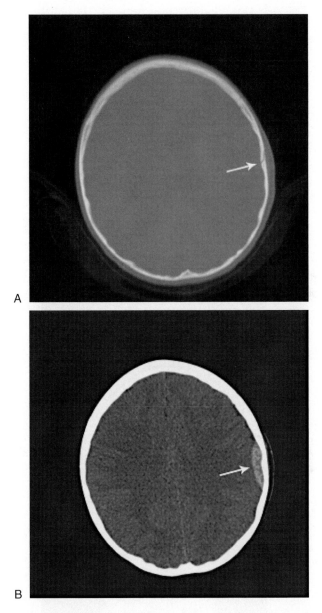

FIGURE 2.1. Head trauma: 9-yr-old boy struck in the head by a knee during soccer practice. An unenhanced head CT was obtained and demonstrated a nondisplaced linear fracture of the left parietal bone **(A, arrow)** with a small subjacent epidural hematoma **(B, arrow)**.

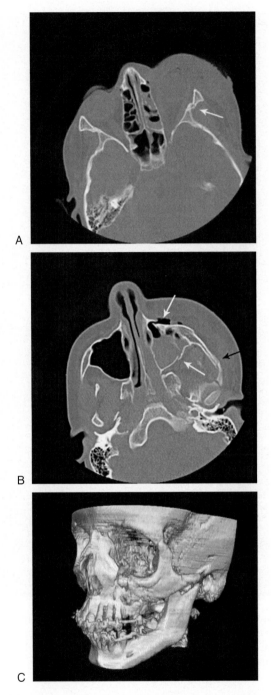

FIGURE 2.2. Facial trauma: 11-yr-old boy involved in a snow skiing accident. Axial images from a maxillofacial CT demonstrate fractures of the lateral wall of the left orbit **(A, arrow)**, the anterior and posterior walls of the left maxillary sinus **(B, white arrows)**, and the zygomatic arch **(B, black arrow)**, which is consistent with a zygoma complex ("tripod") fracture. A three-dimensional image **(C)** clearly shows the fracture and assists in surgical planning.

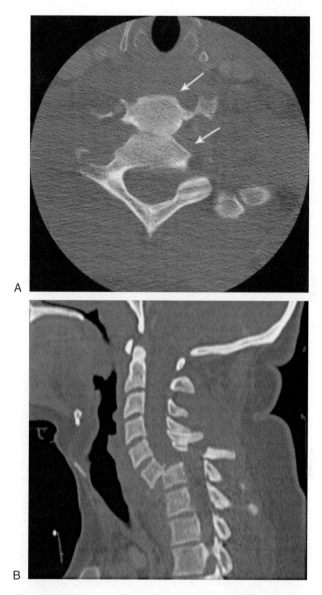

FIGURE 2.3. Cervical spine trauma: 18-yr-old male who struck a pole while snow skiing. An axial image through the lower cervical spine **(A)** shows the C6 and C7 vertebrae on the same image (arrows), which is consistent with a subluxation. A midline sagittal reformatted image **(B)** confirms this finding, which was secondary to bilateral interfacet dislocation.

in conjunction with frontal and lateral views, the latter of which demonstrates any associated spondylolisthesis. Alternatively, a bone scan with SPECT can be performed, demonstrating abnormal uptake of the radiopharmaceutical in the pars interarticularis (11). CT is usually reserved for assessing the size of the defect, to assess the need for possible surgical intervention, and to evaluate the healing of the pars fracture after treatment.

Chest and Abdomen

Injury to the chest or abdomen in children and adolescents is most commonly the result of bicycle accidents or sports-related trauma. The most concerning injuries are parenchymal contusions or lacerations (including the lung, liver, spleen, kidneys, or pancreas) and pneumothorax (Figure 2.4). Injuries to the chest are best evaluated initially with radiographs to assess for a pneumothorax, which would require immediate chest tube placement, after which CT may be performed in cases of suspected mediastinal or vascular injury. Trauma to the abdomen or pelvis, on the other hand, is best evaluated initially with ultrasound or CT. Though ultrasound can depict

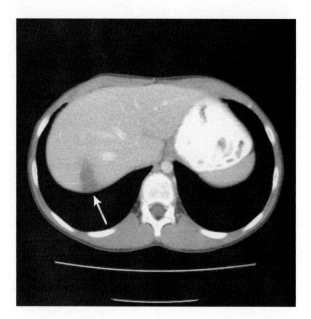

FIGURE 2.4. Abdominal trauma: 14-yr-old boy who fell from his bicycle. An axial image of the upper abdomen from an abdominal CT with oral and intravenous contrast demonstrates a laceration of the posterior dome of the right lobe of the liver (arrow).

parenchymal injury or abnormal fluid collections, it is user dependant and may miss clinically important injuries. As a result, CT is most commonly performed for the evaluation of trauma in these patients (12).

Extremity Injuries

Fractures

By 16 years of age, 42% of boys and 27% of girls have sustained a fracture, with 6–30% of fractures involving the growth plate (13). Growth plate fractures are characterized using the Salter–Harris classification, where the higher the numerical type, the greater the risk of subsequent growth arrest (14). Radiographs are most commonly utilized for the initial and follow-up imaging evaluation of fractures. Nuclear medicine bone scan and MRI are more sensitive, but rarely clinically indicated. A bone scan demonstrates increased uptake at the site of fracture, usually within 24 hours of the injury. CT clearly demonstrates the path of the fracture, including involvement of the growth plate, and scan data may be used to create three-dimensional images for surgical planning. Immediately after the injury, MRI demonstrates local marrow edema and, often, the path of the fracture, including its course through the growth plate, if it is involved (15). MRI may be of diagnostic and prognostic value in growth plate fractures, particularly those involving the knee, where there are frequently associated meniscal and ligamentous injuries and a high incidence of posttraumatic growth disturbance.

Avulsion Injuries

In adolescents, the ligaments, tendons, and capsular tissues are stronger than the growth plates at or near their attachments, thereby predisposing them to avulsion injuries, which are quite common in this age group (16). Avulsions around the hip and pelvis are most common and are best diagnosed on radiographs (Figure 2.5). Initial radiographic changes may be subtle, but follow-up radiographs frequently demonstrate prominent new bone formation at the site of avulsion. Imaging with other modalities, including CT, MRI, and bone scan, is rarely necessary, except when the radiographic findings are atypical and suggest other pathology, such as neoplasia.

Internal Derangement

In general, the nonosseous tissues of a joint (including ligaments, tendons, muscles, cartilage, and capsular tissue) are best evaluated with MRI or MR arthrography (Figure 2.6) (17). Many joints, such as the knee,

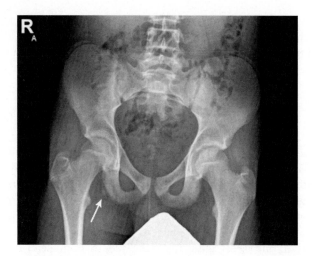

FIGURE 2.5. Tendon avulsion: 16-yr-old male with right groin pain after weightlifting. A frontal radiograph of the pelvis demonstrates a crescent-shaped fragment of avulsed bone adjacent to the right ischial tuberosity (arrow), which is consistent with a hamstring avulsion.

ankle, and elbow, are adequately imaged with MRI alone; however, other joints, such as the shoulder and hip, are better evaluated with intraarticular contrast. The decision to perform an MR arthrogram frequently depends on the suspected injury. For example, evaluation of the shoulder for a rotator cuff tear is usually adequate using MRI alone, but evaluation for a labral tear is best done with MR arthrography.

Chronic Physeal Injury

Repetitive stress on growing bone, which commonly affects adolescent athletes, can lead to chronic growth plate injury. Such injury can be a source of pain and weakens the growing bone, predisposing to acute injury and fracture. Examples include "gymnast's wrist," which is secondary to repetitive axial loading of the distal radius, and "little leaguer's shoulder," resulting from repetitive torsion and distraction of the proximal humerus from throwing (18,19). The thickness of the growth plate is normally constant until skeletal maturation. With chronic injury, however, the growth plate becomes widened and irregular, with cartilage extending vertically into the metaphysis and the development of thin bone bridges, without evidence of growth arrest (20). The findings of chronic growth plate injury may be seen on radiographs, but are often more conspicuous on MRI, where cartilage-sensitive sequences

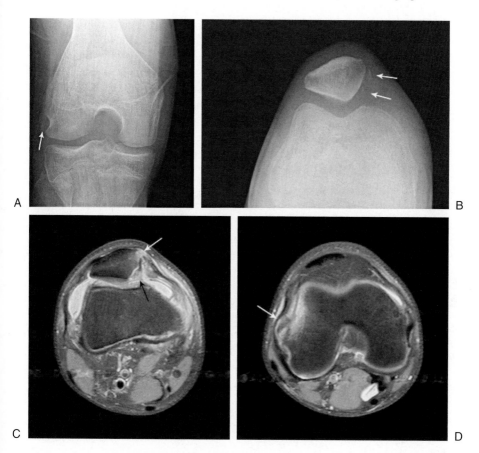

FIGURE 2.6. Internal derangement: 16-yr-old male with right knee pain after falling on the knee during a soccer game. A frontal radiograph of the knee **(A)** demonstrates a bone fragment adjacent to the lateral femoral condyle (arrow), with no clear donor site on the condyle. A sunrise view of the patella **(B)** demonstrates two bone fragments adjacent to the medial patellar facet (arrows), with no clear donor sites identified. MRI of the knee was performed for further evaluation. Axial fat-saturated, fluid-sensitive (proton density) images demonstrate a tear of the medial patellar retinaculum **(C, white arrow)** and a loose osteochondral fragment **(C, black arrow)**. An osteochondral fragment adjacent to the lateral femoral condyle **(D, arrow)** is likely from the medial patellar facet and accounts for the radiographic finding.

clearly demonstrate the characteristic growth plate change. MRI is also useful in the follow-up of these lesions after resting, as these findings can be reversible (21).

Chronic physeal injury may lead to a superimposed acute injury, as in the case of slipped capital femoral epiphysis (SCFE). SCFE is the result of chronic repetitive shear stress at the hip, leading to progressive physeal damage and, ultimately, an acute Salter–Harris type I fracture of the proximal femoral growth plate and subluxation (or "slip") of the epiphysis (22). Radiographs are usually sufficient to demonstrate the injury with subluxation of the epiphysis. Before epiphyseal subluxation, however, radiographs will be normal despite growth plate injury. In such cases, MRI shows findings of chronic growth plate injury (or "pre-slip"), allowing early intervention and prevention of subluxation.

Stress Injuries

Stress injuries include insufficiency type (normal stress on abnormal bone) and fatigue type (abnormal stress on normal bone) injuries. In adolescents, these injuries are nearly all fatigue-type injuries, frequently affecting the lower extremities. Any bone may be involved, but the tibia and femoral neck are most commonly involved and associated with running. Radiographs may be normal early on, but later show periosteal new bone formation or linear sclerosis at the site of fracture. If radiographs are normal, nuclear medicine bone scan or MRI are useful for further evaluation. Bone scan demonstrates normal uptake on flow and blood pool images, with increased uptake on delayed images (Figure 2.7). Images from MRI show prominent marrow edema with a low signal intensity fracture line.

Growth Arrest

Growth arrest most commonly develops because of growth plate injury, affecting approximately 15% of such injuries (23). The risk of growth disturbance after physeal injury is dependant on several factors, including the severity of the injury, the patient's growth potential (i.e., age or skeletal maturity), and the anatomic site involved (24). The mechanism of posttraumatic growth arrest is transphyseal vascular communication between the epiphysis and the metaphysis after the injury, leading to deposition of osteoblast precursors and formation of a bone bridge that tethers together the epiphysis and metaphysis (25). In general, posttraumatic physeal bridge formation is more common in the distal physes of the lower extremities, where there are normal undulating or multiplanar physes (26). For example, the distal femur and the proximal tibia, though uncommon sites of physeal fracture (1.4% and 0.8%, respectively), are frequent sites of posttraumatic bone bridge formation and growth arrest (35 and 16%,

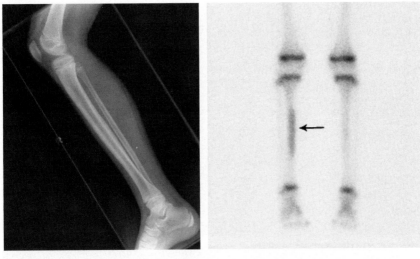

A   B

FIGURE 2.7. Stress injury: A 10-yr-old male soccer player with left leg pain. A lateral radiograph of the left lower leg **(A)** demonstrates subtle thickening of the anterior and posterior cortices of the mid tibia. Images from a nuclear medicine bone scan **(B)** demonstrate segmental increase in radiopharmaceutical uptake in the mid tibia (arrow), which is consistent with stress injury. No discrete fracture was identified on either study.

respectively). The most common site of posttraumatic growth arrest is the distal tibia (27).

Growth recovery lines (or Parks–Harris lines) develop when growth slows down after the fracture and resumes during the process of healing. The line is visible on radiographs and indicates the position of the growth plate at the time of injury, and the distance between the growth plate and the line indicates the amount of growth since the injury. If there is growth arrest, the growth recovery line will either be absent (indicating no growth) or it will not be parallel to the physis (indicating angular deformity). CT with coronal and sagittal reformatted images may be performed to demonstrate the transphyseal bone bridge, but MRI more clearly demonstrates the size and location of transphyseal bridges (28). Sequences that differentiate the growth plate from surrounding bone may be performed and postprocessed to yield a transverse map of the growth plate. This map can then be used to determine the percent of the growth plate that the bridge occupies, as bridges smaller than 50% of the total physeal area may be resected with good clinical result (Figure 2.8).

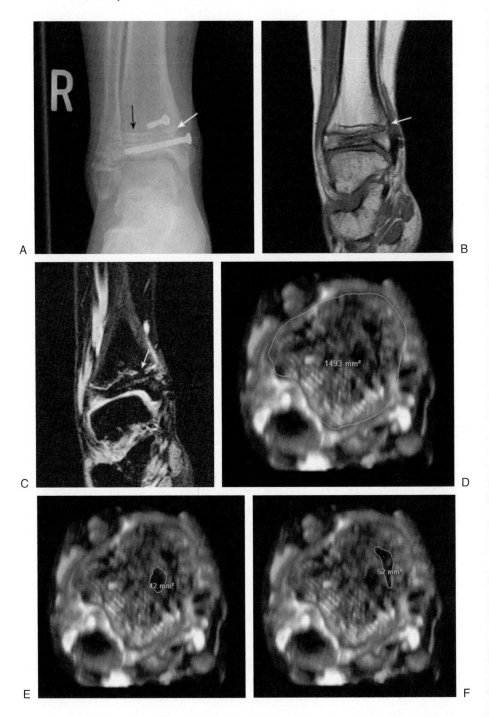

FIGURE 2.8. Growth arrest: 14-yr-old male who twisted his ankle and sustained a Salter IV fracture of the distal tibia during a basketball game. A frontal radiograph of the ankle 1 yr later **(A)** demonstrates screws related to open reduction and internal fixation of the fracture. There is focal sclerosis of the growth plate laterally (white arrow), with a growth recovery line extending medially at an angle from the site of sclerosis (black arrow), which is consistent with a bony bar and growth arrest. Coronal fat-sensitive **(T1-weighted; B)** and fluid-sensitive **(gradient echo; C)** images of the ankle performed 6 mo later, after hardware removal, demonstrate the bony bridge (arrows). Maps of the growth plate show the area of the growth plate **(D)** and the area of two bony bridges **(E and F)**, assisting with surgical planning for resection of the bridges.

◀————————————————————————————————————

Conclusion

Imaging is frequently required in the evaluation of adolescent sports-related injuries. The modalities available for imaging the musculoskeletal system include radiography, CT, MRI, nuclear medicine, ultrasound, and arthrography. Though each modality has associated advantages and disadvantages, it is the nature and site of the injury that frequently determines the most appropriate imaging technique.

References

1. Bushberg JT, Seibert JA, Leidholdt EM, Boone JM. The Essential Physics of Medical Imaging. 2nd ed. Baltimore: Williams and Wilkins; 2002.
2. Fayad LM, Johnson P, Fishman EK. Multidetector CT of musculoskeletal disease in the pediatric patient: principles, techniques, and clinical applications. Radiographics 2005;25:603–618.
3. Brenner DJ, Elliston CD, Hall EJ, Berdon WE. Estimated risk of radiation-induced fatal cancer from pediatric CT. Am J Roentgenol 2001;176:289–296.
4. Hendrick RE. Basic physics of MR imaging: an introduction. Radiographics 1994;14: 829–846.
5. Love C, Din AS, Tomas MB, Kalapparambath TP, Palestro CJ. Radionuclide bone imaging: an illustrative review. Radiographics 2003;23:341–358.
6. Middleton WD, Kurtz AB. Ultrasound: The Requisites. 2nd ed. St. Louis: Mosby; 2003.
7. Poussaint TY, Moeller KK. Imaging of pediatric head trauma. Neuroimaging Clin N Am 2002;12:271–294.
8. Noguchi K, Ogawa T, Seto H, et al. Subacute and chronic subarachnoid hemorrhage: diagnosis with fluid-attenuated inversion recovery MR imaging. Radiology 1997;203:257–262.
9. Turner BG, Rhea JT, Thrall JH, Small AB, Novelline RA. Trends in the use of CT and radiography in the evaluation of facial trauma, 1992–2002: Implications for Current Costs. Am J Roentgenol 2004;183:751–754.

10. Keenan HT, Hollingshead MC, Chung CJ, Ziglar MK. Using CT of the cervical spine for early evaluation of pediatric patients with head trauma. Am J Roentgenol 2001;177:1405–1409.
11. Afshani E, Kuhn JP. Common causes of low back pain in children. Radiographics 1991;11:269–291.
12. Sivit CJ, Eichelberger MR, Taylor GA. CT in children with rupture of the bowel caused by blunt trauma: diagnostic efficacy and comparison with hypoperfusion complex. Am J Roentgenol 1994;163:1195–1198.
13. Landin L. Epidemiology of children's fractures. J Pediatr Orthop B 1997;6: 79–83.
14. Salter R, Harris W. Injuries involving the epiphyseal plate. J Bone Joint Surg Am 1963;45:587–622.
15. Jaramillo D, Kammen BF, Shapiro F. Cartilaginous path of physeal fracture-separations: evaluation with MR imaging–an experimental study with histologic correlation in rabbits. Radiology 2000;215:504–511.
16. Stevens MA, El-Khoury GY, Kathol MH, Brandser EA, Chow S. Imaging features of avulsion injuries. Radiographics 1999;19:655–672.
17. Oeppen RS, Connolly SA, Bencardino JT, Jaramillo D. Acute injury of the articular cartilage and subchondral bone: a common but unrecognized lesion in the immature knee. Am J Roentgenol 2004;182:111–117.
18. Shih C, Chang C, Penn I, et al. Chronically stressed wrists in adolescent gymnasts: MR imaging appearance. Radiology 1995;195:855–859.
19. Fleming JL, Hollingsworth CL, Squire DL, Bisset GS. Little leaguer's shoulder. Skeletal Radiol 2004;33:352–354.
20. Jaramillo D, Shapiro F. Musculoskeletal trauma in children. Magn Reson Imaging Clin N Am 1998;6:521–536.
21. Laor T, Wall EJ, Louis PV. Physeal widening in the knee due to stress injury in child athletes. Am J Roentgenol 2006;186:1260–1264.
22. Umans H, Liebling MS, Moy L, et al. Slipped capital femoral epiphysis: a physeal lesion diagnosed by MRI, with radiographic and CT correlation. Skeletal Radiol 1998;27:139–144.
23. Rogers L, Poznanski A. Imaging of epiphyseal injuries. Radiology 1994;191: 297–308.
24. Peterson HA, Madhok R, Benson JT, et al. Physeal fractures: Part 1. Epidemiology in Olmstead County, Minnesota, 1979–1988. J Pediatr Orthop 1994;14:423–430.
25. Peterson HA. Physeal and apophyseal injuries. In: Rockwood J, Wilkins KE, Beaty JH, eds. Fractures in Children. 3rd ed. Philadelphia: Lippincott-Raven; 1996:103–165.
26. Ecklund K, Jaramillo D. Patterns of premature physeal arrest: MR imaging of 111 children. Am J Roentgenol. 2002;178:967–972.
27. Disler DG. Fat-suppressed three-dimensional spoiled gradient-recalled MR imaging: Assessment of articular and physeal hyaline cartilage. Am J Roentgenol 1997;169:1117–1124.
28. Borsa JJ, Peterson HA, Ehman RL. MR imaging of physeal bars. Radiology 1996;199:683–687.

Section II
Anatomic Regions

3
Traumatic Head Injuries

Laura Purcell

Head injuries are common among children, and they result in a significant number of visits to emergency departments and physicians' offices each year. In children 15 yr old and under, the estimated incidence of traumatic brain injury is 180 per 100,000 children per year, totaling more than 1 million injuries annually in the United States and accounting for more than 10% of all visits to emergency departments (1). A recent study conducted in emergency departments in Canada demonstrated that 3% of all sport-related injuries were head injuries (2). The majority of sport-related head injuries occurred in individuals less than 20 yr of age. Head injuries represented 2.8% of all sport injuries in children less than 10 yr old, 3.7% in 10–14 yr olds, and 4.2% in 15–19 yr olds (2). Head injuries as a result of sport participation include minor injuries such as contusions, lacerations, and superficial hematomas, as well as more serious injuries, including concussions, skull fractures, and intracranial hemorrhages. Head injuries can occur in both organized sports, such as football, hockey, basketball, and soccer, as well as recreational activities, including biking, skiing, skateboarding, and rollerblading.

Anatomy

The brain is enclosed in the bony skull or cranium (Figure 3.1 A). Below the skull, there are three layers of meninges between the skull and the brain. The meninges, or mater, include the outer dura mater, enclosing the venous sinuses; the arachnoid mater, which bridges the sulci on the cortical surface of the brain; and the pia mater, which is a delicate vascular membrane lining the cerebral cortex. There are three potential meningeal spaces: the epidural space between the cranium and the dura; the subdural space between the dura and arachnoid; and the subarachnoid space between the arachnoid and pia, which contains cerebrospinal fluid.

The brain consists of right and left cerebral hemispheres, which are divided into lobes corresponding to the overlying cranial bones: frontal,

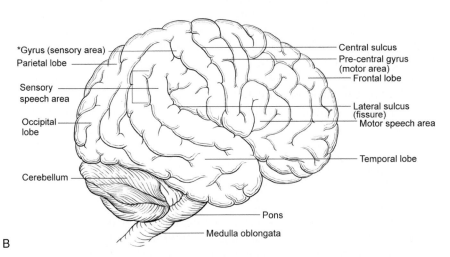

FIGURE 3.1. **(A)** Coronal section of the skull and meninges, including the dura, arachnoid, and pia mater. **(B)** Lateral view of the brain.

parietal, occipital, and temporal (Figure 3.1 B). The cerebral cortex consists of gyri (folds) and sulci (grooves). Posterior and inferior to the cerebral cortex are the cerebellum and the brainstem, consisting of the medulla oblongata, pons, and midbrain.

Clinical Evaluation

The athlete's level of consciousness should guide management priorities (3,4). In an unconscious athlete, a cervical spine injury should be assumed, and appropriate immobilization of the cervical spine should be immediately instituted to protect against potential catastrophic spinal injury (4–6). Management then proceeds through the ABCs (airway, breathing, and circulation) (3–6). A patent airway must be established and protected. If the patient is unable to protect the airway, or if there are signs of neurological deterioration, such as posturing or pupillary abnormalities, the athlete should be intubated and hyperventilated (4–7). If the airway is patent, adequate ventilation must be ensured. Circulation should be monitored and supported as necessary. The athlete should be transported on a spinal board by ambulance to the nearest trauma center as quickly as possible (Table 3.1) (3–7).

An injured athlete who is conscious should be immediately removed from the field of play and taken to an area where medical examination can take place (4). The athlete should not be left alone and should be frequently reassessed for signs and symptoms of deterioration (4,6). The athlete should be assessed by a physician with experience evaluating sport head injuries as soon as possible (8).

History

Information regarding the mechanism of injury should be obtained from the athlete and any witnesses (3,4). The athlete should be asked about symptoms that he or she is experiencing, such as headache, nausea, or difficulty

TABLE 3.1. Indications for immediate transfer to hospital in a head-injured athlete.

Prolonged loss of consciousness (>5 min)
Increasing headache, nausea, vomiting
Decreased level of consciousness (GCS <14)
Unstable vital signs
Unequal pupils
Seizure
Focal neurological deficits/evolving neurological signs

Source: Reprinted with permission from Hunte G, 2005.

concentrating. It should be determined if there was any loss of consciousness and if so, for how long. Amnesia should also be assessed. Athletes may seem dazed or have difficulty answering questions. They may also be irritable, moody, or combative and may not want to answer questions.

Orientation should be evaluated by asking the athlete questions about person, time, and place (4). For example, ask the athlete to identify the opposing team, what position he/she plays, and the score of the game. Assess memory by asking questions regarding events before the injury, such as how the team got to the field of play, the score at halftime, etc. Immediate and delayed memory should be evaluated by giving the patient a list of five words to recall immediately and at the end of the examination (4). Concentration is often affected, and it can be assessed by asking the patient to recite the months of the year backwards or doing serial sevens. Note the athlete's ability to do the test—do they get frustrated or confused, take a long time to answer, or make mistakes?

Physical Examination

ABCs should be assessed initially in all injured athletes. In athletes with an impaired level of consciousness, neurological assessment should proceed with a determination of level of consciousness using the Glasgow Coma Scale (Table 3.2) (3,5–7,9). Any athlete with a Glasgow coma score of 13 or less should be transported to hospital for further evaluation (Table 3.1) (7).

TABLE 3.2. Glasgow coma scale.

Eye Opening	E
Spontaneous	4
to speech	3
to pain	2
no response	1
Verbal Response	V
alert and oriented	5
disoriented conversation	4
speaking but nonsensical	3
moans or unintelligible sounds	2
no response	1
Motor Response	M
follows commands	6
localizes pain	5
movement/withdrawal to pain	4
decorticate flexion	3
decerebrate extension	2
no response	1
Total score = E + V + M	

Source: Teasdale and Jennett, 1994. Reprinted with permission from Elsevier.

Once the athlete has been removed from the field of play, inspection of the head and scalp should be conducted, looking for scalp tenderness, lacerations, hematomas, bleeding from the ear and leakage of cerebrospinal fluid from the nose (3). If the athlete is stable, a baseline neurological exam should be performed, including cranial nerve assessment, gross visual field examination, pupillary and fundoscopic examination, strength and sensation, deep tendon reflexes, and cerebellar testing, as well as gait and Romberg testing (3,4). In the vast majority of cases, the neurological exam is normal. Occasionally, in concussion, balance may be affected and patients may have a positive Romberg (10).

If there are abnormalities on the neurological exam, patients should be transported to hospital for further evaluation (7). However, it is important to note that absence of abnormal signs, particularly early in the course of injury, does not rule out a potentially serious brain injury. Frequent reassessments are necessary to monitor potential deterioration, which may indicate a serious brain injury (4,5).

Diagnostic Tests

On Field/Office Assessment

The Sport Concussion Assessment Tool (SCAT) was developed by the Concussion in Sport Group at the Second International Conference on Concussion in Sport (10). This tool was designed for patient education, as well as physician assessment of sports concussion. It was developed by combining several existing tools, including the Maddocks questions (11) and Standardized Assessment of Concussion (SAC) (12). The SCAT assesses orientation, immediate memory, concentration, and delayed memory, and it is available on www.thinkfirst.ca. To date, this tool has not been formally validated for use in children.

Neuroimaging

If there are any focal or localizing neurological signs, computed tomography (CT) scan or magnetic resonance imaging (MRI) should be obtained to rule out an intracranial injury (Table 3.3) (4,5,8,10,13,14). In cases of concussion, imaging studies are usually normal, and therefore are not routinely ordered (8,10,13,14). In complex concussions (i.e., prolonged symptoms), imaging studies may be appropriate (5,10,14). Magnetic resonance imaging is a more sensitive modality to detect subtle structural injuries, such as contusions and diffuse axonal injury (DAI) (15). There are more specialized imaging techniques, such as single-photon emission computed tomography (SPECT), positron emission tomography (PET), and functional MRI (fMRI), which may be able to demonstrate pathophysiologic and functional abnormalities after concussion (15).

TABLE 3.3. Indications for neuroimaging.

Repeated vomiting (>3 times)
GCS <13
Focal neurological signs
Suspicion of skull fracture
Seizure
Loss of consciousness >5 min

Neuropsychological Testing

After head injury, children may have cognitive functional deficits, such as impaired attention and concentration, mild disorientation, and memory difficulties (12,16,17). There have been numerous studies looking at neuropsychological testing in the athletic population, including traditional pen and paper tests (11,12,16,17) and, more recently, computer-based programs (1,18–20). The SCAT tool (10) combines several existing tools, including the SAC, which has been studied in healthy children aged 9–14 yr and has been found to be a reliable assessment tool in this age group (21). The SCAT has not yet been validated in children.

Neuropsychological tests can help with return to play decisions in athletes who have sustained a concussive head injury. They are most beneficial when baseline data has been obtained before injury (10,14). After a concussive injury, athletes can then be compared to their own baseline to determine any deficits. This is recommended because neuropsychological tests can be affected by many factors, including previous head injury, test anxiety, attention deficit disorder, psychiatric conditions, very high or low cognitive functioning, or learning disabilities (17). In the absence of baseline data, however, neuropsychological tests can still provide objective data to help with return to play decisions (10).

A unique concern regarding neuropsychological testing in the pediatric population is that children are undergoing rapid cognitive development. Computer-based tests have demonstrated that there is a substantial improvement in performance between 9 and 18 yr of age on tests of simple and choice reaction time, working memory, and new learning, with the largest changes in function seen between the ages of 9 and 15 yr (1,20). These developmental changes can potentially confound postinjury assessments, as maturational improvements may offset any cognitive impairment resulting from injury; therefore, baseline testing may need to be done as often as every 6 mo (1).

For most pediatric athletes, universal baseline neuropsychological testing for routine evaluation of concussion is impractical because of lack of availability and cost. However, age-appropriate, validated neuropsychological testing may be helpful to assist with return to play decisions in those athletes who demonstrate prolonged postconcussive symptoms (i.e., complex concussions) (10,17).

Head Injuries

Skull Fractures

Skull fractures (Figure 3.2) are not common in the sport setting, but are serious injuries that may require neurosurgical consultation. Skull fractures are often associated with underlying brain injury and may result in focal neurologic deficits or seizures (22). A CT scan is the best initial study in this setting because it will demonstrate both the fracture and any associated intracranial bleeding (22). Skull fractures are often associated with epidural hematomas or other intracranial hemorrhages (5,6,22,23).

Intracranial Hemorrhage

The leading cause of death from sport-related head injury is intracranial hemorrhage (23). Intracranial hemorrhage includes epidural hematoma, subdural hematoma, intracerebral hematoma, and subarachnoid hematoma. Hematomas of the brain usually cause headache and may result in neurological deficit, depending on what area of the brain is affected. Seizures may be precipitated by the accumulation of blood. Traumatic seizures usually last only 1–2 min. Hemorrhage in the brain can be rapidly fatal, and therefore, prompt, accurate assessment and follow-up after a sport-related head injury is mandatory (23).

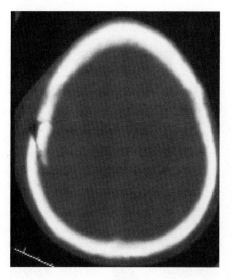

FIGURE 3.2. Depressed skull fracture. (Courtesy of Dr. Anthony L. Alcantara, St. John Hospital and Medical Center, Detroit, MI.)

Epidural Hematoma

Epidural hematomas result from damage to the middle meningeal artery (Figure 3.3), causing blood to accumulate between the skull and the dura of the brain (4–6,22,23). It is often associated with a fracture of the temporal bone (5,22,23). The brain itself is usually uninjured. The mechanism of injury is typically a high-impact event, such as getting hit by a baseball (4). The injured athlete may have a brief period of unconsciousness or being stunned, and then have a lucid period before developing a severe headache

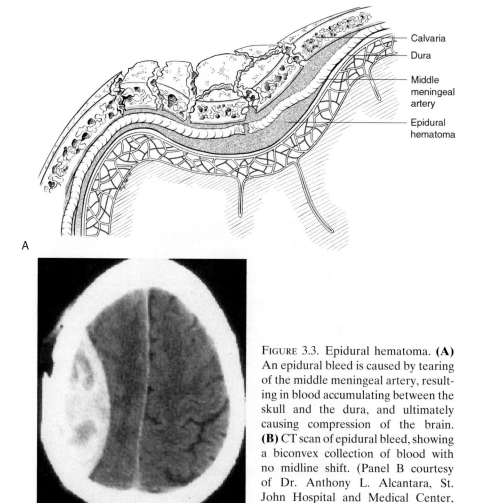

FIGURE 3.3. Epidural hematoma. **(A)** An epidural bleed is caused by tearing of the middle meningeal artery, resulting in blood accumulating between the skull and the dura, and ultimately causing compression of the brain. **(B)** CT scan of epidural bleed, showing a biconvex collection of blood with no midline shift. (Panel B courtesy of Dr. Anthony L. Alcantara, St. John Hospital and Medical Center, Detroit, MI.)

and progressive decline in level of consciousness (4–6,22,23). This deterioration can happen quite quickly, in a matter of minutes to hours after the injury, and can be rapidly fatal if it is missed. It occurs as a result of the accumulation of the clot and resulting increase in intracranial pressure (5,23). It is imperative that these athletes be immediately transferred to a hospital with neurosurgical expertise to prevent death (4,5,23). If the clot can be evacuated promptly, the athlete usually has a complete neurological recovery, as the brain is not injured (5,23).

Subdural Hematoma

Subdural hematomas are three times more common in sport-related head injuries than epidural hematomas (6,22). High-impact injuries to the head can result in damage to the venous structures beneath the dura mater, causing bleeding below the dura (Figure 3.4) (4,23). The mechanism of injury is usually a fall or high-speed collision (4). If a skull fracture is also present, signs and symptoms can evolve rapidly. However, if there is no fracture, signs and symptoms may be delayed for several days (4). This injury typically results in a prolonged loss of consciousness (greater than a few minutes) (5,6,22,23). There is a 30–40% mortality rate from subdural hematomas; there is often significant residual morbidity secondary to brain damage (4,5,22,23).

Intracerebral Hematoma

This usually results from a torn artery, which causes bleeding into the brain itself, usually associated with an extremely severe acceleration injury to the head (5,23). This may also result from congenital vascular lesions, such as aneurysms or arteriovenous malformations (23). Consciousness is usually impaired. Often, these injuries can be rapidly fatal and result in death before transport to hospital is possible (23).

Subarachnoid Hematoma

Bleeding in this instance results from tearing of tiny surface brain vessels, resulting from trauma (Figure 3.5), causing bleeding that is confined to the cerebrospinal fluid space (23). It may also result from a congenital malformation (5). Neurologic deterioration, including death, may be quite rapid (5). Surgery is rarely necessary because the bleeding is superficial.

Malignant Brain Edema Syndrome

Malignant brain edema syndrome is a rare condition that occurs in children as a result of head trauma (4,5,22,23). Brain edema develops rapidly, secondary to loss of vascular autoregulation of the brain's blood supply, with resultant vascular engorgement and increasing intracranial pressure (ICP)

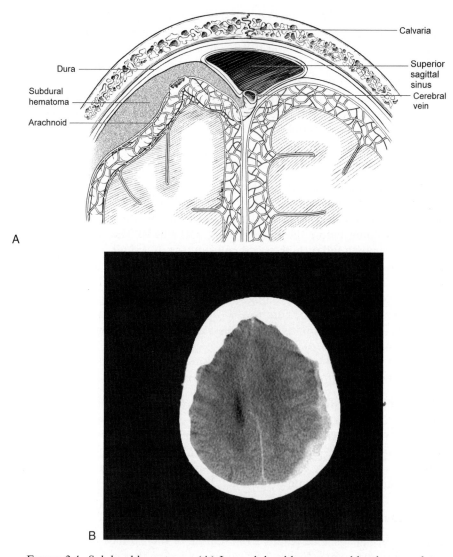

FIGURE 3.4. Subdural hematoma. **(A)** In a subdural hematoma, blood accumulates between the dura and the arachnoid mater, causing midline shift. There is associated underlying brain injury. **(B)** CT image of an acute left frontoparietal subdural hematoma. (Panel B courtesy of Dr. David Pelz, Department of Radiology, London Health Sciences Centre, University Campus, London, Ontario, Canada.)

(5,22,23). As the ICP increases, brain herniation and brainstem compromise occurs, rapidly leading to death in almost 50% of cases (22,23). Death occurs in minutes to hours. This is believed to be the underlying abnormality in second impact syndrome, which occurs rarely when a young athlete returns to competition while still symptomatic from a head injury and sustains another injury (4,5,22).

Diffuse Axonal Injury

This is an uncommon injury in sports because it requires severe trauma (6). It results from severe shearing forces on the brain, causing the disruption of axonal connections (5,6). There is no hematoma associated. The athlete

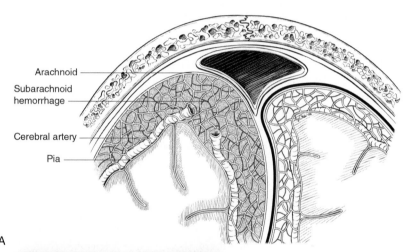

Arachnoid
Subarachnoid
hemorrhage

Cerebral artery

Pia

A

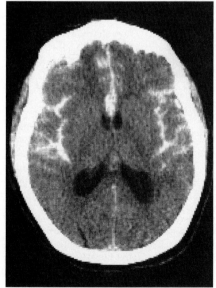

B

FIGURE 3.5. Subarachnoid hemorrhage. **(A)** Blood accumulates between the pia mater and arachnoid layers, accumulating in the fissures and sulci. **(B)** CT scan showing a subarachnoid hemorrhage. (Panel B is from Cochrane Miller J, Headache—when is neuroimaging needed? Radiology Rounds. September 2003. http://www.mghradrounds.org/index.php?src=gendocs&link=2003_September. Copyright 2003 MGH Department of Radiology.)

is deeply comatose. This condition generally results in long-term neurologic deficits. It is the most common cause of persistent vegetative state resulting from a head injury (6).

Concussion

Concussions are the most common head injury in children participating in sports. However, there is still a lot of controversy surrounding this injury, particularly in the pediatric population. The newest definition of concussion was proposed by the Concussion in Sport Group, which defines concussion as "a complex pathophysiological process affecting the brain, induced by traumatic biomechanical forces" resulting "in the rapid onset of short-lived impairment of neurological function that resolves spontaneously" (10,14). Concussion does not result in a structural injury to the brain; rather, the injury is at the functional level. Concussion may be sustained by a direct blow to the head, face, or neck, or by a blow to somewhere else on the body that transmits an impulsive force to the head (10,14,24).

Concussion can be difficult to diagnose and can present a management challenge to many physicians who care for these children (25–27). Diagnosis is often challenging because signs and symptoms of concussion can be quite subtle, and thus may not be easily identified (Table 3.4). There is also

TABLE 3.4. Features of concussion.

Cognitive features	Symptoms	Signs
• General confusion • Difficulty determining time, date, place • Unaware of time of game, opposing team, score of game • Amnesia—retrograde; posttraumatic/anterograde • Loss of consciousness	• Headache • Dizziness • Feeling dazed • Feeling "dinged" or stunned; "having my bell rung" • Seeing stars or flashing lights • Ringing in the ears • Sleepiness • Loss of vision • Double vision/blurry vision • Nausea	• Poor coordination or balance • Vacant stare/glassy eyed • Vomiting • Slurred speech • Slow to answer questions or follow directions • Easily distracted, poor concentration • Unusual or inappropriate emotions • Personality changes • Inappropriate playing behavior (i.e., moving in the wrong direction) • Decreased playing ability

Source: McCrory et al., 2004; Kissick et al., 2000. Reprinted from Canadian Paediatric Society, Healthy Active Living Committee [Principal author: Laura Purcell]. Identification and management of children with sport-related concussion. Paediatr Child Health 2006; 2006; 11(7):420–428. Also available at http://www.cps.ca/english/statements/HAL/HAL06–01.htm (Version current at June 4, 2007).

TABLE 3.5. Classification of concussion.

Simple	Complex
• most common • usually resolve in 7–10 d • no sequelae	• persistent symptoms >10 d, including recurrence with exertion • prolonged LOC (>1 min) • symptoms may last weeks to months • permanent deficits/cognitive impairment • multiple concussions, with less impact force

Source: McCrory et al., 2004; reprinted from Canadian Paediatric Society, Healthy Active Living Committee [Principal author: Laura Purcell]. Identification and management of children with sport-related concussion. Paediatr Child Health 2006; 2006; 11(7):420–428. Also available at http://www.cps.ca/english/statements/HAL/HAL06–01.htm (Version current at June 4, 2007).

a tendency for athletes to minimize or not recognize signs/symptoms of concussion, and therefore to underreport injuries (28,29).

There have been many grading systems for concussion published in the literature (5,6,10,14). These systems used loss of consciousness or amnesia as an indication of injury severity. Evidence suggests that brief losses of consciousness (less than 1 min) and amnesia do not correlate with severity of sporting concussive injury (10,14). It is now recognized that the severity of concussions can best be determined retrospectively, once all symptoms and signs have resolved (10).

A simplified system of classification was proposed in the 2005 Prague guidelines, which classify concussion into "simple" and "complex" forms (Table 3.5) (10). Simple concussions usually resolve within 7–10 d, with no sequelae. Complex concussions have prolonged signs and symptoms lasting for weeks to months, sometimes with permanent deficits (10). Athletes who have complex concussions should be managed by physicians with specific concussion expertise and may require a multidisciplinary management team, possibly including a neurologist, neurosurgeon, sport medicine physician, and a neuropsychologist (8,10).

Management

The first priority in any injured athlete is to rule out serious head or spinal injury. If the athlete is unconscious, a spinal injury should be assumed and appropriate cervical spine precautions must be taken before transport to hospital (4–6). Structural head injuries such as skull fractures and intracranial hemorrhages require neurosurgical evaluation (5,22).

The majority of head injuries do not result in a loss of consciousness. A conscious athlete who is suspected of having sustained a head injury should be immediately removed from the game and not allowed to return to play that day (4–6,8,10,14). A physician should evaluate the athlete as soon as possible. A player should never return to sport if symptomatic (4–8,10,14,24). They often will have decreased attention, slower response times, and memory deficits, which may impair an athlete's ability to avoid dangerous situations, thus putting them at risk for further injury. *If in doubt, sit them out!*

In athletes who have sustained a concussive injury, the most important aspect of management is *rest* for as long as the athlete remains symptomatic (4–6,8,10,13,14). After physician assessment, most athletes can be observed at home by a responsible caregiver who has been instructed on signs of neurological deterioration (3,13). Signs of neurological deterioration warrant urgent transport to the hospital for reexamination by a doctor and imaging studies. Consultation with neurosurgery may be necessary (3–5,13).

As long as the athlete is symptomatic, he/she should not play sports, exercise, or participate in recreational activities such as riding a bike or wrestling with friends or siblings (8,10,14). Cognitive rest is also important (8,10). This may necessitate avoiding daily activities that require mental concentration, such as reading, computer work, and video games. Athletes may need to miss school while symptomatic because the concentration and attention required to perform schoolwork may make symptoms worse and prolong recovery. Once symptoms have resolved, children should try going back to school half-days. If they do not have worsening/recurring symptoms, they may return full time.

Activity can be resumed once all concussive symptoms have resolved. Return to play should follow a medically supervised stepwise process, outlined below (8,10,14,24). It is important that a physician with experience treating concussions guides the return to play process. Each step should take at least 24h. Athletes may progress to the next step as long as they remain asymptomatic. If symptoms recur, athletes should rest for 24–48h and attempt to progress again, starting at the level where their symptoms recurred. The time required to progress through these steps may be variable, depending on the severity of concussion and the individual athlete's concussion history (8,10,14,24).

Stepwise Process (8,10,14,24):

1. Complete rest, no activities such as exercising, riding a bike, computer work, video games, etc. Once all symptoms have resolved, athletes can proceed to step 2. Athletes should be asymptomatic for several days before proceeding to step 2.
2. Light aerobic exercise such as walking or stationary cycling for 10–15min. No resistance training.

3. Sport-specific activity (i.e., skating in hockey, running in soccer) with NO CONTACT for 20–30 min.
4. Noncontact training drills.
5. "On field" practice with body contact, once cleared by a physician.
6. Game play.

Prevention

Head injuries may be prevented by wearing the appropriate protective equipment for a specific sport (10,14,22,24,30–34). Approved helmets should be worn for all contact sports and for recreational activities with a risk of head injury (i.e., cycling, skateboarding, or in-line skating) (10,14,22,24,34,35) The equipment should be worn properly and be well maintained (36,37). Any damaged equipment should be replaced promptly.

   Athletes, coaches, and parents should realize that there is no such thing as a "concussion-proof" helmet. Risk compensation, whereby players feel they are not at risk for head injury if wearing their helmet and therefore play more aggressively, may actually put athletes at greater risk of injury (10,14,38). To minimize risk of head injury, athletes should respect the rules of their sport and practice fair play.

   Coaches and trainers are important in reducing the incidence of head injuries in sport. They must ensure that athletes learn the proper sport techniques, such as correct body checking technique in hockey, correct tackling technique in football, and correct heading technique in soccer. Neck muscle strengthening programs may help reduce concussions by reducing the impact forces transmitted to the brain, although evidence for this is lacking at present (14,34).

   Sport rule changes and rule enforcement can also decrease head injuries in sport (10,14,34,38). Padded goal posts in soccer and football, and the banning of spearing in football have reduced the number of head injuries in these sports (34,38,39). Head injuries in hockey may be reduced by limiting checking in boy's hockey (less than 16 yr), banning checking from behind, and banning fighting (8,10,14). Discouraging enrollment in sports where intentional head injury is encouraged may also decrease sport-related head injury in children and adolescents (8).

Return to Play

Certain conditions preclude return to sport after a head injury (Table 3.6) (5). After an intracranial hematoma requiring surgery, return to contact sport is not encouraged. Return to noncontact sports is not contraindicated if recovery has been complete. Athletes with an intracranial hemorrhage

TABLE 3.6. Conditions that preclude participation in contact sports.

Permanent neurological deficits
Persistent postconcussion symptoms
Hydrocephalus
Spontaneous subarachnoid hemorrhage

Source: Cantu, 1998. Modified by permission of Elsevier.

that did not require surgery, or with an epidural hematoma without brain injury, who have a complete recovery may return to contact sport, in selected cases, a year or longer after the injury; however, extreme deliberation with the athlete and family should occur before return (5). *No athlete should participate in sports if symptomatic from a head injury.*

Return to sport after a concussion continues to be a controversial area, particularly in the pediatric age group. Current recommendations are largely anecdotal, based on recommendations for adults but urging more caution in children and adolescents. One point of consensus is that an athlete with a concussive injury should not be allowed to return to activity until ALL signs and symptoms have resolved (4–6,10,14,22–24). It is important that athletes do not return to play the day of an injury because even if initial symptoms resolve quickly, they may recur later that day or evening.

After a period of rest, during which all postconcussive symptoms have resolved, the athlete should follow a medically supervised stepwise approach to return to their sport, as previously outlined (8,10,14,24). Each step should take at least 24h, and athletes may progress through the steps as long as they remain asymptomatic. If symptoms recur, athletes should rest for 24–48h and attempt to progress again, starting at the step where their symptoms recurred.

Clinical Pearls

- Head injuries occur frequently in sport.
- Athletes, trainers, coaches, officials, parents should recognize symptoms of a head injury and the need to seek prompt medical attention in the event of a head injury.
- Any head injury should be considered serious.
- In an unconscious athlete, a cervical spine injury should be assumed and appropriate immobilization of the cervical spine should occur before transport to hospital.
- There is potential for players to get worse over time; therefore, they should not be left alone.
- Any athlete who sustains a head injury should be assessed by a physician as soon as possible.

- No player should return to sport while symptomatic. **IF IN DOUBT, SIT THEM OUT!**
- Concussed athletes should rest until completely symptom free.
- Return to play after a concussion should follow a step-wise progression of exertion, guided by a physician knowledgeable in the management of sport-related concussion.

References

1. McCrory P, Collie A, Anderson V, Davis G. Can we manage sport-related concussion in children the same as in adults? Br J Sports Med 2004;38: 516–519.
2. Kelly KD, Lissel HL, Rowe BH, Vincenten JA, Voaklander DC. Sport and recreation-related head injuries treated in the emergency department. Clin J Sport Med 2001;11:77–81.
3. Emergency Paediatrics Section, Canadian Paediatric Society. The management of children with head trauma. CMAJ 1990;142(9):949–952. Reaffirmed January 2002.
4. Smith BW. Head Injuries. In: Anderson SJ and Sullivan JA, eds. Care of the Young Athlete. American Academy of Pediatrics and American Academy of Orthopedic Surgeons; 2000:171–178.
5. Cantu RC. Return to play guidelines after a head injury. Clinics in Sport Med 1998;17(1):45–60.
6. Warren WL, Bailes JE. On the field evaluation of athletic head injuries. Clinics in Sport Med 1998;17(1):13–26.
7. Hunte G. Sporting emergencies. Brukner P and Khan K, eds. In: Clinical Sports Medicine. 2nd ed. Roseville NSW; McGraw-Hill: 2001:713–725.
8. Canadian Paediatric Society, Healthy Active Living Committee [Principal author: Laura Purcell]. Identification and management of children with sport-related concussion. Paediatr Child Health 2006;11(7):420–428. Also available at http://www.cps.ca/english/statements/HAL/HAL06-01.htm (Version current at June 4, 2007).
9. Teasdale G, Jennett B. Assessment of coma and impaired consciousness. A practical scale. Lancet 1974;2:81–84.
10. McCrory P, Johnston K, Meeuwisse W, et al. Summary and Agreement Statement of the 2nd International Symposium on Concussion in Sport, Prague 2004. Clin J Sports Med 2005;15(2):48–55.
11. Maddocks DL, Dicker GD, Saling MM. The assessment of orientation following concussion in athletes. Clin J Sport Med 1995;5:32–35.
12. McCrea M, Kelly JP, Randolph C, et al. Standardized Assessment of Concussion (SAC): On-Site Mental Status Evaluation of the Athlete. J Head Trauma Rehab 1998;13:27–36.
13. Committee on Quality Improvement, American Academy of Paediatrics. The management of minor closed head injury in children. Peds 1999;6:1407–1415.
14. Aubry M, Cantu R, Dvorak J, et al. Summary and Agreement Statement of the 1st International Symposium on Concussion in Sport, Vienna 2001. Clin J Sports Med 2002;12:6–11.

15. Johnston KM, Ptito A, Chankowsky J, Chen JK. New frontiers in diagnostic imaging in concussive head injury. Clin J Sport Med 2001;11:166–175.
16. Yeates KO, Luria J, Bartkowski H, Rusin J, Martin L, Bigler, ED. Postconcussive symptoms in children with mild closed head injuries. J Head Trauma Rehabil 1999;14(4):337–350.
17. Grindel SH, Lovell, MR and Collins, MW. The assessment of sport-related concussion: The evidence behind neuropsychological testing and management. Clin J Sport Med 2001;11(3):134–143.
18. Collie A, Maruff P, Makdissi M, McCrory P, McStephen M, Darby D. CogSport: Reliability and correlation with conventional cognitive tests used in postconcussion medical evaluations. Clin J Sport Med 2003;13:28–32.
19. Janusz JA et al. Construct validity of the ImPACT post-concussion scale in children. Poster presentation at the 2nd International Symposium on Concussion in Sport. Prague November 5–6, 2004.
20. Gioia GA, Gioia GA, Gilstein K, Iverson G. Neuropsychological management of concussion in children and adolescents: Effect of age and gender on ImPACT. Poster presentation at the 2nd International Symposium on Concussion in Sport. Prague November 5–6, 2004.
21. Valovich McLeod TC, Perrin DH, Guskiewicz KM, Shultz SJ, Diamond R, Gansneder BM. Serial administration of clinical concussion assessments and learning effects in healthy young athletes. Clin J Sport Med 2004;14(5): 287–295.
22. Putukian M, Harmon KG. Head injuries. In: Birrer RB, Griesemer BA, Cataletto MB, eds. Pediatric Sports Medicine for Primary Care. Philadelphia: Lippincott Williams and Wilkins; 2002:266–290.
23. Proctor MR, Cantu RC. Head and neck injuries in young athletes. Clin Sport Med 2000;19(4):693–715.
24. Kissick J, Johnston K. Position statement: Guidelines for the assessment and management of sport-related concussion. Clin J Sports Med 2000;10(3):209–211.
25. Bazarian JJ, Veenema T, Brayer AF, Lee E. Knowledge of concussion guidelines among practitioners caring for children. Clin Peds 2001;40(4): 207–212.
26. Genuardi FJ, William DK. Inappropriate discharge instructions for youth athletes hospitalized for concussion. Peds 1995; 95(2):216–218.
27. Poirier MP, Wadsworth MR. CME review article: Sports-related concussions. Ped Emerg Care 2000;16(4):278–283.
28. Kaut KP, DePompei R, Kerr J, Congeni J. Reports of head injury and symptom knowledge among college athletes: Implications for assessment and educational intervention. Clin J Sport Med 2003;13:213–221.
29. Delaney JS, Lecroix VJ, Leclerc S, Johnston KM. Concussions among university football and soccer players. Clin J Sport Med 2002;12:331–338.
30. LeBlanc JC, Huybers S. Improving bicycle safety: The role of paediatricians and family physicians. Paediatr Child Health 2004;9(5):315–318.
31. Cook A, Sheikh A. Trends in serious head injuries among English cyclists and pedestrians. Injury Prevention 2003;9:266–267.
32. Thompson DC, Rivara FP, Thompson RS. Effectiveness of bicycle safety helmets in preventing head injuries: A case-control study. JAMA 1996;276: 1968–1973.

33. Thompson RS, Rivara FP. Protective equipment for in-line skaters. N Engl J Med 1996;335:1680–1682.
34. McCrory P. Minor head injury in sport. In: Brukner P and Khan K, eds. Clinical Sports Medicine. 2nd ed. Roseville NSW: McGraw-Hill; 2001: 189–194.
35. In favour of legislation for mandatory use of helmets by participants of all ages and for manually operated wheeled activities including bicycles, skateboards, in-line skates and roller skates on streets, roads, trails and parks in all provinces and territories of Canada. Position statement from ThinkFirst Foundation of Canada, June 2007. Available at www.thinkfirst.ca.
36. ThinkFirst helmet guide. June 2007. Available at www.thinkfirst.ca.
37. Bernhardt DT. Football: A case-based approach to mild traumatic brain injury. Pediatric Annals 2000;29(3):31–35.
38. Hagel B, Meeuwisse W. Risk compensation: A "side effect" of sport injury prevention? Clin J Sport Med 2004;14:193–196.
39. Landry GL. Central nervous system trauma: Management of concussions in athletes. Pediatr Clin N Am 2002;49:723–741.

4
Cervical and Thoracic Spine Injuries

Pierre d'Hemecourt and Jessica Flynn Deede

Cervical spine injuries are very common in contact sports such as wrestling, football, hockey, and rugby. It has been estimated that up to 15% of football athletes suffer from some cervical spine injury. The National Center for Catastrophic Sports Injury reported over the 12-yr period between 1982 and 1994 there were 450 catastrophic injuries, and 75% involved the cervical spine (1). Although thoracic spine injuries are less frequently involved in catastrophic injury, they do occur in the adolescent athlete participating in hockey, football, gymnastics, and wrestling, as well as other contact sports.

Noncontact sports also produce overuse injuries to the cervical and thoracic spine. In the adolescent athlete, this may produce spinal deformity such as kyphosis, as well as adult pattern injury. The physician involved in sports medicine must understand the different injury patterns of specific sports, as well as the evaluation of the athlete for these injuries. The cervical and thoracic spine contains the spinal cord. Consequently, a full understanding of anatomy is important. The physician must also understand the assessment of mechanical and neurologic stability at the initiation and completion of treatment. A safe return to sports participation also requires an understanding of injury prevention with proper conditioning, sports technique, and equipment.

Anatomy

The cervical and thoracic spine are structurally critical for motion and support. The thoracic spine serves to transfer forces between the upper and lower extremities, and the cervical spine provides support and motion for the skull. Together, these two upper spinal segments act as a conduit for the central nervous system and are prone to injury in the athlete. This includes both acute and chronic overuse injuries.

The cervical spine is a flexible structure between the head and more rigid thoracic spine. This mobility imparts a greater risk for injury to the discs and osseous structures. In contrast, the thoracic spine is more rigid and protected with the rib attachments. However, the lower two ribs are free floating and allow some increased motion in the lower thoracic spine. Consequently, traumatic and overuse injury patterns are more frequent in these transition zones of flexibility at the lower cervical and lower thoracic spine.

The cervical vertebrae can be divided into two distinct areas of the upper and lower cervical spine. The lower portion, C3 through C6, has a typical appearance, with vertebral bodies separated by the intervertebral disc. Furthermore, the superiorlateral aspects of the body have a projection of the uncus that articulates with the convex inferior endplate of the cephalad vertebrae. In late childhood, this developmentally becomes an articulation, the joint of Luschka. This articulation forms an anterior border of the neuroforamina and, with degeneration, may contribute to foraminal stenosis. The facet joints form the posterior border of the foramina. These facets are in a more horizontal plane and progress to a more vertical coronal plane in the thoracic spine. The horizontal orientation allows rotation. The transverse process contains the foramen for the vertebral artery (2). The lower cervical spine is primarily responsible for flexion and extension. Lateral flexion is coupled with rotation (3).

The upper cervical spine is comprised of the occiput to C1, as well as the C1–2 articulation. The atlas, C1, has a smaller anterior arch and a larger posterior arch connected by the lateral masses. The axis, C2, contains the odontoid process that articulates with the anterior arch of the atlas and is constrained by the transverse ligament. Between the occiput-C1 and C1–2 articulations, 40% of cervical flexion and extension occurs, whereas 60% of rotation occurs, at these levels (4).

The thoracic vertebrae gradually increase in size from T1 through T12. This region is unique because of the facets on the vertebral bodies for the heads of the ribs and the facets on the transverse processes, which articulate with the tubercle of the rib (Figure 4.1). The thoracic facet joints are in a more coronal orientation to allow for lateral flexion. However, there is a transition of the upper and lower thoracic vertebrae, with the upper vertebrae configured in a more cervical morphology, whereas the lower vertebrae resemble the lumbar vertebrae (5). All of these articulations have been associated as pain generators. A further confounding structure to the thoracic spine is the scapula. This triangular shaped bone lies between the 2nd and 7th ribs. It projects 30–40 degrees to the frontal plane. Bony ridges or osteophytes may rub against the ribs. Furthermore, several bursae assist with scapulothoracic articulation. There are several at the superior medial angle and one at the inferior corner (Figure 4.2). Each of these is subject to inflammation and pain.

From C3 through T12, as well as the lumbar spine, each functional unit of motion acts as a tripod, with the disc anterior and the facet joints posterior. Anteriorly, the intervertebral disc is composed of the anulus, with ligamentous layers encompassing the gelatinous nucleus pulposus. The

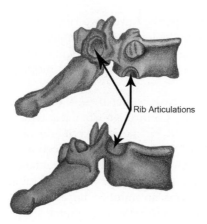

FIGURE 4.1. Thoracic vertebrae.

Rib Articulations

anulus, comprised of 10–20 layers of concentric, obliquely oriented ligamentous lamellae, provides for torsional stability (6). The outer layers of
the anulus are innervated by the sinuvertebral nerves posteriorly and by
the gray ramus communicans anteriorly. Mechanical and chemical irritation
from the nucleus pulposus may produce pain.

The growing spine has some unique considerations. The anulus is attached
to the growth cartilage of the epiphysis and apophyseal ring. The vertebral
body is bound on the superior and inferior borders by the epiphyseal
growth plate with its overlying cartilaginous endplate and its contiguous
ring apophysis (Figure 4.3). This growth cartilage is the weak link. Injury
to the growth zone has been demonstrated with both flexion and extension

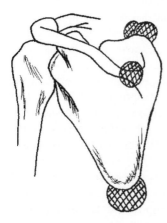

FIGURE 4.2. The scapula is a triangular shaped
bone that lies between the 2nd and 7th ribs.

FIGURE 4.3. Adolescent endplate.

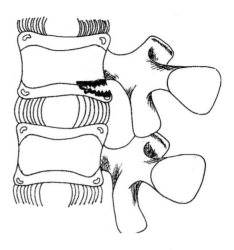

and an applied compression load, which may be a factor with pain and increased kyphosis in the adolescent spine (7). During adolescent growth, there is a normal increase of approximately 10 degrees of thoracic kyphosis (8). Repetitive flexion and extension during this growth period has been shown to accentuate this kyphosis (9).

There are numerous paraspinal muscles of the thoracic and cervical spine inherently associated with the lumbopelvic musculature. Each of these may be involved in myotendonopathies and acute contusions and strains. Functionally, the anterior and middle scalene muscles are important, as they arise from the anterolateral cervical spine and attach to the first rib. The brachial plexus traverses between these in its passage through the thoracic outlet and is subject to impingement here, as well as between the clavicle and first rib.

Clinical Evaluation

History

When assessing an athlete with a neck or back complaint, whether on the athletic field or in the office, it is crucial to obtain a detailed history of the inciting event and pattern of symptoms. When there is suspicion of a traumatic spinal injury, appropriate measures must immediately be taken to immobilize and protect the spinal column until further evaluation with radiographic assistance can be undertaken in the hospital setting. Airway management should be closely coordinated with immobilization and transport. This should always be well rehearsed before the event.

The demographics of gender, age, and type of sport or occupation are relevant. Gender may be important, with males having more spondyloarthopathies, whereas females have more osteoporosis issues. Younger athletes are predisposed to growth cartilage injury, whereas the young adult may be more predisposed to discogenic issues. The type of sport can predispose to certain patterns of injury. For instance, participants in gymnastics have a high prevalence of thoracolumbar disc and endplate injury (10).

The history should include mechanism of injury, onset of pain (sudden or insidious), location of pain, and associated neurologic symptoms (including transient paresthesias, paralysis, or weakness). Cervical pain may radiate to the interscapular region, as well as into the upper extremity. Thoracic pain may radiate to the anterior trunk or to the lower extremities. With the cervical and thoracic spine, myelopathic symptoms must be elicited. These include an unstable gait, weak or fumbling hands, and bowel or bladder incontinence. One should also inquire about previous evaluation and treatment. Previous medical problems are elicited, such as Down syndrome or Klippel–Feil syndrome with cervical instability.

In the setting of trauma, the mechanism of injury and position of the head during impact can aid in determining the distribution of forces in the injured spine. Hyperflexion injuries are the most common and can cause compression fractures of the anterior vertebral body and disruption of the posterior spinal ligaments. Hyperextension injuries can cause the opposite, with compression of the posterior elements and disruption of the anterior longitudinal ligament. Axial loading can cause compression or burst fractures of the vertebral bodies. Rotational injuries may cause injury to the facet joints.

Neurologic symptoms are very important to elicit when taking a sideline history. Whether these symptoms persist or have resolved, they will give clues to the location of possible spinal cord involvement. A classic injury observed in football players is the "burning hands" syndrome, in which transient burning dysesthesias in the hands are associated with hyperextension of the cervical spine and central cord contusion (11). Loss of consciousness may imply more serious closed head injury, with possible shearing injury to the cervical spinal cord and brainstem.

Common red flags include ages > 55 or < 18 yr old, night pain, trauma, and history of cancer and immunosuppression, which may be seen with use of systemic steroids, HIV, or drug abuse. Further considerations include trauma, weight loss, systemic symptoms, crescendo pain, structural deformity, gait disturbance, and inflammatory symptoms, such as prolonged morning joint stiffness for greater than 1 h. Finally, Cauda equina syndrome is considered and manifested by difficulty with micturition, incontinence of bowel or bladder, loss of anal sphincter tone, and saddle anesthesia (12). This is a surgical emergency.

Physical Examination

Examination of the spine begins with inspection for obvious deformities, sites of impact, or postures that may predispose to injury. Next, palpation of the posterior elements is conducted from the base of the skull to the sacrum. Posterior element fracture or ligamentous disruption may be suggested by tenderness to palpation over the corresponding spinous processes. Palpation of the surrounding musculature in the neck and upper back may reproduce pain that is consistent with muscle spasm.

Range of motion of the spine should be examined. Active range of motion should be tested before passive range of motion. Flexion and extension of the neck is tested by asking the patient to put their chin to their chest and look up at the ceiling. This is followed by side-to-side flexion, which is established by having the patient put their right ear to their right shoulder, and then repeat this task on the left. Normal range of motion on lateral bending is approximately 40 degrees. Finally, lateral rotation of the neck is tested by asking the patient to turn their chin to the left and then right. Normal range of rotation is 60–80 degrees (13). Range of motion of the thoracic spine is tested in the standing position. The patient is asked to bend forward with their chin to their chest and touch their toes. If this causes or is limited by pain, injury to the anterior elements of the spine should be suspected, such as a disc injury or vertebral body fracture. Extension of the thoracic spine is tested by asking the patient to bend back while the examiner stabilizes the patient's hips. Pain with this maneuver may be suggestive of posterior element injury, such as facet injury.

The examination should then turn to provocative maneuvers of the neck, which may help to identify the etiology of neck or upper extremity symptoms. The Spurling test is used to look for cervical root compression caused by pathology of the root or narrowing of the exiting foramen. The patient's neck is extended and rotated toward the symptomatic side as a simultaneous gentle axial load is applied. This position narrows the foramen of the exiting nerve and may reproduce symptoms. This test is highly specific for cervical nerve root compression, but has very poor sensitivity (14). The axial compression test is similar. The examiner applies a compressive force on the head of the patient in the axial plane, therefore narrowing the intervertebral space and foramina. This may reproduce pain caused by disc disease or foraminal narrowing. The final provocative test of the cervical spine is the distraction test, in which vertical traction is carefully applied to the patient's head. If this relieves symptoms, the pain may have been caused by increased pressure or compression at the intervertebral disk or facet joints.

Neurologic examination of the upper and lower extremities is imperative in evaluating the athlete with neck or back pain. If the cervical spine is affected, neurologic examination should also include cranial nerve testing. Neurologic exam should begin with muscle strength testing. Weakness in a specific muscle group may direct you to the level of spinal cord injury. Muscle tone is also important to assess. Flaccid muscle tone would indicate lower motor neuron injury or spinal shock, whereas increased muscle tone would be indicative of either muscle spasm or upper motor neuron injury.

Deep tendon reflexes should then be tested in the upper and lower extremities, followed by sensation testing. The dermatomal distribution of the sensory defect should be established to localize the level of injury. The ipsilateral posterior spinal tract is tested with light touch, vibration, and proprioception. The lateral spinal tract is tested with contralateral thermal and pain perception.

Imaging

There are many options available for imaging the cervical and thoracic spine. Each study has its own strengths in evaluating different elements of the spine. However, the clinician must remember that radiologic studies of the spine may often have findings that are not associated with the patient's symptoms (15–17). Therefore, it is imperative that the imaging method of choice is specific and localized to the area of suspected injury. The four major methods of radiographic imaging are x-ray, computed tomography (CT) scan, magnetic resonance imaging (MRI), and bone scan.

Radiographs are best used to evaluate the bony structures of the spine and their spatial relationships to each other. They can be used as a screening tool in the cervical and thoracic spine for congenital malformations and injuries such as dislocations, compression fractures, and posterior element fractures.

In the cervical spine, the lateral view is often the first view, especially in the trauma setting. All seven cervical vertebrae from C1 through the top of T1 should be visualized. Arm traction or a swimmers view with one arm elevated may enhance the visualization of the C7-T1 junction. At times, a CT may be needed to see this area. On the lateral view, several bony relationships are carefully reviewed with the understanding that the child has some variations from the adult (Figure 4.4). First, four lines are considered: the anterior vertebral line, the posterior vertebral line, the spinolaminar line, and the tips of the spinous processes. All of these should have an even contour with parallel facets. A widened interspinous space greater than 10 mm may indicate instability (18). In the child, there is increased ligamentous laxity, along with a more horizontal facet joint. This imparts a common pseudosubluxation at C2 through C3 and, less commonly, at C3 through C4. In the child, this pseudosubluxation is acceptable up to 4–5 mm. In the adult, a translation of only 3 mm is acceptable at every level. However, acceptable sagittal plane angulation at any level should be less than 11 degrees in both the child and adult (19). The atlantodens interval (ADI) is also assessed on the lateral view. This should be less than 3 mm in the adult and less than 4 mm in the child under 8 yr of age. Atlantoaxial instability is a feature in approximately 15% of adolescents with Down Syndrome, with an ADI of up to 5 mm. Retropharyngeal soft tissue swelling may also indicate spinal injury on the lateral view. Acceptable levels of swelling in the adult are 6 mm of soft tissue swelling at C2 and 22 mm at C6. In the child,

FIGURE 4.4. The child has some variations from the adult's lateral cervical spine radiograph.

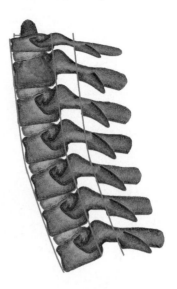

this can equate to 7mm in the retropharyngeal space and 14mm in the retrotracheal space (20). A patient active flexion and extension dynamic view is controversial in the acute setting, but may help distinguish instability.

The AP view aids in assessing for scoliosis, congenital malformations, and lytic lesions. In the traumatic setting, an offset spinous process may indicate a facet dislocation (21).

A third view that should always be obtained when evaluating for a cervical spine injury is the open-mouth odontoid view (Figure 4.5). On this view, one looks for an odontoid fracture and signs of C1–C2 instability manifested by greater than 7mm (total of both sides) of lateral mass overhang or asymmetric position of the dens between the lateral masses.

In the thoracic spine, the anterior–posterior (AP) view will assess scoliosis and congenital vertebral malformation. It may also detect paravertebral soft tissue swelling. The lateral view will assess for kyphosis and Scheuermann changes. The normal thoracic kyphosis has an upper range of 45–50 degrees. Scheuermann's disease involves multiple endplate changes of the thoracic spine, which are discussed later in this chapter.

CT scan is the best study for assessing osseous injury in detail. CT scan is often used in a trauma situation to assess the spine for stability, particularly in the patient with mental status changes or with persistent symptoms and subtle findings, such as soft tissue swelling. A CT is useful in assessing facet arthroses, as well as unclear degenerative disc–osteophyte complexes seen on MRI. Lytic or sclerotic lesions seen on x-ray may also be better defined.

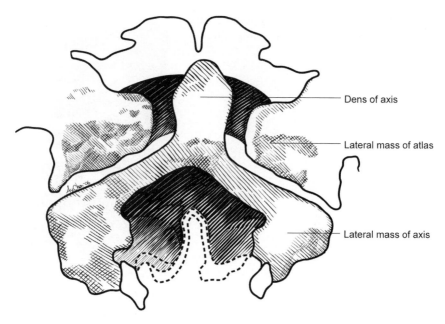

Dens of axis

Lateral mass of atlas

Lateral mass of axis

FIGURE 4.5. The open mouth odontoid view is necessary to obtain information for cervical spine injury.

MRI is excellent for evaluating soft tissues, and offers good bone resolution without ionizing radiation. With the trauma assessment of the child, the upper cervical spine is often involved and is well assessed with an MRI. Any patient with neurologic complaints or findings on exam that may be consistent with spinal cord or nerve root injury should be evaluated with MRI. This is superior for assessing detail of the spinal cord and its exiting nerve roots, as well as the intervertebral disc. Disc herniations are well defined on MRI, and may be further classified as protruded (contained by the outer anulus), extruded (uncontained by the outer anulus), and sequestrated (separated from the disc). Signal changes may also be noted in the corresponding vertebral bodies, which indicates increased load to those osseous structures secondary to loss of disc shock absorption. Increased T2 signal in the endplates of the vertebral bodies in an immature skeleton may indicate endplate apophysitis, which is a common cause of back pain in the young athlete. And finally, when investigating for infection, active tumor, and syringomyelia, gadolinium intravenous injection may enhance visualization.

MRI often picks up subtle spinal column and cord changes that are missed on x-ray and CT scan. MRI is readily available in most medical centers and has resulted in a decrease in the prevalence of a particular type of spinal injury specific to the pediatric population. In 1982, spinal cord injury without radiographic abnormality (SCIWORA) was defined as myelopathy on exam after a traumatic injury without positive findings on plain films, flexion-extension films, or CT scan (22). It occurs with greater severity in children less than 8 yr of age. The existence of SCIWORA is an important reminder that children can have significant spinal cord injuries in the absence of detectable osseous injury.

Bone scan is a study of the metabolic activity of the skeletal system. Lesions associated with increased activity on bone scan are fractures, tumors, infection, stress reactions, and oftentimes, arthritis. However, it is important to remember that any area with increased bone formation or destruction may "light up" on bone scan, and in the skeletally immature patient, that includes the growth plates. SPECT bone scan is often used in assessing for pars interarticularis stress and spondylolysis, although these injuries are most often located in the lumbar spine.

Acute Injuries

Burners

Burners (also called stingers) are nerve injuries to the brachial plexus or cervical nerve roots caused by a direct blow or traction injury. These are the most common cervical injuries seen in football and other contact sports, such as rugby and hockey, but also have been described in wrestling and gymnastics. Injury results from either compression or traction of the upper trunk of the brachial plexus or, less commonly, cervical nerve roots C5 and C6. Brachial plexus traction injury occurs when the shoulder is held in a depressed position and the neck is distracted toward the opposite side, therefore stretching the ipsilateral brachial plexus (23,24). Compression of the brachial plexus occurs with either neck hyperextension combined with ipsilateral flexion or from a direct blow to the supraclavicular fossa (25,26). Cervical nerve root injuries may be predisposed by cervical neuroforaminal stenosis or spinal canal stenosis, conditions seen more commonly in the older college and professional athletes. It is thought that the neuroforaminal space is narrowed with neck extension and rotation; this crowding is even more pronounced in athletes with anatomically narrowed foramina or canals.

The most common mechanism of injury for burners is tackling. The player will report that immediately after contact, he or she developed a burning pain in the upper extremity. This pain will often start in the supraclavicular fossa and progress down the ipsilateral arm in a diffuse, nondermatomal pattern. Sometimes the player will also report sensations of numbness or weakness in the extremity as well. These symptoms usually resolve within 1–2 min, but may progress for days or weeks (27). Physical exam should begin with making sure that the athlete has not incurred a head or neck injury during the play. Attention should then be turned to the affected arm. It is common for the athlete to shake the affected arm immediately after injury to relieve the burning or numbness. Inspection should be followed by palpation of the arm and shoulder to assess for other possible injuries, such as muscle rupture, contusion, or fracture. Range of motion of the shoulder should be assessed to rule out dislocation, followed by a careful neurologic exam of the upper extremity.

Burners usually affect the upper trunk of the brachial plexus, which consists of nerve fibers from the C5 and C6 nerve roots. These nerves primarily supply innervation to the biceps brachii, deltoid, supraspinatus, infraspinatus, and pronator teres muscles. Therefore, strength in these muscles should be assessed during the exam. It is very important to reexamine the patient within 24 h of injury because although most weakness resolves within minutes of injury, there are times when neuropraxia is delayed in its presentation.

Diagnosis of burners depends mostly on history and physical exam; often, further testing is not necessary. It is critical to exclude any bilateral or associated leg symptoms that would indicate a more central cause, such as transient quadriparesis. In such cases, or with repetitive injury or chronic symptoms, further evaluation may be helpful in confirming the diagnosis. Plain x-rays of the cervical spine, including flexion and extension lateral views, and an MRI may be indicated in these cases. Electromyelogram (EMG) studies evaluate the conduction of electric impulse from nerve to muscle unit, and can often help pinpoint the area and degree of nerve injury. However, there is usually at least a 3–4 wk delay between injury and the onset of changes in nerve conduction that are perceptible by EMG (28).

Treatment of burners consists of rest and regular reexamination until pain and neurologic symptoms have resolved. Because this injury is so common in tackling sports and often recurs, prevention of repeat injury is very important. This is accomplished by adjusting tackling technique, protective equipment, and a conditioning program that emphasizes cervical and upper trunk strength for a "chest-out posture."

Fractures and Traumatic Instability

Trauma from athletics is an important cause of acute cervical and thoracic spine fractures. Although these fractures are relatively uncommon, they can have devastating neurologic consequences. Therefore, knowledge of the diagnosis and management of these fractures is critical in limiting progression of neurologic injury.

Acute cervical fractures are more frequently associated with serious neurologic injury; therefore, any athlete with acute neck pain must be promptly evaluated and immobilized on the athletic field. Athletes should remain in their pads and helmet to maintain spine position. However, any facemask equipment should be removed to allow quick access to the airway if necessary. Although most of these fractures occur in sports such as diving, and high-velocity winter sports such as snowmobiling and ice hockey, they may occur in any contact sport.

Injuries to the cervical spine may be divided into upper and lower (subaxial) spine. Upper injuries refer to the occiput, C1, and C2 levels, whereas the subaxial spine involves C3 and below. Injuries to the atlantooccipital juncture are uncommon, but occur more frequently in children because of the incompletely developed articulation here (29). These are frequently life threatening at the scene.

Jefferson fractures involve the ring of C1 and result from axial loading injury (30). These fractures may involve the anterior and posterior arch (Figure 4.6). If the transverse ligament is involved, this will be demonstrated on the open mouth odontoid view with greater than 7 mm of lateral mass overhang. These fractures may also be seen on the lateral view, along with widening of the predens space. Posterior arch fractures are the more common type of Jefferson fracture and usually heal with a bony or fibrous union. Burst fractures are less stable fractures and consist of fractures of both the anterior and posterior arches with involvement of the transverse ligament. Because these fractures are unstable, they may lead to both neurologic and vascular compromise. Management of stable atlas fractures is usually nonsurgical, with the implementation of bracing. Follow-up flexion and extension views of the atlantodens interval are necessary to establish the integrity of the transverse ligament. Unstable fractures or those progressing to nonunion may require surgical stabilization and permanent removal from contact sports.

Axis (C2) fractures are most commonly of the odontoid or the dens, and they account for approximately 20% of all cervical spine fractures (31). This usually occurs from an extension injury mechanism. The dens is the superior portion of the axis, which protrudes upwards and articulates with the atlas (C1). Fractures of the dens occur at the apex (type I), the body (type II), or basilar (type III) aspect of the vertebral body and are usually a result of direct trauma to the head in contact sports (Figure 4.7). Type II fractures are associated with a higher rate of nonunion. Most commonly, the

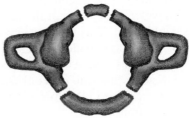

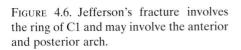

FIGURE 4.6. Jefferson's fracture involves the ring of C1 and may involve the anterior and posterior arch.

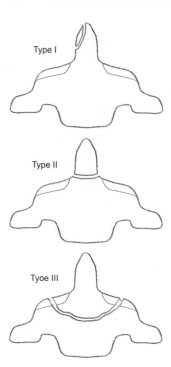

Type I

Type II

Tyoe III

FIGURE 4.7. Odontoid fracture is a result of direct trauma to the head in contact sports.

fractured fragment will displace anteriorly with posterior angulation of the dens (32). Stable dens types I and III fractures are often managed nonsurgically with traction followed by halo or hard cervical collar immobilization for 8–12 wk (type I) or 6 wk (type III). Type II is somewhat more controversial, but if there is any displacement or if there is any failure to maintain stability, surgical stabilization is needed (33).

The Hangman's fracture is another type of axis (C2) fracture, which is also caused by a hyperextension and compression injury to the pedicle or pars interarticularis of C2 (Figure 4.8). It is therefore more appropriately termed a traumatic spondylolisthesis. This injury is less common in children who are more likely to sustain a dens fracture through the synchondrosis of the dens. This fracture is most commonly a result of forced hyperextension with compression of the neck, such as diving and motor vehicle windshield impact. This fracture may cause an anterior displacement of C2 on C3. Diagnosis is made with plain radiographs (particularly the lateral view), followed by CT scan of the cervical spine. Stable undisplaced fractures may be treated with 3 mo of semirigid collar immobilization (Miami J or Philadelphia collar) (34). Unstable fractures are treated with halo or surgical stabilization.

FIGURE 4.8. Hangman's fracture is caused by a hyper-extension and compression injury to the pedicle or pars interarticularis of C2.

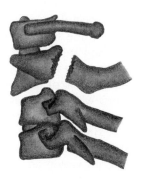

Subaxial cervical and thoracic compression fractures may be classified using the Denis three-column theory (Figure 4.9) (35). The anterior column consists of the anterior longitudinal ligament with the anterior half of the vertebral body including anulus fibrosus. The middle column consists of the posterior half of the vertebral body with the anulus. The posterior column comprises the posterior arch and stabilizing ligaments. Involvement of a single column indicates stability, whereas two-column involvement (any middle column involvement) would indicate instability. This may involve neurologic instability and/or mechanical instability with deformity progression. Plain lateral x-rays that demonstrate an anterior compression fracture of 25% or less would indicate stability. It is also important to carefully assess the middle and posterior columns, where only a widening of the interspinous space may indicate three-column involvement and severe instability. As the compression approaches 50%, involvement of the posterior arch is more likely and best demonstrated on a CT scan.

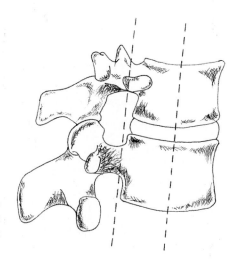

FIGURE 4.9. Subaxial cervical and thoracic compression fractures may be classified using the Denis three-column theory.

Cervical flexion injuries may be subdivided into compression and distraction mechanisms. Cervical compression-flexion fractures are the most common fractures of the cervical spine, and are caused by axial loading forces applied to the head, often with neck flexion. These comprise approximately 36% of lower cervical injuries (35). This injury is seen in tackling sports where the head is used to tackle, as well as in sports such as diving. Compression fractures are classified as stages I through V. Stage I fractures have simple rounding of the anterior superior vertebral body (Figure 4.10). Stage II fractures are more compressed, with a beaking appearance of the anterior vertebrae. Stage III represents an anterior inferior teardrop type of fracture and may indicate instability. Stage IV and V represent the teardrop fracture with increasing displacement (36). These injuries are demonstrated on the lateral radiograph. However, a CT will help define the extent of a fracture. An MRI is useful with stage III injuries to define disc and ligament components of instability. Stable stage I and II lesions, as well as some stage III lesions, may be immobilized in a rigid cervical collar for 10–12 wk. Before discontinuing the collar, healing should be demonstrated on radiographs, including flexion and extension views, to assess stability. Stage IV and V, as well as some stage III injuries, will require traction and either halo immobilization or surgical stabilization.

Flexion distraction injuries comprise a spectrum of injuries with variable amounts of flexion and distraction, as well as rotation. A simple flexion distraction injury will demonstrate posterior element ligamentous disruption with widening of the spinous processes or facet subluxation. This will be demonstrated on lateral x-rays with subtle spinous process widening, the occult injury of McSweeney. When flexion is combined with rotation, a unilateral facet dislocation may occur. This is often stable and demonstrated on a lateral radiograph with 25% displacement of the vertebral

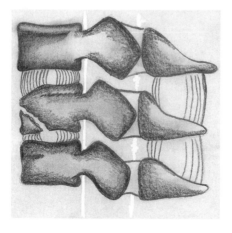

FIGURE 4.10. Compression flexion injuries. Stage I fractures have simple rounding of the anterior superior vertebral body.

body, along with nonparallel facet joints at the same motion segment. This may be seen in a full nelson maneuver in wrestling. A more extensive flexion-distraction injury is a bilateral facet dislocation with 50% displacement of one vertebral body at the motion segment, with parallel facets demonstrated on the lateral radiograph (37). This is unstable, with involvement of the anterior anulus and posterior ligamentous structures.

Treatment for a simple flexion-distraction injury with mild widening of the interspinous space may be treated with a rigid cervical orthosis for 6 wk, with care to assess flexion and extension stability before discontinuation of the collar (38). Unilateral and bilateral facet dislocations require immediate reduction with traction and, often, surgical stabilization. An MRI may be considered before reduction if there are signs of disc herniation, which could worsen neurologic injury during the maneuvers (39).

Compression fractures with a direct axial load produce burst fractures, with fracture fragments possibly being displaced into the spinal canal. This is a classic catastrophic football and hockey injury that occurs when the head is slightly flexed and an axial load is applied, as seen with spearhead tackling in football or a hockey check into the boards. This type of unstable fracture may result in permanent neurologic sequelae, and thus should be immobilized promptly pending surgical evaluation (40–42). Prevention of this injury is paramount by banning spearhead tackling and maintaining a heads up posture in hockey (43).

Extension injuries may occur with compression, as well as distraction, and may produce injuries to the pedicles, articular pillars, and laminae. These may be associated with anterior ligamentous injury to the anulus, rendering them more unstable. Stable unilateral posterior arch fractures with no anterior involvement may be treated with a cervical orthosis. More extensive injuries involving the soft tissue supports should be considered for halo or surgical stabilization (44).

Thoracic vertebral compression fractures are also associated with axial loading of the spine, usually when it is in flexion. Although the neurologic complications are often less frequent than in cervical compression fractures, it remains important to immobilize the spine with a backboard until the diagnosis can be confirmed. Athletes with thoracic vertebral compression fractures may present with upper back pain with or without paresthesias of the trunk or upper extremities.

If a thoracic compression fracture results in less than 25% loss of vertebral body height, the fracture is usually stable. However, as the fracture approaches 50%, the likelihood of posterior arch involvement increases and should be assessed with a CT scan (45). If there are any neurologic symptoms, even transient, an MRI is useful to assess cord and soft tissue injury. Minimal compression injuries with no posterior arch involvement may be immobilized in a thoracolumbosacral orthosis (TLSO) for 6–12 wk until pain free. Return to sports, however, is delayed until the bracing period is completed and the athlete has regained full strength and range of motion, with attention to extension strengthening. More severe compression fractures, which are associated with instability and neurologic deficits, may require longer immobilization or surgical intervention. Athletes with no neurologic deficits and mild vertebral compression may return to contact sports when healed. If internal fixation is employed to stabilize the fracture, contact sports are often contraindicated.

Cervical and Thoracic Disc Disease

Cervical disc disease accounts for approximately 36% of all spinal disc disease (46). This may be an acute soft tissue herniation of the disc or more of a degenerative disc–osteophyte complex at the neuroforamina. Acute soft tissue cervical disc herniations are less common than degenerative disc disease in the athletic population, particularly in the adult. The anulus is quite deficient at the posterolateral corner near the uncovertebral joint, which disrupts the normal lamellae of the anulus. This is anterior to the neuroforamina. As such, the well-hydrated nucleus in the younger individual may violate the attenuated anulus during rapid flexion or rotation that is accentuated with an axial load. This may occur with noncontact and contact sports, particularly tackling sports, as well as wrestling. Acute minor protrusions may cause an acute torticollis or wryneck, whereas a more significant herniation will produce a frank radiculopathy.

Conversely, a degenerative disc with osteophyte formation at the uncovertebral joint, and subsequent zygapophyseal joint degenerative changes, may also produce radicular symptoms. This is referred to as a hard disc herniation (47). This may occur with repetitive coupled lateral flexion and rotation, as well as flexion and extension (48). The most common levels are the C5 through C6 and C6 through C7 levels.

MRI imaging is quite good at defining the spacial soft tissue relations of a disc herniation. However, a CT scan can be quite helpful in defining the elements of the hard disc involvement. It is also helpful in the patient that is unable to have an MRI. However, the interpretation must carefully correlate with the clinical symptoms. Approximately 15% of 20 yr olds and about 85% of 60 yr olds will demonstrate some disc degeneration (49). An EMG may be helpful in delineating the level of neuroimpingement, as well as detecting comorbid peripheral impingement.

Cervical disc herniations can be managed conservatively with rest, nonsteroidal antiinflammatory drugs, short courses of tapering corticosteroids, and analgesics. A soft cervical collar can be used for temporary pain relief and to remind the athlete to rest. Early therapy centers on pain control with traction, modalities, and postural biomechanics. When neurologic symptoms and pain have improved, a gentle, progressive physical therapy program can be instituted to restore range of motion and improve cervical stabilization. At times, a cervical epidural injection may be quite helpful to reduce radicular symptoms (50). As the athlete progresses, the sports-specific phase of rehabilitation addresses the full, closed-chain upper trunk and cervical stabilization musculature, along with the biomechanics of the sport. This conservative management course is most often quite successful in managing cervical radiculopathy (51). Nonetheless, surgical intervention is indicated in cases with refractory radicular pain, a progressive motor deficit, or signs of spinal cord involvement. Most often this is an anterior discectomy with fusion (52). Return to sport will be discussed later in the chapter.

Thoracic disc herniations are uncommon and represent approximately 1% of all symptomatic disc herniations (53). The lower thoracic spine (T8–11) is more prone to herniation because this is the transition zone from the less flexible upper thoracic spine, with fixation of the rib cage, to the more flexible lower thoracic spine, with free-floating ribs. These patients often present with acute onset of midline thoracic pain, with or without radicular symptoms in the chest or abdomen. MRI is the study of choice to assess the degree of disc protrusion. The clinician must have a high index of suspicion for a herniation because as many as 11–13% of adults have asymptomatic thoracic disc herniations (54). As with the cervical spine, the clinician must ascertain the safety of the cord. In the absence of progressive neurologic symptoms, treatment is conservative. Extension strengthening is started as tolerated by the athlete. Return to play is allowed when the athlete is pain-free and strength and flexibility are fully restored. Follow-up is indicated to ensure that myelopathy does not develop.

Other Causes of Acute Neck and Upper Back Pain

The most common cause of acute-onset neck and upper back pain in the adolescent athlete is muscle strain or contusion. This type of injury is often the result of either a direct blow to the muscle mass, resulting in contusion and spasm, or an abrupt isometric contraction of a muscle, resulting in muscle tear. Although these injuries can initially be debilitating, most may be managed conservatively with rest, moist heat, gentle massage, muscle relaxants, and nonsteriodal antiinflammatory drugs. Athletes may return to play when pain symptoms resolve. It is important that the clinician recognize that muscle spasm may be a sign of further underlying spinal injury. Therefore, patient education about reasons to return for evaluation, such as neurologic symptoms or persistent pain, is imperative.

Chronic Injuries

Cervical Disc Degeneration

Cervical disc disease was previously addressed, along with acute disc herniation. However, one specific pattern of overuse in the football athlete should be recognized. Repetitive axial loading of the cervical spine is seen in football players who repeatedly tackle using the top of the head as the initial point of impact, the now illegal maneuver called "spear tackling." This leads to a more insidious injury pattern of narrowing of the cervical spinal canal and loss or reversal of normal cervical lordosis, predisposing the athlete to permanent neurologic impairment. Athletes with spear tackler's spine should be kept out of contact sports until the normal lordosis is restored, neck pain or neurologic symptoms resolve, and there is no demonstrated spinal stenosis (55).

Cervical Facet Syndrome

Cervical facet pain is common in the general population. It represents about 25% of axial neck pain as verified by selective injection techniques (56). It has been demonstrated to cause pain in 54% of whiplash patients (57). Asymmetrical motions in sports may acutely or chronically impact the hyaline cartilage surface of these joints. Football impact, such as a tackle to a wide receiver, may mimic the motion of whiplash. Certain ballet dance patterns may repetitively load these joints. Since the facet joints couple lateral flexion and rotation to the ipsilateral side, any cyclical motion to the side may overload the joint's resilience. Another mechanism of injury may occur in a cyclist with an improperly fitted bike, causing hyperextension of the neck to maintain road visibility. This hyperextension will also overload the facet joint complex. These patients will present with posterior cervical pain, along with possible radiation to the interscapular region or occipital region. Examination will elicit facet and paraspinal tenderness. Spurling extension maneuvers will produce axial neck pain. Plain films with oblique views may demonstrate osteophytes from the facets. An MRI may demonstrate capsular and ligamentum flavum hypertrophy.

Treatment should be initiated with antiinflammatory medication, gentle pain-free range of motion, and modalities such as ice, electrical stimulation, and ultrasound. Muscle activation techniques and joint mobilization may also be helpful. As the acute pain subsides, the athlete should initiate isometric, followed by dynamic, exercises that emphasize the chest out posture for the upper trunk. Finally, a full resistive cervical strengthening program with attention to the chin-back posture is undertaken. Infrequently, a cervical facet injection may temporarily reduce the pain to allow better rehabilitation (58). Highly resistant symptoms may benefit from a radiofrequency ablation of the medial branch innervating the facet joints. This has been shown to be 71% effective in the treatment of whiplash patients (59).

Scheuermann's Kyphosis

In the adolescent athlete, rhythmic flexion of the thoracolumbar spine may cause Scheuermann's kyphosis, which may result in a painful deformity. This abnormality is defined as 3 contiguous vertebrae with 5 degrees of anterior wedging, irregular endplates, and a Cobb angle of at least 45 degrees. When this occurs in the thoracolumbar region, the athlete may present with thoracolumbar kyphosis and lumbar hypolordosis. This is often called atypical Scheuermann's or lumbar Scheuermann's. This is thought to occur because of repetitive flexion forces applied to the soft growth cartilage of the vertebral epiphyseal endplate. This is a fixed deformity, in contrast to juvenile roundback deformity, which is flexible and responds to an extension-strengthening program. This has been particularly noted in the young athlete participating in 400h per year of many sports, but especially gymnastics, swimming, and wrestling (60). These deformities are best detected on physical examination, while having the athlete forward flex the thoracolumbar spine.

In the adolescent athlete with Scheuermann changes, bracing is quite effective if there is spinal growth remaining. This can be assessed by a Risser score of the iliac crest apophysis. For thoracic involvement with curves less than 50 degrees, observation and extension exercises are indicated. Bracing is initiated for curves greater than 45–50 degrees. At 60–70 degrees, surgical intervention is considered. For curves above T7, a Milwaukee brace is used. A TLSO with upper chest support is utilized for curves with an apex below this level. Thoracolumbar Scheuermann's may be treated with a TLSO brace in 15 degrees of extension.

Scoliosis

Adolescent idiopathic scoliosis is common in the young female athlete. Scoliosis is classified according to the age when it was identified. Infantile scoliosis presents before 3yr of age. Juvenile scoliosis manifests between 3 and 10yr of age. Adolescent idiopathic scoliosis presents between 10yr of age and skeletal maturity (61). Minimal curves have equal gender frequency. However, more severe curves have a female to male ratio of 4:1 (62,63). Adolescent scoliosis occurs in 2–3% of the population. However, minor curve asymmetries have been noted more often in some sports such as ballet, with a reported 24% prevalence in young dancers (64). Repetitive asymmetric torque forces may contribute to this phenomenon. This may also be seen in swimming, serving, and throwing sports, and in rhythmic gymnastics (65). Other factors contributing to this sports curve asymmetry may include delayed menarche, small body habitus, and intense prepubertal training (66).

Adolescent scoliosis should not initially be ascribed as the cause of back pain. Other etiologies must be considered that may coexist with or cause the scoliosis. Consideration should be given to tethered cord, tumors, spondylolysis, syrinx, and disc herniation (67). This may indicate the need for a spinal-screening MRI. However, curves that present in later adolescence with Risser scores over 2 have been associated with back pain (68). The Risser score refers to the plain x-ray finding of the AP pelvis in regard to the maturation of the iliac crest apophysis, which appears from lateral to medial. The score refers to the most advanced quadrant of ossification, with Risser 1 being the first quadrant, Risser 2 the second, Risser 3 the third, and Risser 4 showing complete apophyseal cap ossification. A Risser 5 refers to the fusion of the cap to the ileum.

The Risser score, along with the curve magnitude, age, and maturity, indicate the risk of curve progression. For example, a curvature of less than 20 degrees and a Risser score of 0–1 has a 22% risk of progression. Conversely, the mature patient with the same curve has a 1.6% risk of progression (69). Other risk factors for curve progression include magnitude of curve at presentation, premenarche, and the presence of double curves (70).

Consideration should be given to a limb length discrepancy causing a nonfixed curve, which corrects with a lift. If a minor curve is felt to be secondary to sports participation, the athlete may benefit from cross training and core stabilization. Although exercises are not accepted as solo treatment, an investigation has demonstrated the benefit of trunk strengthening with attention to rotary exercises (71). At the very least, core strength and flexibility may prevent mechanical injury.

Those curves less than 25 degrees are observed with repeat x-rays every 4–6 mo, unless they manifest sudden changes. The immature athlete with a curve of 25 degrees is usually treated with a brace, such as the Boston brace, which is worn 16–23 h per day. The Charleston brace is a nighttime brace. The Boston brace has shown less curve progression in some studies (72). The athlete may opt to play without the brace for a couple of hours. Curves that exceed 40–45 degrees have a high risk of progression and should be considered for surgical intervention. With instrumentation and fusion, much athletic activity is allowed and encouraged. However, contact sports are contraindicated.

Congenital Anomalies

Klippel–Feil Syndrome

Klippel–Feil syndrome refers to a spectrum of congenital abnormalities associated with fusion masses of the cervical spine. These fusions are often incidentally detected but require some consideration for involvement in contact sports. This syndrome may be classified into three categories. Type I involves a massive cervical spine fusion. Type II involves a one or two level fusion. Type III includes both types I and II, with associated thoracic or lumbar spine. Other associated congenital abnormalities include hearing disorders (both conductive and sensorineural), cardiac abnormalities, such as ventricular septal defects, and urologic defects (73). Scoliosis and Sprengel's deformity are often associated. Sprengel's deformity involves an osteocartilaginous connection of the scapula to the cervical spine.

Although the classic triad is a short neck, low hairline, and decreased range of motion, this only occurs in about 40% of cases. Often, this will present incidentally or with mild motion loss, which usually involves the axial rotation component. In respect to contact sports, the major issues are instability and stenosis. Instability is most severe with fusions that involve the craniocervical and C1–C2 junction. Stenosis is often a concern at a free level between 2 fusion masses (74).

Evaluation should include lateral flexion and extension views to detect instability. An MRI is very useful in defining the amount of stenosis and associated craniocervical involvement such as basilar impression. A flexion and extension MRI may be useful in borderline cases to define functional stenosis. Thoracic and lumbar plain radiographs will detect fusion masses at these lower levels. Other evaluations include audiometric, renal ultrasound, and cardiac auscultation (further evaluation as indicated).

Direct contact sports are contraindicated with C1–C2 fusions, craniocervical fusions, and any associated fusions with instability or significant stenosis. Consideration should be given to avoiding involvement in sports that require repetitive extreme motion, as the free disc spaces may be predisposed to premature degeneration.

Os Odontoideum

Os odontoideum is a nonunion of the dens to the axis at the level of the synchondrosis. Although originally thought to be a congenital abnormality, it is now considered a nonunion from previous overuse stress at the level of the synchondrosis, which is at the base of the dens (75). Because atlantoaxial stability is largely maintained by the transverse atlantal ligament behind the dens, this integrity is violated and represents a contraindication to contact sports participation. This should not be confused with a small benign apical ossicle, the ossiculum terminale, which is above the transverse atlantal ligament.

Radiographic evaluation should include lateral flexion and extension views with attention to three findings of instability (76). A posterior atlantodens interval (PADI) of less than 13 mm indicates instability and neurologic decline. Two other findings between C1 and C2 include greater than 5 mm of translation or 20 degrees of angular rotation. Surgical stabilization should be performed in these circumstances. MRI imaging is very useful in determining cord compression (77).

Other odontoid abnormalities include rare aplasia and hypoplasia and associated ligamentous laxity. These may be associated with Down syndrome, Morquio syndrome, and other skeletal dysplasias. Full imaging evaluation, as previously discussed, is indicated to evaluate neurologic compromise.

Return to Play Guidelines

The team physician is often called upon to clear an athlete to return to sports after a specific injury to the cervical and thoracic spine. As a rule, the athlete must be pain free without neurologic symptoms and demonstrate a full range of motion and strength. However, there may be structural defects that the physician must assess for appropriateness to participate in contact sports. Watkins has created risk categories that are very helpful in determining return to play. He has classified these as minimal risk, moderate risk, and extreme risk (78). Minimal risk implies little more risk than the sport would normally involve. Moderate risk implies a reasonable possibility of recurrent injury and neurologic injury. Extreme risk implies a high risk of permanent damage; therefore, athletes should be discouraged from participating in contact sports.

Extreme risk injuries include a Jefferson fracture, unless it is completely healed with no demonstrated instability on dynamic radiographs and no symptoms. A partially or fully ruptured transverse ligament of the axis, unhealed odontoid fracture, unhealed hangman's fractures, and unhealed flexion injuries of the interspinous ligaments with separation on flexion radiographs are all examples of extreme risk injuries. Also included are fractures or dislocations that have demonstrated incomplete bony healing, ligamentous instability, neurologic deficit, pain, stiffness, or residual spinal stenosis. Other conditions include cervical myelopathy, occiput-C1 fusions, C1–C2 fusions, C1–C2 rotary instability, basilar invagination, Arnold–Chiari malformation, multilevel Klippel–Feil fusions, 2 episodes of cervical neuropraxia, symptomatic disc herniation, 3 level spine fusion, cervical involvement of ankylosing spondylitis, rheumatoid arthritis, or diffuse idiopathic skeletal hyperostosis (DISH).

Moderate risk injuries include disc herniations that demonstrate symptomatic radiculopathy, previous single episode of cervical neuropraxia that is symptom free, a healed posterior single-level fusion, three or more burners, and a healed two-level anterior fusion.

Minor risk injuries include healed undisplaced fractures, asymptomatic disc herniations without central spinal stenosis, single-level Klippel–Feil, or healed surgical fusion and two previous burners.

Another difficult aspect of decision making is the return of an athlete to contact sports who has suffered a transient neurologic deficit and demonstrates some central spinal stenosis. Watkins developed a rating system to assist in this decision-making process. The rating takes into account the amount of canal narrowing, extent of neurologic deficit, and the length of symptoms (Table 4.1).

By adding these three scores, a total number of 6 or less would be a mild episode; a score of 6–10 would indicate a moderate risk episode; and a score of 10–15 would indicate a severe episode (61). This is a guideline in manag-

TABLE 4.1. Watkins neurologic deficit rating system for return to play.

Canal narrowing	Rating
>12 mm	1
>10 mm and <12 mm	2
10 mm	3
8–10 mm	4
<8 mm	5
Neurologic deficit	
Single arm symptomatic	1
Bilateral upper extremities	2
Hemi arm and leg symptoms	3
Transient quadriparesis	4
Transient quadriplegia	5
Duration of Symptoms	
<5 min	1
<1 h	2
<24 h	3
<1 wk	4
>1 wk	5

Source: Rogala et al., 1978.

ing the return to play decision. Any neurologic deficit would preclude the athlete from returning to sport, regardless of score.

Prevention

Prevention revolves around conditioning, sports technique, and proper equipment. Cervical spine and upper trunk strengthening are important to absorb the forces in contact sports. It is generally felt that upper back postural strength imparts a chest out posture for better cervical stability. Isolated cervical strengthening for the longus colli, extensor, and rotational stabilizers are important. Attention to sports technique has been demonstrated to diminish severe cervical spine injuries. Specifically, this was shown with the abolishment of spearhead tackling. Heads-up hockey also accomplishes this by avoiding impact on a straightened spine. Proper equipment may help with burners in football. Well-fitted shoulder pads that prevent lateral flexion may be useful to avoid recurrent burners.

Clinical Pearls

- The cervical and thoracic spine house the central spinal cord.
- The clinician treating injuries to these areas should have a full understanding of the anatomy and the implications of injury to the various areas.

- Neurologic and mechanical stability must always be assessed.
- Sport-specific biomechanical loads to the spine must be understood to determine injury patterns.
- Preseason conditioning and specific sports techniques can help prevent injury, such as avoiding spearhead tackling in football and encouraging heads-up hockey.
- Any neurological symptoms should preclude return to sport.
- Athletes with extreme risk injuries or conditions, such as incompletely healed fractures or spinal stenosis, are at high risk for permanent injury and should be discouraged from participating in contact sports.

References

1. Clarke KS. Epidemiology of athletic neck injury. Clin Sports Med 1998;17(1): 83–97.
2. Lang J. Clinical anatomy of the cervical spine. New York: Thieme Medical Publishers; 1993.
3. Panjabi MM, Summers DJ, Pelker RR, et al. Three-dimensional load displacement curves of the cervical spine. J Ortho Res 1986;4:152.
4. Ghanayem AJ, Paxinos O. Functional anatomy of joints, ligaments and discs. In: The Cervical Spine Research Society, eds. The Cervical Spine. 4th ed. Philadelphia: Lippincott-Raven; 2005.
5. Bogduk N. The zygapophyseal joints. Clinical Anatomy of the Lumbar Spine. 3rd ed. London; Churchill Livingston; 1997:333–341.
6. Bogduk N. The inter-body joints and intervertebral discs. In: Bogduk N, ed. Clinical Anatomy of the Lumbar Spine and Sacrum. 3rd ed. London; Churchill Livingston; 1997:13–31.
7. Baranto A, Ekstrom L, Hellstrom M, et al. Fracture patterns of the adolescent porcine spine: an experimental loading study in bending-compression. Spine 2004;30(1):75–82.
8. Akin C, Muharrem Y, Akin U, et al. The evolution of sagittal segmental alignment of the spine during childhood. Spine 2004;30(1):93–100.
9. Wojtys EM, Ashton-Miller JA, Huston LJ, et al. The association between athletic training time and the sagittal curvature of the immature spine. Am J Sp Med 2000;28:490–498.
10. Goldstein JD, Berger PE, Windler GE. Spine injury in gymnasts and swimmers. An epidemiologic investigation. Am J Sports Med 1991;19:463–468.
11. Maroon JC. "Burning hands" in football spinal cord injuries. JAMA 1977;238: 2049.
12. Overmeer T, Linton SJ, Holmquist L, et al. Do evidence-based guidelines have an impact in primary care? A cross-sectional study of Swedish physicians and physiotherapists. Spine 2005;30(1):146–151.
13. Tachdjian MO. The neck and upper limb. In: Clinical Pediatric Orthopedics: The Art of Diagnosis and Principles of Management. Stamford, CT: Appleton and Lange; 1997:263.
14. Viikari-Juntura E, Porras M, Laasonen R. Validity of clinical tests in the diagnosis of root compression in cervical disc disease. Spine 1989;14:253.

15. Boden SD, Davis DO, Dina TS, et al. Abnormal magnetic resonance scans of the lumbar spine in asymptomatic subjects: a prospective investigation. J Bone Joint Surg Am 1990;72:403–408.
16. Weisel SW, Tsourmas N, Feffer HL, et al. A study of computer assisted tomography: I. The incidence of positive CAT scans in an asymptomatic group of patients. Spine 1984;9:549–551.
17. Hitselberger WE, Witten RM. Abnormal myelograms in asymptomatic patients. J Neurosurg 1968;28:204–206.
18. Pennecot GF, Gouraud D, Hardy JR, et al. Roentgenographical study of the stability of the cervical spine in children. J Pediatr Orthop 1984;4:346–352.
19. Panjabi MM, White AA, Keller D, et al. Stability of the cervical spine under tension. J Biomech 1978;11:189–197.
20. Wholey MH, Bruwer AJ, Baker HLJ. The lateral roentgenogram of the neck (with comments on the atlanto-odontoid-basion relationship). Radiology 1958;71:350–356.
21. Graber MA, Kathol M. Cervical spine radiographs in the trauma patient. Am Fam Physician 1999;59:331.
22. Pang D, Wilberger, JE, Jr. Spinal cord injury without radiographic abnormalities in children. J Neurosurg 1982;57:114.
23. Sallis RE, Jones K, Knopp W. Burners, offensive strategy for an underreported injury. Phys Sportsmed 1992;20:47.
24. Hershman EB. Injuries to the brachial plexus. In: Torg JS, ed. Athletic Injuries to the Head, Neck, and Face. 2nd ed. St. Louis, MO: Mosby-Year Book, Inc.; 1991.
25. Markey KLO, Di Benedetto M, Curl WW. Upper trunk brachial plexopathy. The stinger syndrome. Am J Sports Med 1993;21:650.
26. Watkins RG. Neck injuries in football players. Clin Sports Med 1986;5:215.
27. Speer KP, Bassett FH, III. The prolonged burner syndrome. AM J Sports Med 1990;18:591.
28. Di Benedetto M, Marhkey K. Electrodiagnostic localization of traumatic upper trunk brachial plexopathy. Arch Phys Med Rehabil 1984;65:15.
29. Avellino AM, Mann FA, Grady MS, et al. Why acute cervical spine injuries are "missed" in infants and children: 12-year experience from a level 1 pediatric and adult trauma center. International Society for Pediatric Neurosurgery Abstracts, 1999.
30. Panjabi MM, Oda T, Crisco JJ, et al. Experimental study of atlas injuries. I. Biomechanical analysis of their mechanisms and fracture patterns. Spine 1991 Oct;16(10 Suppl):S460–S465.
31. Schatzker J, Rorabeck CH, Waddell JP. Fractures of the dens (odontoid process). An analysis of thirty-seven cases. J Bone Joint Surg Br 1971 Aug;53(3):392–405.
32. Loder RT. The cervical spine. In: Morissy RT, Weinstein, SL, eds. Lovell and Winter's Pediatric Orthopaedics. 5th ed. Philadelphia: Lippincott Williams Wilkins; 2001;799.
33. Rao G, Apfelbaum RI. Dens fractures. In: The Cervical Spine Research Society, eds. The Cervical Spine. 4th Ed. Philadelphia: Lippincott-Raven; 2005:614–628.
34. Levine MM, Edwards CC. The management of traumatic spondylolisthesis of the axis. J Bone Joint Surg Am 1985 Feb;67(2):217–226.

35. Allen BL, Ferguson RL, Lehmann TR, et al. A mechanistic classification of closed, indirect fractures and dislocations of the lower cervical spine. Spine 1982 Jan-Feb;7(1):1–27.
36. Anderson DG, Vaccaro AR. Classification of lower cervical spine injuries. In: The Cervical Spine Research Society, eds. The Cervical Spine. 4th Ed. Philadelphia: Lippincott-Raven; 2005.
37. Crawford, NR, Duggal N, Chamberlain RH. Unilateral Cervical Facet Dislocation: Injury Mechanism and Biomechanical Consequences. Spine 2002;27(17):1858–1863.
38. Vives MJ, Garfin SE. Flexion injuries In: The Cervical Spine. 4th Ed. The Cervical Spine Research Society, eds. Philadelphia: Lippincott-Raven; 2005:660–670.
39. Eismont FJ, Arena MJ, Green BA, et al. Extrusion of an intervertebral disc associated with traumatic subluxation or dislocation of cervical facets. Case report. J Bone Joint Surg Am 1991;73(10):1555–1560.
40. Allen BL, Jr., Ferguson RL, Lehmann TR, O'Brien RP. A mechanistic classification of closed, indirect fractures and dislocations of the lower cervical spine. Spine 1982;7:1.
41. Zmurko MG, Tannoury TY, Tannoury CA, Anderson DG. Cervical sprains, disc herniations, minor fractures, and other cervical injuries in the athlete. Clin Sports Med 2003;22:513.
42. Mazur JM, Stauffer ES. Unrecognized spinal instability associated with seemingly "simple" cervical compression fractures. Spine 1983;8:687.
43. Pashby T, Carson J, Ordogh D, et al. Eliminate head-checking in ice hockey. Clin J Sport Med 2001;11(4):211–213.
44. Vives MJ, Garfin SE. Extension injuries. In: The Cervical Spine Research Society, eds. The Cervical Spine. 4th ed. Philadelphia: Lippincott-Raven; 2005:671–682.
45. Keene JJ. Thoracolumbar fractures in winter sports. Am J Sports Med 1987;216:39.
46. Kramer J. Intervertebral Disk Diseases. Causes, Diagnosis, Treatment and Prophylaxis. George Thieme Verlag, Stuttgart Year Book, Medical Publishers Inc; 1981.
47. Ellenberg MR, Honet JC, Treanor WJ. Cervical radiculopathy. Arch Phys Med Rehabil Mar 1994;75(3):342–352.
48. White AA, Panjabi MM. Clinical Biomechanics of the Spine. 2nd ed. Philadelphia, PA: JB Lippincott; 1991:85–125.
49. Matsumoto M, Fujimura Y, Suzuki N, et al. MRI of cervical intervertebral discs in asymptomatic subjects. J Bone Joint Surg Br Jan 1998;80(1):19–24.
50. Slipman CW, Lipetz JS, Jackson HB, et al. Therapeutic selective nerve root block in the nonsurgical treatment of atraumatic cervical spondylotic radicular pain: a retrospective analysis with independent clinical review. Arch Phys Med Rehabil Jun 2000;81(6):741–746.
51. Saal JS, Saal JA, Yurth EF. Nonoperative management of herniated cervical intervertebral disc with radiculopathy. Spine Aug 15 1996;21(16):1877–1883.
52. Palit M, Schofferman J, Goldthwaite N. Anterior discectomy and fusion for the management of neck pain. Spine 1999;24(21):2224–2228.
53. Arce CA, Dohrmann GJ. Herniated thoracic disks. Neurol Clin 1985 May; 3(20):383–392.

54. Awwad EE, Martin DS, Smith KR, Jr. Asymptomatic versus symptomatic herniated thoracic discs: their frequency and characteristics as detected by computed tomography after myelography. Neurosurgery 1991 Feb;28:(2):180–186.
55. Cantu RC, Bailes JE, Wilberger JE, Jr. Guidelines for return to contact or collision sport after a cervical spine injury. Clin Sports Med 1998;17:137.
56. Bogduk N, Aprill C. On the nature of neck pain, discography and cervical zygapophysial joint blocks. Pain 1993;54(2):213–217.
57. Barnsley L, Lord SM, Wallis BJ, Bogduk N. The prevalence of chronic cervical zygapophyseal joint pain after whiplash. Spine 1996;20(1):20–25.
58. Roy DF, Fleury J, Fontaine SB, Dussault RG. Clinical evaluation of cervical facet joint infiltration. Can Assoc Radiol J 1988;39(2):118–120.
59. McDonald GJ, Lord SM, Bogduk N. Long-term follow-up of patients treated with cervical radiofrequency neurotomy for chronic neck pain. Neurosurgery 1999;45(1):61–67; discussion 67–68.
60. Wojts EEM, Ashton-Miller JA, Huston LJ, et al. The association between athletic training time and the sagittal curvature of the immature spine. Am J Sports Med 2000;28(4):490–498.
61. Rogala EJ, Drummond DS, Gurr J. Scoliosis: incidence and natural history. A prospective epidemiologic study. J Bone Joint Surg 1978;60A:173–176.
62. Brooks HL, Azen SP, Gerberg E, et al. Scoliosis: a prospective epidemiologic study. J Bone Joint Surg Am 1975;57:968–972.
63. Miller NH. Adolescent idiopathic scoliosis: etiology. In: The Pediatric Spine. Philadelphia, PA: Lippincott Williams and Wilkins; 2001:347–354.
64. Warren MP, Brooks-Gunn J, Hamilton LH, et al. Scoliosis and fractures in young ballet dancers. Relationship of delayed menarche and secondary amenorrhea. N Eng J Med 1986;314:1348–1353.
65. Tanchev PI, Dzherov AD, Parushev AD, et al. Scoliosis in rhythmic gymnasts. Spine 2000;25(11):1367–1372.
66. Warren MP. The effects of exercise on pubertal progression and reproduction in girls. J Clin Endocrinol Metab 1980;51:1150.
67. Schwend RM, Hennrikus W, Hall JE, et al. Childhood scoliosis: Clinical indications for MRI. J Bone Joint Surg 1995;77A:46–53.
68. Ramirez M, Jonsston CE, Browne RH. The prevalence of back pain in children who have idiopathic scoliosis. J Bone Joint Surg 1997;79A:364–368.
69. Lonstein JE, Carlson JM. The prediction of curve progression in untreated idiopathic scoliosis during growth. J Bone Joint Surg Am 1984;66:1061–1071.
70. Weinstein SL. Adolescent idiopathic scoliosis: Natural history. In: The Pediatric Spine. Philadelphia, PA: Lippincott Williams and Wilkins; 2001:355–370.
71. Mooney V, Gulick J, Pozos R. A preliminary report on the effect of measured strength training in adolescent idiopathic scoliosis. J Spinal Disord 2000;3(2):102–107.
72. Emans JB, Kaelin A, Bancel P, et al. The Boston bracing system for idiopathic scoliosis. Follow-up results in 295 patients. Spine 1986;11:792–801.
73. Hensinger RN, Lang JE, MacEwen GD. Klippel-Feil syndrome; a constellation of associated anomalies. J Bone Joint Surg Am 1974 Sep; 56(6): 1246–1253.
74. Baba H, Maezawa Y, Furusawa N, et al. The cervical spine in the Klippel-Feil syndrome. A report of 57 cases. Int Orthop 1995;19(4):204–208.
75. Fielding JW, Hensinger RN, Hawkins RJ. Os odontoideum. J Bone Joint Surg Am 1980;62(3):376–383.

76. Hosono N, Yonenobu K, Ebara S, Ono K. Cineradiographic motion analysis of atlantoaxial instability in os odontoideum. Spine 1991; 16(10 Suppl):S480–S482.
77. Hughes TB Jr, Richman JD, Rothfus WE. Diagnosis of Os odontoideum using kinematic magnetic resonance imaging. A case report. Spine 1999;24(7):715–718.
78. Watkins RG, Williams L, Watkins RG IV. Cervical Injuries in Athletes. In: The Cervical Spine Research Society, eds. The Cervical Spine. 4th Ed. Philadelphia: Lippincott-Raven; 2005:567–586.

5
Lumbar Spine Injuries

Merrilee Zetaruk

As children are increasingly involved in highly competitive sports and training at a greater intensity, new patterns of injury are emerging (1–4). Low back pain is identified in 10–15% of participants in youth sports in general (5,6), with this percentage being even higher in certain sports. Studies reveal that 27% of college football players (7), nearly 50% of young artistic gymnasts (8,9), and up to 86% of rhythmic gymnasts (10) complain of low back pain.

The etiology of low back pain in young athletes differs significantly from that seen in the adult population (4,6). Injuries to the pars interarticularis are more common in the younger population (6). Although disc-related problems are prevalent among adults, only 11% of children and youth with back pain have symptoms referable to the disc (11). The discs in children are well hydrated, firm, and solidly attached to the adjacent vertebral end plate (4,12), leading to a different pattern of injuries.

Structural problems are relatively common in adolescent athletes; therefore, earlier and more thorough investigations may be indicated in this age group, compared with adults presenting with low back pain (13,14). Idiopathic pain is much less common among younger athletes than among adults (15,16). In one series of physically active individuals between 12 and 18 yr of age who presented with low-back pain, only 6% had symptoms caused by lumbosacral strain, compared with 27% of adults (11). Physicians who hastily attribute persistent low back symptoms in young patients to simple "back strains" run the risk of delaying the diagnosis of more severe injuries, such as spondylolysis or spondylolisthesis (3).

Injuries in all age groups occur either as a result of acute traumatic events or from repetitive microtrauma (3,4). In younger athletes, more sinister causes of low back pain, such as infection, neoplasm, inflammatory conditions, and visceral dysfunction, need to be considered as well (1,3). Trauma is still the most common cause of low back pain, with high-energy contact sports such as football or rugby producing acute injuries, and sports such as gymnastics, figure skating, and dance resulting in overuse injuries from repetitive flexion, extension, and torsion (4).

Anatomy

The lumbosacral spine typically consists of 5 lumbar segments, 5 fused segments of the sacrum, and 4 fused segments of the coccyx (12). Common anatomic variants include a sacralized 5th lumbar vertebra or a lumbarized 1st sacral segment (17,18). A common developmental defect seen in the lumbar spine is spina bifida occulta, which is usually of little clinical relevance in isolation and may be considered a normal variant (19).

Each lumbar vertebra can be divided into anterior and posterior elements. The anterior elements include the vertebral body, intervertebral discs, and vertebral end plates (2). The portions of the vertebrae between the superior and inferior articular facets are referred to as the posterior elements (14). The posterior elements include the facet joints and pars interarticularis (2). These structures are injured when extension and torsion forces are applied to the spine (2).

Figure 5.1 shows the anatomic structure of the discovertebral joint. The intervertebral disc consists of a central core called the nucleus pulposis. This gel-like substance is contained by the anulus fibrosus, which makes the disc resilient to compressive forces and able to function as a shock absorber (12,14). The cartilaginous epiphyseal plates or "end plates" form the inter-

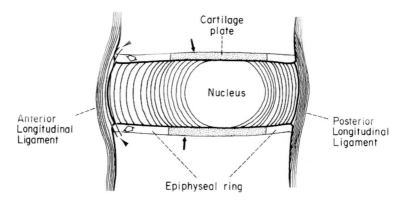

FIGURE 5.1. Intervertebral disc and adjacent vertebral bodies. Concentric fibers of the anulus fibrosus surround the nucleus pulposis. Solid arrows indicate subchondral bone plate beneath the cartilaginous end plates. Open arrows indicate attachment of the anulus fibrosus to the bony rim that is formed by fusion of the epiphyseal ring (ring apophysis). The anulus fibrosus also attaches to the vertebral body cortex via strong Sharpey's fibers (arrowheads). (Reprinted with permission from Resnick D. Degenerative diseases of the vertebral column. Radiology 1985;156:3–14.)

face between the disc and vertebral body (3,12,18). A cartilage ring apophysis, which is present on the vertebral bodies and circumscribes the end plates, eventually fuses with its vertebral body (20). Disc herniation through the apophysis may prevent this fusion from occurring, resulting in a limbus vertebra (20).

The sacroiliac joints, which form part of the pelvic ring (21), have a synovial portion and a ligamentous portion (22,23). The anterior inferior portion is a true synovial joint, whereas the superior posterior portion has no cartilage, synovium, or capsule; rather, this portion of the joint is traversed with ligaments (22,23).

Clinical Evaluation

History

A complete history and physical examination are necessary when evaluating a young athlete with pain in the lumbar region. Although trauma (acute or overuse) is most frequently encountered in young athletes with low back pain, other conditions including infection, tumor, and rheumatologic disorders, must be considered as well (2,11). Key points on history will help determine the nature of the injury, or may give clues to the presence of a more serious underlying condition.

Onset of symptoms should differentiate between acute trauma and a more gradual, insidious onset of pain. Duration, location, quality, and severity of pain should be determined, along with associated neurologic symptoms and aggravating factors. "Red flag" symptoms, which may be associated with more sinister causes of low back pain such as infection, tumor, or arthritis, include fever, malaise, weight loss, morning joint stiffness, and night pain (14,24).

The type of sport or physical activity must be determined, along with the volume of training or level of competition (13). History of disordered eating, menstrual irregularities, and previous stress fractures may suggest an associated diagnosis of "Female Athlete Triad," which places the athlete at increased risk of stress fractures (25).

A past or family history of HLA-B27–associated conditions, such as (juvenile) ankylosing spondylitis, psoriatic arthritis, inflammatory bowel disease, or Reiter's syndrome, may be enlightening (26). Review of systems may identify symptoms suggestive of a visceral or systemic etiology of low back pain.

Physical Examination

Physical examination should begin with observation of gait and posture. The patient should be observed in both flexion and extension of the spine. Pain in the lumbar region on flexion may suggest muscle spasm or strain, or may indicate injury to the anterior elements of the spine. Extension of the spine will provoke pain in posterior element injuries and SI joint conditions. FABER (Flexion-Abduction-External-Rotation) test, also known as Patrick's test, and Gaenslen's test can aid in localizing the pain to the SI joint (Figure 5.2). Areas of tenderness should be noted.

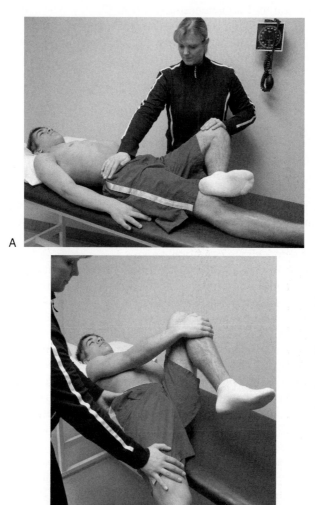

A

B

FIGURE 5.2. **(A)** FABER test: With the athlete supine on the examining table, the leg is placed in a "figure 4" position and pressure is applied to the knee and contralateral ASIS. **(B)** Gaenslen's test: With the patient lying supine at the edge of the examining table, one knee is flexed maximally and the other leg is extended over the edge of the table. Both tests assess sacroiliac joint symptoms.

A screening neurologic exam, including sensation, strength, and reflexes of the lower extremities, should be conducted. Slump test and straight leg raise test for neural tension should be performed. Pain in the lumbar region, which radiates down the leg on the affected side, is consistent with nerve root irritation or impingement caused by disc herniation (27) or spondylolisthesis (28).

Low back pain is much more frequently associated with structural abnormalities in children than in adults. In the young athlete, muscle spasm or tenderness should never be attributed simply to muscle strain until other etiologies have been ruled out. Finally, if history is suggestive of visceral pathology, abdominal examination should be performed, and costovertebral angle tenderness evaluated.

Risk Factors

Several factors distinguish growing athletes from adults. Many experts feel that during rapid growth, soft tissues are unable to keep pace with the rate of bone growth. This results in muscle imbalances and a reduction in flexibility (3,4), both of which place the young athlete at greater risk of injury.

Growth cartilage, which is present only in the skeletally immature individual, is particularly vulnerable to injury (6). With repetitive flexion, the intervertebral disc of the young athlete may herniate through the anterior portion of the ring apophysis (4), which is a secondary center of ossification, circumscribing the vertebral end plates. The presence of growth cartilage along the iliac crest apophyses may also produce symptoms of low back pain.

The variability in size and skeletal maturation among children of the same chronological age poses additional risks to young athletes (4). Most youth sports teams group children by age. As a result, on the same Bantam Hockey team, ages 13–14, the skeletal age and physical development may range from 11–16 yr (29). The smaller, skeletally less mature participants face significant risk from contact with bigger players (3).

The volume of training influences the risk of injury. Gymnasts who train 15 h or more per week have a much higher prevalence of spine abnormalities on magnetic resonance imaging (MRI) (57%) compared with those who train less than 15 h per week (13%) (30). It is difficult to determine the optimum amount of training for young athletes, because variability in rate of development may also represent variability in risk of injury. All members of the same sports team may not tolerate equivalent volumes of training. Certain overuse injuries present with greater frequency in athletes undergoing a rapid growth spurt (31,32). This suggests that as a young athlete grows and matures, the volume and intensity of training that his or her body can tolerate may vary. Additionally, poor technique, which is a risk factor for injury at any age, may be of particular concern among younger athletes whose muscular development may be more advanced than neurologic development (33).

Other risk factors for low back injury include hip flexor tightness, increased femoral anteversion, thoracolumbar fascia tightness, abdominal weakness, genu recurvatum, and increased thoracic kyphosis. Each of these contributes to low back injury by increasing lumbar lordosis and placing additional stress on the posterior elements of the spine (6). Hamstring tightness has also been associated with increased incidence of low-back pain in general (34) and, more specifically, with spondylolysis (14).

Injuries of the Posterior Elements of the Spine

Sports that involve repetitive extension and torsion of the spine, such as gymnastics, figure skating, and dance, place the athlete at increased risk of injury to the posterior elements. Weightlifting and contact sports, such as football and ice hockey, also have an increased association with posterior element injuries (27,35).

Athletes with injuries, either acute or overuse, which involve the posterior elements of the spine, typically present with pain on extension. Twisting motions may also precipitate pain in these patients. The athlete may describe tightness in the low back or hamstrings. The pain may be diffuse over the lumbar region, particularly in the setting of significant associated muscle spasm, or the athlete may be able to localize the pain to one side of a single vertebral level. Associated neurologic symptoms such as weakness, numbness, or tingling in the lower extremities may also be present. Any young athlete, particularly one involved in a high-risk sport, who presents with extension pain in the lumbar region requires a thorough history and physical examination, as well as early investigations to rule out significant pathology such as spondylolysis or spondylolisthesis.

Spondylolysis and Spondylolisthesis

Spondylolysis, from the Greek words "spondylos" (spine) and "lysis" (break), refers to a defect of the pars interarticularis. Although congenital or developmental defects ("dysplastic spondylolysis") exist, most cases of spondylolysis and spondylolisthesis are isthmic (36) in adolescence. These are stress fractures caused by repetitive extension and torsion of the lumbar spine. In a study of 327 high-school rugby players, 72.5% of those with radiographic evidence of spondylolysis had co-existing low back pain (37), which supports the contention that pars defects are not innocuous. In one study, 47% of athletes presenting with back pain to Boston Children's Hospital were found to have spondylolysis (11). The most common level of involvement is L5 (38,39).

Spondylolisthesis is the forward translation of one vertebra on the next caudal segment (36). The grade of spondylolisthesis is based on the percentage of slip of one vertebral body in respect to the next caudal segment. A slip of 0–25% is grade I, 25–50% is grade II, 50–75% is grade III, and >75% is classified as grade IV (40). Athletes are at a low risk for progression of spondylolisthesis. This clinical entity is less common than simple spondylolysis (41). Unilateral spondylolysis may lead to increased stress and possible fracture of the contralateral side (42). When bilateral pars defects are present, there is limited restraint to forward motion of the affected vertebral segment, resulting in a slip. The peak age for development of a slip is during the adolescent growth spurt. Slips rarely progress after age 20 (41,43). Slip angle is determined by drawing a line along the posterior border of the sacrum. The angle between the inferior border of L5 and a line drawn perpendicular to the posterior border of the sacrum forms the slip angle (44). An increased slip angle (>45–55 degrees), representing the degree of kyphosis at the lumbosacral junction, is associated with greater risk of progression (36,44).

Risk Factors

There is a genetic predisposition for spondylolysis among certain ethnic groups. Whereas the prevalence is reported to be approximately 5% by 7 yr of age (41) and 6% in the adult population in general (36), the prevalence of spondylolysis among the Inuit in Northern Canada is reported to be high as 20–50% (41).

Upright posture and repetitive loading of the posterior elements of the spine through extension and torsion appear to place the athlete at increased risk of spondylolysis (36). Sports that involve repetitive extension of the spine have been shown to have a high prevalence of spondylolysis among athletes complaining of low back pain (45,46). Among female competitive gymnasts, the rate of spondylolysis is 11% (47). In a 1998 study by Perugia and Rossi of athletes with low back pain, 42% of divers, 28% of wrestlers, and 16% of gymnasts were shown to have spondylolysis on plain radiographs (45).

Factors that increase lumbar lordosis and increase stresses on the posterior elements of the spine place the young athlete at greater risk of spondylolysis and spondylolisthesis. Tight hip flexors tilt the pelvis by contracting the anterior portion of the hip joint (Figure 5.3). Young dancers with increased femoral anteversion may "cheat" by increasing their lumbar lordosis to augment the degree of turnout of the lower extremities (Figure 5.4) (6,48). Athletes with weak abdominal musculature will have difficulty stabilizing the lumbar spine in neutral. A tight thoracolumbar fascia may produce a tethering effect in the lumbar region, resulting in increased lordosis. An increased thoracic kyphosis is frequently accompanied by lumbar hyperlordosis. Genu recurvatum will tilt the pelvis into a hyperlordotic

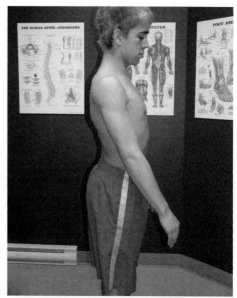

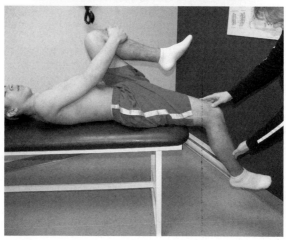

FIGURE 5.3. **(A)** Increased lumbar lordosis increases risk of lumbar spine injury. **(B)** Tight hip flexors may increase lordosis.

posture (6). Finally, there is an association between spina bifida occulta and spondylolysis (43).

Presentation

Young athletes with spondylolysis characteristically present with pain on spine extension (49). Onset is usually insidious, with symptoms increasing over months (36). Affected athletes may have a milder degree of discomfort on spine flexion associated with a sense of tightness in the lumbar muscles. There is frequently an associated reduction in flexibility of the ipsilateral hamstrings described by the patient (49,50). This is particularly true among dancers and gymnasts, who are often very aware of any changes in flexibility. Affected individuals may complain of pain with impact, for example during running or jumping activities, or with body contact in football or hockey. There may be accompanying radicular symptoms, such as radiating pain, numbness, or weakness (24,51). These symptoms may make the diagnosis of spondylolysis more difficult because they may also be present in the setting of disc herniation.

Clinical Examination

Typical features of spondylolysis and spondylolisthesis on examination include lumbar hyperlordosis, ipsilateral paraspinal muscle spasm, and mild discomfort with tightness of the hamstrings on forward flexion of the spine (50). There is focal pain on provocative hyperextension of the spine. Pain on extension localizes the pathology to the posterior elements, whereas single-leg extension, which is a very sensitive test for spondylolysis, further localizes it to the affected side (Figure 5.5) (13).

Radicular signs are less common in the younger athlete, but may accompany injuries to the pars (44). Strength, sensation, and reflexes of the lower extremities must be evaluated. Abnormal findings may be detected in the setting of nerve root irritation associated with spondylolysis, or more

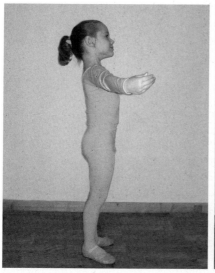 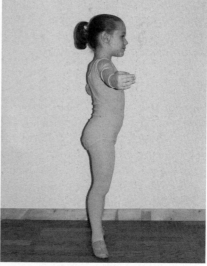

A   B

FIGURE 5.4. **(A)** A young dancer with good lumbar posture. **(B)** Same dancer who is now increasing apparent hip turnout by increasing lumbar lordosis.

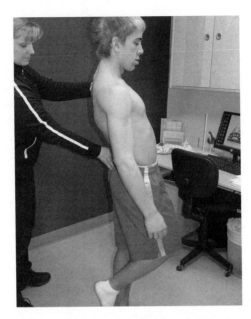

FIGURE 5.5. Single leg extension helps to localize pain to the side of the spondyloly-sis when standing on the ipsilateral leg.

frequently, with spondylolisthesis. Neural tension signs may also be present.

Focal tenderness over the site of the bony lesion is usually present. Over-lying paraspinal muscle spasm may make localization of tenderness more difficult; however, the point of maximal tenderness usually corresponds with the level and side of the spondylolytic lesion. A step-off at the lumbo-sacral junction may be palpable in the presence of a slip (36).

Investigations

Lumbar pain that has been present in the young athlete for at least 3 wk warrants further investigations (6). Imaging with plain radiographs is the initial step in investigating a possible spondylolysis (24). X-rays, including anteroposterior (AP), lateral ± coned lateral, and oblique views, are often recommended. The AP view most commonly identifies other anatomic variants or developmental defects, which may be associated with greater incidence of spondylolysis. Spina bifida occulta (Figure 5.6), although clini-cally insignificant in isolation, is seen more frequently in patients with spondylolysis (4,43). Transitional vertebrae (sacralization of L5 or lumbari-zation of S1) may also be seen in spondylolysis (4). The lateral view may demonstrate a lytic lesion or spondylolisthesis (Figure 5.6) (24). Coned lateral x-ray at the level of the suspected lesion will identify some lesions missed on regular lateral view (36,52). Oblique views demonstrate the pars interarticularis (Figure 5.6). Some authors (6) discourage the use of oblique views, which demonstrate spondylolysis in only 1/3 of cases because of the orientation of the x-ray beam to the lesion (53).

After plain radiographs, a single-photon emission computed tomography (SPECT) bone scan should be obtained. This diagnostic tool identifies bony lesions in which active bone turnover is occurring (50). A simple planar bone scan may fail to identify an active spondylolytic lesion. Twice as many cases of abnormal uptake within the pars interarticularis will be detected on SPECT scan compared with simple planar views (Figure 5.7) (54, 55).

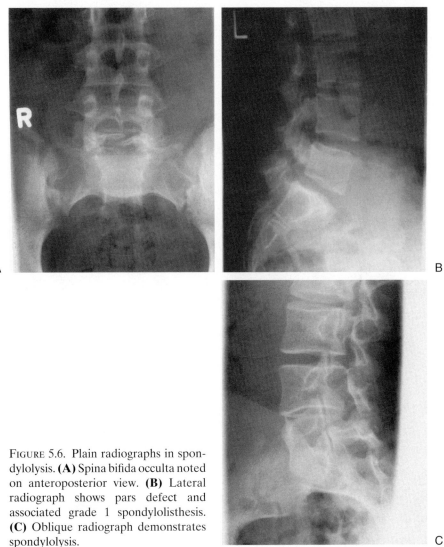

A

B

FIGURE 5.6. Plain radiographs in spondylolysis. (A) Spina bifida occulta noted on anteroposterior view. (B) Lateral radiograph shows pars defect and associated grade 1 spondylolisthesis. (C) Oblique radiograph demonstrates spondylolysis.

C

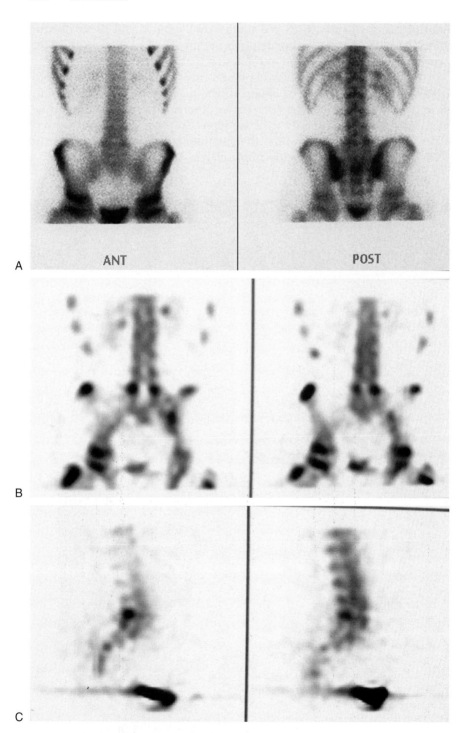

FIGURE 5.7. Technetium-99 bone scan in spondylolysis. **(A)** Abnormality may be missed on planar images. **(B and C)** SPECT images clearly reveal abnormal uptake in posterior elements.

McCormack and Athwal (56) described a "spondylolysis mimic," which is a vertebral articular facet fracture, in a young gymnast. The clinical presentation was identical to that of spondylolysis. Although planar bone scan was normal, SPECT images revealed abnormal uptake in the posterior elements of the spine. Only on CT scan were the authors able to determine that the pathology was localized to the facet, rather than the pars interarticularis.

Some clinicians elect to perform CT scans on all patients with abnormal uptake on SPECT scan (38). CT is very sensitive in identifying true stress fractures of the pars interarticularis (54), but may fail to identify very early lesions, which are considered "stress reactions." Some sclerosis may be identified in this circumstance; however, CT may be entirely normal (38). Because of the additional radiation involved in CT scanning, the author's practice is to subject only those patients who are not responding to treatment to CT scanning. In this setting, the CT scan is used to identify the persistence of a lytic defect and to gather additional information regarding further healing potential. Spondylolytic lesions with sclerotic, well-corticated margins are unlikely to progress to further bony union; however, some experts have found external electrical stimulation to be of benefit in this situation (57,58).

MRI, because of the lack of ionizing radiation involved, would appear to be a desirable investigation for young athletes; however, the sensitivity of MRI to detect pars defects is low, ranging from 57–86% (59,60). Although recent studies suggest that MRI may be a useful tool in the evaluation of spondylolysis (60–62), further investigations are needed.

Management

For the young athlete with low back pain caused by a metabolically active spondylolysis, initial management is activity modification. Any activities that provoke pain must be avoided. These activities may include running, jumping, extension, torsion of the spine, and body contact. A program of daily home exercises should begin immediately. This program should include strengthening of the abdominal muscles, hip flexor, and hamstring stretches, and antilordotic exercises for the lumbar spine (39). Physiotherapy may be necessary to ensure exercises are performed correctly. Improper techniques, such as increasing lumbar lordosis to increase turnout in ballet, must be corrected as well.

The use of bracing incites debate among specialists, because no prospective, randomized controlled trials have directly compared bracing versus nonbracing in spondylolysis. Some authors recommend early use of custom thoracolumbar orthoses to protect the injured spine by limiting extension and rotation (6,25,50,55). Anderson (63) studied intensity of uptake on SPECT scan and timing of brace use in spondylolysis with respect to symptom resolution, and concluded that earlier implementation of bracing in the more active stage of spondylolysis (greater intensity of uptake) is associated with better resolution of symptoms (63). Others feel that spondylolysis can be treated successfully with simple activity restriction in conjunction with physiotherapy without mandatory rigid bracing (64), or with bracing being reserved for those not responding to activity restriction alone (44).

d'Hemecourt et al. (39) found that 80% of young athletes treated with a rigid thoracolumbar orthosis and structured physiotherapy program were able to return to full sports participation without a brace and with no, or only occasional, pain associated with vigorous activity (39). The brace, typically at zero degrees of lordosis, helps prevent spine extension and torsion. Although evidence suggests that such bracing may not actually immobilize the lumbosacral junction (65), the brace does serve to limit extension and rotation, which are movements that can exacerbate the condition. Athletes are permitted to return to training in the brace as soon as pain subsides. The brace prevents the athlete from performing techniques with spine extension, such as "laybacks" in figure skating or "walkovers" in gymnastics, or minimizes the degree of extension in dance techniques such as arabesques. Only pain-free activities in the brace are permitted.

Recent attention has been given to external electrical stimulation to assist healing of nonunited spondylolysis. In a small series of only two patients, one group of investigators (58) found that application of an external electrical stimulator during sleep allowed for bony union of spondylolytic lesions that were previously unhealed by a full course of bracing and activity modification. Further research is necessary in this area before electrical stimulation can be recommended on a more routine basis for recalcitrant spondylolytic lesions (66).

It is difficult to determine the point at which healing of a spondylolysis has taken place. At this time, no single investigation can definitively provide this information. Bone scans remain positive for some time, even after healing has occurred. CT may help determine the stage of healing (13,24). MRI may also prove to be useful in the future, but at this point, the best indicator of healing is clinical assessment. A patient who has resumed full activities out of any brace used in treatment and without recurrence of pain should be considered clinically healed. Patients with spondylolisthesis should be monitored until skeletal maturity to ensure no further slip occurs. Coned lateral x-rays every 3–4 mo during rapid growth will detect any progression of the condition. All patients who experience a recurrence of pain after treatment has concluded should be re-evaluated immediately to assess the status of the spondylolysis or spondylolisthesis.

Cauda Equina Syndrome

One potential complication of spondylolisthesis is cauda equina syndrome, a compression of nerve roots below L1 (67). Other conditions, such as dislocations of the spine or large posterocentral intervertebral disc herniations, may also lead to cauda equina syndrome (67). This syndrome is characterized by lower motor neuron deficits with variable sensorimotor, reflex, bladder, bowel, and sexual dysfunction (67). Symptoms suggestive of cauda equina syndrome, such as "saddle anesthesia" with bowel or bladder dysfunction, necessitate immediate surgical intervention (24).

Posterior Element Overuse Syndrome

Once spondylolysis has been ruled out, the diagnosis of posterior element overuse syndrome should be considered. This is not, in fact, a single clinical entity, but represents injury to one or more of the following posterior elements of the spine: muscle–tendon units, ligaments, joint capsules, and facet joints (4,25). The inferior articular facets of one vertebra articulate with the superior articular facets of the next caudal segment to form the facet joints, which are also known as apophyseal joints. Posterior element overuse syndrome is also referred to by other names, including spondylogenic back pain (5), hyperlordotic back pain (11), mechanical low back pain (3,4), and lumbar facet syndrome (68).

Risk factors for posterior element overuse syndrome include weak abdominal muscles, tight hamstrings, tight thoracolumbar fascia, limited lumbar motion, and poor training technique (4,69).

Presentation and Clinical Examination

Young athletes with this condition present with symptoms and signs similar to those of spondylolysis. They complain primarily of pain on extension or rotation of the spine. Common physical findings include pain on rising from flexion (70) and pain on provocative hyperextension. Paraspinal muscle tenderness may be present (4,70). Nerve root signs are not typical features of posterior element overuse syndrome. Focal tenderness is present over the lower lumbar spine, adjacent to the midline. Transitional vertebrae, with pseudoarthrosis between the lateral spinous process and the iliac wing (Bertolotti's syndrome), may result in focal pain and tenderness, which may mimic spondylolysis (6).

Management

Treatment consists of a daily home exercise program that, in more recalcitrant cases, is carried out under the supervision of a physiotherapist. Abdominal strength exercises, antilordotic exercises, and stretches of the hamstrings and thoracolumbar fascia should be included in the rehabilitation program (4). Ice and nonsteroidal antiinflammatories (NSAIDs) may help reduce pain and associated inflammation. Pain-free activities are permitted. This typically excludes extension of the spine. In the case of persistent pain, despite the aforementioned measures, use of a soft lumbar support brace or an antilordotic brace may provide some relief (3,25).

Low Back Pain Related to Injuries of the Pelvis

Sacroiliac Joint Dysfunction

The sacroiliac, or SI, joint is a frequent site of discomfort in active individuals. The SI joint dissipates the forces between the trunk and the lower extremities (6). Motion within the SI joint is quite limited, but excessive or reduced motion (6) can lead to pain in the joint. Altered mechanics in the lumbar region, which result from other lumbar pathology, can apply stress to the SI joints if muscle spasm is present. Leg length discrepancies may also contribute to SI joint pain (6).

Inflammation of the SI joint occurs in various conditions: the HLA-B27 seronegative spondyloarthropathies, such as juvenile ankylosing spondylitis, Crohn's disease, and psoriatic arthritis, as well as infectious causes, such as Reiter's syndrome. The differential diagnosis of SI dysfunction also includes stress fracture of the sacrum (6,50).

Presentation and Clinical Examination

Athletes with SI joint pain present with symptoms similar to those of spondylolysis. Pain is usually exacerbated with spine extension, and the onset is often insidious (13). Physical examination findings confirm pain in the lower lumbar or buttock region with extension, often localizing to the affected SI joint on single-leg extension. Poor pelvic stability may be noted on Trendelenburg testing. Weakness of the gluteus medius muscles allows the pelvis to rock side to side with ambulation, thereby placing additional stress across the SI joints. Tests for SI joint mobility may detect hyper- or hypomobility of the joint, leading to increased pain. FABER (Patrick's) test and Gaenslen's test may be positive (Figure 5.2). Hopping on the affected side produces pain in the presence of a sacral stress fracture (71).

With the athlete prone, focal tenderness may be elicited over the affected SI joint. Careful distinction must be made between SI joint tenderness and tenderness of the posterior elements of the lumbar spine. The pseudoarthrosis between the lateral spinous process and the iliac wing in Bertolotti's syndrome may result in focal pain and tenderness near the superior portion of the SI joint (6).

Investigations

If symptoms persist for more than 3 wk, plain radiographs of the lumbar spine and pelvis may be warranted. Anatomic variants that place the SI joints under additional stress may be detected (e.g., transitional vertebrae). Abnormalities of the SI joint related to sacroiliitis associated with seronegative spondyloarthropathy include erosions, pseudowidening of the joints, and sclerosis (72).

Technetium-99 bone scan will detect the rarer stress fractures of the sacrum (50,71) and may detect abnormal uptake associated with sacroiliitis. Some caution should be exercised in interpreting the results because the SI joints may have some degree of increased uptake in the skeletally immature individual. Bone scan should be able to differentiate between Bertolotti's syndrome and spondylolysis (6).

MRI may be useful in distinguishing between SI joint dysfunction/inflammation and sacral stress fractures by more precisely defining the anatomic location of the abnormality. It has the added ability over bone scan to rule out bone or soft tissue tumors, and lacks ionizing radiation (71). In a series of 21 runners with sacral stress fractures, 15 subjects underwent MRI, all of whom had abnormalities at the site of the fracture (9 were full stress fractures, 6 showed marrow edema only) (71).

In the appropriate setting, blood work may be warranted to screen for sacroiliitis resulting from one of the seronegative spondyloarthropathies. Erythrocyte sedimentation rate (ESR) and c-reactive protein (CRP) will be elevated, whereas rheumatoid factor (RF) and antinuclear antibodies (ANA) will be negative. HLA-B27 may be positive because the seronegative spondyloarthropathies are frequently associated with this histocompatibility antigen (72,73).

Management

Treatment of SI joint dysfunction involves ice, NSAIDs, bracing, activity modification, and physiotherapy. Physiotherapy may involve mobilizing a hypomobile SI joint (74) or stabilizing the pelvis in the setting of a hypermobile joint. Pelvic stabilization is essential, particularly if weakness of the gluteus medius is present. Hip girdle and lower abdominal strengthening exercises may attenuate forces transmitted to the affected area, while improving running mechanics (71).

Ice and NSAIDs will help reduce pain and any associated inflammation present in the region. Bracing of the SI joints will assist with stabilization of the joints temporarily and may reduce stress across the joints. Activities should be limited to those that do not provoke pain. Treatment may take a few weeks to a few months until the athlete becomes asymptomatic. Leg length discrepancies should be corrected, to reduce abnormal stresses across the SI joints (6).

For sacral stress fracture, some authors suggest a period of nonweight-bearing until ambulation is pain free (1–2wk), followed by nonimpact activities for 6wk (71), whereas others recommend a period of partial weightbearing for 4–6wk (6). In Fredericson's series, all 21 athletes with sacral stress fractures began a return-to-running protocol within 8–12wk of diagnosis, and returned to full preinjury training levels by 3–6mo (71).

Iliac Crest Apophysitis

Growth cartilage is present along the crest of the ilium in the skeletally immature athlete. Low back pain in the adolescent may be caused by traction of the gluteus medius and oblique abdominal muscles on the iliac crest apophysis (21). Pain may be localized to one area of the iliac crest or may be more diffuse. Resisted contraction of the abdominal oblique muscles on the affected side will reproduce pain when symptoms extend laterally and anteriorly along the iliac crest. Treatment of this condition involves application of ice for pain relief and reduction of associated inflammation. Exercises to stretch and strengthen the core trunk muscles will help prevent recurrence of symptoms. The athlete may continue pain-free activities (31).

Injuries of the Anterior Elements of the Spine

Lumbar (atypical) Scheuermann's

Scheuermann's disease, first described in 1920 (6,75,76), refers to a thoracic kyphosis in which three or more consecutive vertebral segments are wedged 5 degrees or more anteriorly (77). Other radiographic findings include Schmorl's nodes, which are caused by herniation of the intervertebral disc through the vertebral end plates and irregularity of the vertebral end plates (6, 76).

In sports involving rapid flexion, such as gymnastics, injuries of the vertebral end plates may occur in the region of the thoracolumbar junction (4,25,49,78). In contrast with classic Scheuermann's disease, lumbar or "atypical" Scheuermann's is associated with a flat back (6,25). Although there is no associated anterior wedging of the vertebral bodies (76), atypical Scheuermann's has other features in common with the classic form: end plate fractures, Schmorl's nodes, and vertebral apophyseal avulsions (6), as well as wedging of the vertebral bodies and disc-space narrowing (77).

Presentation

Typically, athletes presenting with lumbar Scheuermann's are involved in sports with repetitive flexion, such as gymnastics (4,6,25,49,78), weight lifting, American football (14), rowing, and diving (4,78). Pain is exacerbated with forward flexion (14,49,78).

Clinical Examination

On examination, young athletes with atypical Scheuermann's demonstrate a reduced lumbar lordosis and thoracic kyphosis ("flat back") (3,4,6,25), tightness of thoracolumbar fascia and hamstrings, and pain on forward flexion of the spine (4,6,25,78). Diagnosis of atypical Scheuermann's is based on the clinical findings described above and is confirmed on plain lateral radiographs.

Management

Once the diagnosis is made, the young athlete should begin a rehabilitation program to improve spinal stabilization and stretch tight hamstrings and thoracolumbar fascia (6,25). Bracing at 15 degrees or more of lordosis to unload the affected vertebral elements can facilitate return to play, sometimes within 1–2 mo, as long as the athlete remains pain free (3,6,25,49). Bracing continues until there is evidence of bony healing on x-ray (3,49) and symptoms have resolved (up to 9–12 mo at 18–23 h per day in the brace) (3).

Vertebral Body Apophyseal Avulsion Fracture

Injury to the ring apophysis may occur as a result of repetitive flexion and extension of the spine. Compression forces caused by flexion lead to pain at the thoracolumbar junction, whereas traction from repetitive extension may result in separation of the anterior portion of the ring apophysis (79). Fracture through the cartilage of the ring apophysis may occur. The fractured cartilaginous apophyseal ring may displace posteriorly into the spinal canal, along with a portion of the intervertebral disc (78,80,81). Typically, it is a central disc herniation that is associated with this "slipped vertebral apophysis" (78).

Presentation

Avulsion occurs most frequently in sports that require repetitive lumbar flexion, such as wrestling, gymnastics, weightlifting, and volleyball (78,79). Apophyseal avulsion fracture may present with features similar to a disc herniation (78,81), although numbness and paraesthesias are usually absent (78). Patients typically complain of lumbar pain with spine flexion.

Clinical Evaluation

Physical findings in an athlete with an apophyseal avulsion fracture are similar to those seen in disc herniation (78,81). There is limited lumbar flexion and extension. Paraspinal muscle spasm is often present, but neurologic exam is typically normal (78).

Investigations

Lateral radiographs may reveal an ossified fragment in the canal (78). Additional tests include CT and MRI. CT will better identify the fractured apophysis and its adjacent piece of bone, which may be missed on MRI (78).

Management

Rest, heat, analgesia, and massage may be used for symptomatic pain relief (78). In the presence of significant neural compression, surgical excision of bony fragments or hinged fibrocartilage flap may be required (78,80).

Disc Herniation

The intervertebral disc is subject to compressive, rotational, and shear forces (2). In the adult, a common cause of low back pain is tearing of the anulus fibrosus as the nucleus pulposis herniates through the weakest point of the anulus (70). The intervertebral discs in the young active individual are well hydrated, in contrast to the discs of adults. Whereas adults typically develop herniation of the nucleus pulposis through the anulus in response to applied forces, children are more likely to herniate through the cartilaginous end plates (3), which are firmly affixed to the disc, and into the underlying cancellous bone. This produces the typical "Schmorl's nodes" seen in classic and atypical Scheuermann's disease. In children, herniation of the disc into cancellous bone beneath the ring apophysis may also occur (3).

Disc herniations similar to those seen in the adult population do occur in young athletes, but these make up a much smaller proportion of all low back pain in children and adolescents (3). Disc herniations are more commonly encountered in adolescents than in children (78). The incidence in the active young athlete appears to be increasing (3). Sports that involve repetitive flexion may predispose the athlete to disc herniation.

Presentation

Athletes with disc herniation present with low back, buttock, or hip pain exacerbated by forward flexion of the spine and often aggravated by cough or sneeze, which increases the intradiscal pressure (2,3,78). If the disc herniation impinges upon an adjacent nerve root, sciatic symptoms may be present. In this situation, pain will radiate from the lumbar region into the ipsilateral buttock and, possibly, the posterior thigh region. In young athletes, symptoms are more likely to be restricted to the hip and buttock compared with adults who more frequently experience sciatic symptoms radiating down the leg (3,78). There may be associated weakness or numbness in the lower extremity of the affected side.

Clinical Examination

Clinical findings of disc herniation include limited trunk flexion caused by pain that may radiate down the affected leg, weakness of specific muscle groups in myotomal distribution, and numbness in the involved dermatome; however, altered reflexes, muscle weakness, and atrophy are rare findings in the adolescent with disc herniation (4). The nerve root affected

FIGURE 5.8. Slump test: One knee is extended and the neck is flexed, reproducing lumbar pain with radiation into the extended leg if nerve root impingement is present.

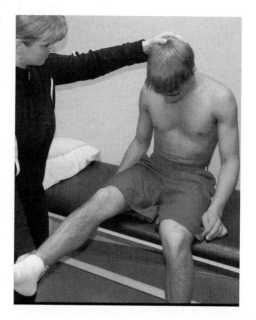

is usually one inferior to the disc that is herniated (78). Slump test and straight leg test will reproduce symptoms (Figure 5.8). Muscle spasm and an antalgic gait may be noted (4). Scoliosis caused by muscle spasm may be present (6,49). Asymmetry of hamstring flexibility may be noted as well (3,6,78).

Investigations

Investigations should include plain radiographs of the lumbosacral spine. Although the degenerative changes and disc space narrowing associated with disc disease in adults are not typical features in young patients, other osseous abnormalities are more commonly encountered (3,78). Avulsion fracture of the vertebral end plate may be seen in young athletes with radicular symptoms (3). More commonly, plain radiographs assist in differentiating between the clinical picture of disc herniation with nerve root impingement and spondylolisthesis with nerve root impingement. Because treatment of these two conditions is very different, this is an important distinction to make. Noninvasive tests, such as CT and MRI can help determine if neurocompressive lesions in the canal are present (3,78).

Management

Treatment of disc herniation necessitates rest from vigorous physical activity, with a particular caution against spine flexion and heavy lifting. Proper back mechanics for lifting must be reviewed with the patient. Ice and

NSAIDs can help reduce pain and inflammation (78). Physiotherapy in the acute stage is aimed at reducing pain, inflammation, and secondary muscle spasm. Modalities and lumbar traction may be of benefit. Symptoms usually improve within a few weeks (3). Once acute symptoms have abated, exercises may be added to the regimen. Hamstring stretches and core strength and stability are essential elements of treatment. Strong, well-conditioned trunk musculature appears to be associated with reduced stress on the discs (82). Although immobilization with bracing is discouraged in the adult population, a rigid polypropylene thoracolumbar orthosis at 15 degrees of lordosis may help unload the affected disc and reduce associated muscle spasm in young athletes who are not responding to other conservative measures (3). This often facilitates an earlier return to light training (3); however, only 50% of young athletes who are braced are able to return to full training within the first year (3,83). In the young athlete with documented discogenic back pain, vigorous physical activity should not be resumed for 6–12 mo (3).

As in the adult population with discogenic back pain, clinical signs and symptoms of impending cauda equina syndrome, such as saddle anesthesia, bowel or bladder dysfunction, or severe motor loss, necessitate emergent referral for surgical intervention (3,78).

Other Causes of Low Back Pain

Low back pain in the young athlete is not always caused by injury. Inflammation, infection, and neoplasm can present with low back pain. Visceral disorders can also present with pain in this region (78). "Red flags" such as fever, weight loss, night pain, and malaise in a patient with low back pain should lead the clinician to rule out more sinister causes for the symptoms (6).

Seronegative Spondyloarthropathies

The seronegative spondyloarthropathies are a group of inflammatory conditions that may affect the spine and SI joints. "Seronegative" refers to the absence of rheumatoid factor. HLA-B27 is often positive in these conditions (72,73). The seronegative spondyloarthropathies encountered in young patients include juvenile ankylosing spondylitis, psoriatic arthritis, and enteropathic arthritis. Reiter's syndrome, which is a reactive arthritis, falls within this category as well.

Presentation

Affected individuals present with low back pain and stiffness that is worse in the morning (4). Pain is often localized to the SI joints. There may be a history of pain at the insertion points of tendons (entheses). Other systemic conditions may be present on history, such as psoriasis or inflammatory bowel disease. A family history of psoriasis, inflammatory bowel disease, or ankylosing spondylitis may also be present (72).

Clinical Examination

Physical examination features include tenderness over the SI joints, positive SI joint stress tests (FABER test and Gaenslen's test), and pain on extension of the spine. A modified Schober's test assesses decreased lumbar mobility. This test is performed by placing a tape measure against the lumbar spine. The 10-cm mark is placed at the level of the PSIS, with marks made on the skin at 0 and 15 cm. The patient is asked to flex the spine. In a normal spine, there should be at least a 5-cm increase between the skin marks with flexion. Skin should be examined for evidence of psoriasis. Patients with SI joint pain should be examined for tenderness caused by inflammation of the Achilles tendon, patellar tendon, and planter fascia insertions to bone (enthesitis). In individuals with seronegative spondyloarthropathy, pain at these sites previously may have been attributed to apophysitis, such as Sever's apophysitis or Osgood–Schlatter apophysitis. Apophysitis is an overuse injury that affects the growth cartilage at the insertion of tendons in skeletally immature individuals. Because enthesitis and apophysitis may be clinically difficult to differentiate, additional imaging, such as ultrasound or MRI, may be of diagnostic benefit (26). Chronic effects of persistent enthesitis include bone edema and overgrowth, formation of enthesophytes, bone bridging, subcortical bone cysts, and erosions at tendon insertions (26).

Investigations

Laboratory investigations should include CBC, ESR, and CRP. Rheumatoid factor is absent. Over 90% of patients with ankylosing spondylitis are positive for HLA-B27 (73); however, because this test is expensive and quite time-consuming, it should not be used as a screening test for all patients who present with SI joint pain.

Plain radiographs may be normal, or may show abnormalities of the SI joints. Erosions, pseudowidening, and sclerosis may be detected (72). Bone scan will typically reveal increased radionuclide uptake within the affected SI joints.

Management

In most cases, children or adolescents with suspected juvenile ankylosing spondylitis should be referred to a pediatric rheumatologist for ongoing management. Other referrals that may be appropriate include ophthalmology, to assess for uveitis, and gastroenterology, if there is suspicion of inflammatory bowel disease.

Discitis

Low back pain associated with systemic symptoms, particularly fever, in a young athlete should prompt consideration of discitis or tumor (81). Discitis, or inflammation of the intervertebral disc, may present with low back pain, which is exacerbated on forward flexion of the spine. Young children may refuse to bear weight (84,85). Although severe back pain, high fever, and signs of bacteremia may accompany discitis (86), the typical presentation is much less dramatic.

Investigations

Plain radiographs may demonstrate disc space narrowing with sclerosis or erosions of the adjacent vertebral end plates (81,85–87); however, these findings are often absent at initial presentation (86,87). Bone scan and MRI can detect the presence of discitis early in the course of the disease (86), often within 1–2 d of onset of symptoms (87). ESR and CRP are generally elevated, whereas white blood cell counts may be normal or only mildly elevated (81,86,87).

Management

Although *Staphylococcus aureus* is the most commonly encountered organism in discitis (84), both blood cultures and disc space needle aspiration often yield negative cultures (81,87); therefore, empiric treatment for *S. aureus* is often initiated after blood cultures alone (81). Bracing and/or bed rest can help reduce pain (27,81,87), and most young athletes may resume exercise in 4–6 wk if they are asymptomatic (78).

Vertebral Osteomyelitis

Hematogenous spread of bacteria to the vertebral body can lead to osteomyelitis of the spine. Infection may also spread directly from discitis (85). Transdiscal spread may result in involvement of two adjacent vertebral bodies (87). The mean age of presentation of vertebral body osteomyelitis is 7.5 yr (88). The clinical presentation is similar to that of discitis in children; however, fever may be more significant.

Investigations

Imaging with plain radiographs may show rapid loss of disc height and adjacent lysis of bone (87). Bone scan demonstrates increased uptake within the affected vertebra. MRI and CT have also been used to detect vertebral osteomyelitis (87). The positive predictive value of MRI is comparable to that of bone scan in the acute setting; however, MRI has the advantage of clearly distinguishing between discitis and vertebral osteomyelitis (89).

Management

As in discitis, *S. Aureus* is the most common infectious agent implicated in vertebral osteomyelitis. Treatment with antibiotics should continue for at least 4–6wk (85), until ESR has normalized (90,91).

Spinal Neoplasms

Although an infrequent cause of low back pain in children and adolescents, tumor should be considered in the differential diagnosis (49,90), particularly when "red flag" symptoms are present. Intractable back pain, pain at night, fever, malaise, and weight loss should prompt the clinician to look for more sinister causes of low back pain, including benign and malignant tumors (27, 49).

Benign lesions that may affect the spine include osteoid osteoma, osteoblastoma, eosinophilic granuloma, and aneurysmal bone cyst (27,86). Primary malignancies such as osteogenic sarcoma and Ewing's sarcoma can present with lesions in the spine (86). Metastatic lesions seen most frequently in the spine include neuroblastoma and rhabdomyosarcoma (92). Other metastatic lesions such as lymphoma, leukemia, and Wilms' tumor, may present with low back pain (27).

Investigations

Screening laboratory investigations, including CBC, ESR, and urinalysis, should be considered where there is clinical suspicion of tumor as a cause of low back pain in the young athlete (81). Radiographic findings that suggest a malignant process include thinning and destruction of pedicles, vertebral body collapse, and expansile lesions with a soft-tissue mass (93). Bone scan will detect bony abnormalities, including those caused by osteoid osteoma and other neoplasms (27,49,93). Further imaging with CT scan or MRI is needed to better identify and localize the lesion (49). Referral to oncology for further work-up and management is necessary.

Scoliosis

Idiopathic scoliosis does not typically cause back pain in the young athlete. Conditions that may be associated with a painful scoliosis include osteoid osteoma, osteoblastoma, disc herniation, spondylolisthesis, infection, and intraspinal tumors (3). Scoliosis caused by nerve root irritation may also occur (3,94). Individuals in whom the scoliosis is reversed (i.e., convex right in the lumbar region) should be more closely evaluated for other causes for the curvature. Such conditions include muscle spasm caused by underlying lumbar injury or spinal neoplasms.

Prevention

The key to prevention of overuse injuries of the lumbar spine is the recognition of risk factors. These risk factors may be identified during preparticipation evaluations. A child who experiences a rapid growth spurt may be more vulnerable to certain conditions of the lumbar spine; therefore, a decrease in training at such times may reduce the risk of injury. Although there is no set volume of training that is safe for all young athletes at all stages of development, parents and coaches should watch for increasing complaints of pain, which may suggest that the athlete's body is unable to tolerate the present levels of stress imposed by the sport.

The nature of certain sports increases the risk of lumbar spine injury in young athletes. Walkovers in gymnastics and laybacks in figure skating place a considerable stress on the posterior elements of the spine. Children involved in such sports should be advised to limit the number of repetitions of movements involving back hyperextension during practices if they begin to experience low back pain. To assist this group of athletes, a core-strengthening program may be beneficial. Athletes with lumbar hyperlordosis should begin an exercise program aimed at reducing their lordosis. This may involve posture exercises, as well as stretches for tight hip flexors. Athletes should be instructed to stretch tight hamstrings to reduce the risk of low back pain.

Proper technique may prevent some injuries of the lumbar spine. For example, young male dancers should be instructed on proper techniques for lifting their partners, to prevent discogenic low back pain. Figure skaters should be instructed to extend through their entire spine, rather than "hinging" in the lower lumbar region to help prevent spondylolysis.

Finally, an important factor in prevention of lumbar spine injury is the recognition that low back pain is not simply "a part" of some sports. Low back pain is not "normal"—it most frequently indicates the presence of stress on the tissues. If this stress is not reduced and the lumbar spine is not allowed to recover, more serious overuse injuries may ensue.

Return to Play Guidelines

Lumbar pain in young athletes may be caused by a wide variety of etiologies, and the stresses placed on the lumbar spine vary from sport to sport. Return-to-play recommendations must take into account the specific diagnosis, the type of sport or physical activity, the age and skeletal maturity of the child, and the level of cooperation of the coaches and parents in providing modified activities for the young athlete.

In general, very few overuse injuries of the lumbar spine and sacrum require complete rest from physical activities. In most situations, young athletes may continue to participate to some degree in their chosen sports, as long as they avoid movements or activities that aggravate symptoms or continue to apply undue stress at the site of injury. For younger children who may not maintain a pain-free level of activity on their own, or for those athletes who notice pain only after cessation of their activities, more specific restrictions may be advised.

For injuries of the posterior elements, including spondylolysis, spondylolisthesis, and posterior element overuse syndrome, athletes may continue modified, pain-free sport participation. For these athletes, extension, spine torsion, and impact activities are often curtailed until symptoms subside. It is the author's practice to use bracing (custom thoracolumbar orthoses for spondylolysis/spondylolisthesis; off-the-shelf lumbar support braces for posterior element overuse syndrome) to facilitate earlier return-to-play. Sport participation gradually increases as healing progresses and symptoms abate. Once the athlete is at full, pain-free sport participation in the brace, with a benign clinical examination, bracing is weaned. This may be after 3–6 wk for posterior element overuse syndrome, or 3 mo or longer in the case of spondylolysis or spondylolisthesis (25).

Pain originating from the sacroiliac joint and iliac crest apophyses may be managed with modified activities and progression to full training as symptoms permit; however, sacral stress fractures require an initial period of partial- or nonweightbearing. These individuals can generally begin a graded running program within 8–12 weeks and return to full training by 3–6 mo (71).

Symptoms will help guide return-to-play recommendations in young athletes with injuries to the anterior spinal elements. As described for posterior element injuries, bracing may assist in returning athletes to training when rest and avoidance of inciting activities are unsuccessful. Atypical Scheuermann's may take up to 9–12 mo for bony healing to occur, as seen on plain radiographs; however, once bracing has been initiated, the athlete may return to full activities in the brace, as long as they remain pain free (3,95).

After disc herniation, activities are often significantly restricted for a few weeks until the acute symptoms of pain and secondary muscle spasm have subsided. Use of a rigid polypropylene thoracolumbar orthosis at 15 degrees of lordosis may help the adolescent athlete resume daily activities and light training (3,6,78). Bracing may also decrease the number of missed school days because of discogenic pain (3). Because recovery from a disc herniation may be prolonged, and recurrence of symptoms frequently accompanies a premature return to sports, some experts recommend a period of 6–12 mo before initiating vigorous sport activity (3). Affected athletes must have a full, pain-free range of motion with normal strength before returning to full sport participation (78).

Clinical Pearls

- The young athlete who presents with lumbar symptoms should be taken very seriously, as there is a greater likelihood of associated structural pathology in younger individuals.
- "Lumbar strain" or other nonspecific conditions should only be entertained as diagnoses of exclusion.
- The etiology of low back pain in skeletally immature athletes is different from that of adults, and management of specific conditions often differs. Even the clinical presentation of the same condition and response to treatment may be dramatically different in younger athletes compared with adults.
- The sport and intensity of training responsible for development of symptoms may give clues to the underlying etiology of low back pain.
- When dealing with young athletes, the physician must also consider more serious, atraumatic conditions in the differential diagnosis of low back pain. "Red flags" for such conditions include fever, weight-loss, morning joint stiffness, and night pain.

References

1. Gross ML, Mandelbaum BR. Spondylolysis and spondylolisthesis. In: Reider B, ed. Sports Medicine: The School Age Athlete. 2nd ed. Philadelphia: W.B. Saunders; 1996:169–184.
2. Anderson SJ. Sports injuries. Dis Mon 2005;51:438–542.
3. Yancey RA, Micheli, LJ. Thoracolumbar spine injuries in pediatric sports. In: Stanitski DL, DeLee JC, Drez DD Jr, ed. Pediatric and adolescent sports medicine. Vol 3. Toronto: W.B. Saunders; 1994:162–174.
4. Kocher MS, Micheli LJ. Upper extremity and trunk injuries. In: Armstrong N, van Mechelen W, eds. Pediatric sport and exercise medicine. Oxford: Oxford University Press; 2000:428–436.
5. Micheli LJ. Back injuries in gymnastics. Clin Sports Med 1985;4:85–93.
6. d'Hemecourt PA, Gerbino PG, Micheli LJ. Back injuries in the young athlete. Clin Sports Med 2000;19:663–679.
7. Semon RL, Spengler D. Significance of lumbar spondylolysis in college football players. Spine 1981;6:172–174.
8. Szot Z, Boron Z, Galaj Z. Overloading changes in the motor system occurring in elite gymnasts. Int J Sports Med 1985;6:36–40.
9. Kolt GS, Kirkby RJ. Epidemiology of injury in elite and subelite female gymnasts: a comparison of retrospective and prospective findings. Br J Sports Med 1999;33:312–318.
10. Hutchinson MR. Low back pain in elite rhythmic gymnasts. Med Sci Sports Exerc 1999;31:1686–688.
11. Micheli LJ, Wood R. Back pain in young athletes: significant differences from adults in causes and patterns. Arch Pediatr Adolesc Med 1995;149:15–18.
12. Snell RS. The back. In: Snell RS, ed. Clinical Anatomy for Medical Students. 3rd ed. Toronto: Little, Brown and Company; 1986:919–954.

13. Kraft DE. Low back pain in the adolescent athlete. Pediatr Clin N Am 2002;49: 643–653.
14. Baker RJ, Patel D. Lower back pain in the athlete: common conditions and treatment. Prim Care Clin Office Pract 2005;32:201–229.
15. Patel DR, Nelson TL. Sports injuries in adolescents. Med Clin North Am 2000;84:983–1007.
16. Clifford SN, Fritz JM. Children and adolescents with low back pain: a descriptive study of physical examination and outcome measurement. J Orthop Sports Phys Ther 2003;33:513–522.
17. Keats TE, Anderson MW. The sacrum. In: Keats TE, Anderson MW, eds. Atlas of Normal Roentgen Variants that May Stimulate Disease. 7th ed. Toronto: Mosby; 2001:333–345.
18. Anderson JE. The back. In: Anderson JE, ed. Grant's Atlas of Anatomy. 8th ed. Baltimore: Williams & Wilkins; 1983:5.1–5.5.
19. Tehranzadeh J, Andrews C, Wong E. Lumbar spine imaging: normal variants, imaging pitfalls, and artifacts. Radiol Clin North Am 2000;38:1207–1253.
20. Resnick D. Degenerative disease of the spine. In: Resnick D, ed. Bone and Joint Imaging. 2nd ed. Toronto: WB Saunders, 1996:355–377.
21. Hutson MA. Pelvic injuries. In: Hutson MA, ed. Sports Injuries: Recognition And Managament. 3rd ed. New York: Oxford University Press; 2001:113–123.
22. Resnick D. Ankylosing spondylitis. In: Resnick D, ed. Bone and Joint Imaging. 2nd ed. Toronto: W.B. Saunders; 1996:246–264.
23. Manaster BJ. Arthritis. In: Manaster BJ, ed. Handbook of Skeletal Radiology. 2nd ed. Toronto: Mosby; 1997:104–170.
24. Moeller JL, Rifat SF. Spondylolysis in active adolescents expediting return to play. Phys Sportsmed 2001;29:27–32.
25. Zetaruk MN. The young gymnast. Clin Sports Med 2000;19:757–780.
26. Burgos-Vargas R. The juvenile-onset spondyloarthritides. Rheum Dis Clin North Am 2002;28:531–560.
27. Payne WK, Ogilvie JW. Back pain in children and adolescents. Pediatr Clin N Am 1996;43:899–918.
28. Solomon R, Brown T, Gerbino PG, et al. The young dancer. Clin Sports Med 2000;19:717–739.
29. Greulich WW, Pyle SI. Radiographic atlas of skeletal development of the hand and wrist. 2nd ed. Stanford: Stanford University Press; 1959.
30. Goldstein JD, Berger PE, Windler GE, et al. Spine injuries in gymnasts and swimmers: an epidemiologic investigation. Am J Sports Med 1991;19:463–468.
31. Kaeding CC, Whitehead R. Musculoskeletal injuries in adolescents. Prim Care 1998;25:211–223.
32. Duri ZAA, Patel DV, Aichroth PM. The immature athlete. Clin Sports Med 2002;21:461–482.
33. Hutchinson MR, Wynn S. Biomechanics and development of the elbow in the young throwing athlete. Clin Sports Med 2004;23:531–544.
34. Sjolie AN. Low-back pain in adolescents is associated with poor hip mobility and high body mass index. Scand J Med Sci Sports 2004;14:168–175.
35. Congeni J, McCulloch J, Swanson K. Lumbar spondylolysis: a study of natural progression in athletes. Am J Sports Med 1997;25:248–253.
36. Herman MJ, Pizzutillo PD, Cavalier R. Spondylolysis and spondylolisthesis in the child and adolescent athlete. Orthop Clin North Am 2003;34:461–467.

37. Iwamoto J, Abe H, Tsukimura Y, et al. Relationship between radiographic abnormalities of lumbar spine and incidence of low back pain in high school rugby players: a prospective study. Scand J Med Sci Sports 2005;15:163–168.

38. Gregory PI, Batt ME, Kerslake RW, et al. Single photon emission computerized tomography and reverse gantry computerized tomography findings in patients with back pain investigated for spondylolysis. Clin J Sport Med 2005; 15:79–86.

39. d'Hemecourt P, Zurakowski D, Kriemler S, et al. Spondylolysis: returning the athlete to sports participation with brace treatment. Orthopedics 2002;25:653–657.

40. Meyerding H. Spondylolisthesis. Surg Gynecol Obstet 1932;54:371–377.

41. Reid DC. Injuries and conditions of the neck and spine. In: Reid DC, ed. Sports injury assessment and rehabilitation. New York: Churchill Livingston Inc.; 1992: 739–837.

42. Sairyo K, Katoh S, Sasa T, et al. Athletes with unilateral spondylolysis are at risk of stress fracture at the contralateral pedicle and pars interarticularis: a clinical and biomechanical study. Am J Sports Med 2005;33:583–590.

43. Fredrickson BE, Baker D, McHolick WJ, et al. The natural history of spondylolysis and spondylolisthesis. J Bone Joint Surg Am 1984;66:699–707.

44. Smith JA, Hu SS. Management of spondylolysis and spondylolisthesis in the pediatric and adolescent population. Orthop Clin North Am 1999;30:487–499

45. Perugia L, Rossi F. Spondylolysis and spondylolisthesis in sport: review of a case series. JTRRE 1998;20:209–212.

46. Trainor TJ, Weisel SW. Epidemiology of back pain in the athlete. Clin Sports Med 2002;21:93–103.

47. Jackson DW, Wiltse LL, Cirincione RJ. Spondylolysis in the female gymnast. Clin Orthop 1976;117:658–673.

48. Brown T, Micheli LJ. Dance: Where artistry meets injury. Biomechanics 1998;5:12–24.

49. Weiker GG. Evaluation and treatment of common spine and trunk problems. Clin Sports Med 1989;8:399–417.

50. Micheli LJ, Curtis C. Stress fractures in the spine and sacrum. Clin Sports Med 2006;25:75–88.

51. Ganju A. Isthmic spondylolisthesis. Neurosurg Focus 2002;13:1–6.

52. Lipton ME. Is the coned lateral lumbosacral junction radiograph necessary for radiological diagnosis? Br J Radiol 1991;64:420–421.

53. Saifuddin A, White J, Tucker S, et al. Orientation of lumbar pars defects: implications for radiological and surgical management. J Bone Joint Surg Br 1998;80: 208–211.

54. Bellah RD, Summerville DA, Treves ST, et al. Low back pain in adolescent athletes: detection of stress injuries to the pars interarticularis with SPECT. Radiology 1991;180:509–512.

55. Akbarnia BA. Pediatric spine fractures. Orthop Clin North Am 1999;30:521–536.

56. McCormack RG, Athwal G. Isolated fracture of the vertebral articular facet in a gymnast: a spondylolysis mimic. Am J Sports Med 1999;27:104–106.

57. Shegog MI, Curtis C, d'Hemecourt P, et al. Spondylolysis in athletes: evaluation of the treatment protocol of division of sports medicine, Children's Hospital Boston. Med Sci Sports Exerc 2005;37:(Supplement)S13 (abstract).

58. Fellander-Tsai L, Micheli LJ. Treatment of spondylolysis with external electrical stimulation: a report of two cases. Clin J Sport Med 1998;8:232–234.
59. Saifuddin A. The value of lumbar spine MRI in the assessment of the pars interarticularis. Clin Radiol 1997;52:666–671.
60. Sherif H, Mahfouz AE. Epidural fat interposition between dura mater and spinous process: a new sign for the diagnosis of spondylolysis on MR imaging of the lumbar spine. Eur Radiol 2004;14:970–973.
61. Campbell RS, Grainger AJ, Hide IG, et al. Juvenile spondylolysis: a comparative analysis of CT, SPECT and MRI. Skeletal Radiol 2005;34:63–73.
62. Ulmer JL, Elster AD, Mathews VP, et al. Lumbar spondylolysis: reactive marrow changes seen in adjacent pedicles on MR images. AJR Am J Roentgenol 1995;164:429–433.
63. Anderson K. Quantitative assessment with SPECT imaging of stress injuries of the pars interarticularis and response to bracing. J Pediatr Orthop 2000;20:28–33.
64. Standaert CJ, Herring SA. Spondylolysis: a critical review. Br J Sports Med 2000;34:415–422.
65. Miller RA, Hardcastle P, Renwick SE. Lower spinal mobility and external immobilization in the normal and pathologic condition. Orthop Rev 1992;21:753–757.
66. Stasinopoulos D. Treatment of spondylolysis with external electrical stimulation in young athletes: a critical literature review. Br J Sports Med 2004;38:352–354.
67. Evans RW, Wilberger JE. Traumatic disorders. In: Goetz CG, ed. Textbook of Clinical Neurology. 2nd ed. Philadelphia: W.B. Saunders; 2003:1129–1154.
68. Harvey J, Tanner S. Low back pain in young athletes: a practical approach. Sports Med 1991;12:394–406.
69. Kujala UM, Taimela S, Oksanen A, et al. Lumbar mobility and low back pain during adolescence: a longitudinal three-year follow-up study in athletes and controls. Am J Sports Med 1997;25:363–368.
70. Watkins RG. Lumbar disc injury in the athlete. Clin Sports Med 2002;21:147–165.
71. Fredericson M, Salamancha L, Beaulieu C. Sacral stress fractures: tracking down nonspecific pain in distance runners. Physiciansportsmed 2003;31:31–32, 38, 40–42.
72. Rheumatology and miscellaneous clinical conditions. Adolesc Med 2003;14:499.
73. Gregersen PK. Genetics of rheumatic diseases. In: Harris ED, Budd RC, Genovese MC, et al, editors. Kelly's Textbook 0f Rheumatology. 7th ed. Philadelphia: W.B. Saunders; 2005:276–294.
74. Rumball JS, Lebrun CM, Di Ciacca SR, et al. Rowing injuries. Sports Med 2005;35:537–555.
75. Scheuermann H: Kyfosis dorsalis juvenilis. Ugeskr Laeger 1920;82:385–393.
76. Lowe TG. Scheuermann's disease. Orthop Clin North Am 1999;30:475–485.
77. Resnick D. Osteochondroses. In: Resnick D, ed. Bone and joint imaging. 2nd ed. Toronto: W.B. Saunders, 1996:960–977.
78. Simon LM, Jih W, Buller JC. Back pain and injuries. In: Birrer RB, Griesemer BA, Cataletto MB, eds. Pediatric Sports Medicine for Primary Care. Philadelphia: Lippincott Williams & Wilkins; 2002:306–325.

79. Sward L, Hellstrom M, Jacobsson B, et al. Vertebral ring apophysis injury in athletes: is the etiology different in the thoracic and lumbar spine? Am J Sports Med 1993;21:841–845.
80. d'Hemecourt PA, Micheli LJ. Back injuries in the young athlete. J Sports Traumatol Allied Sports Sci 1999;1:1–11.
81. King HA. Back pain in children. Orthop Clin North Am 1999;30:467–474.
82. DeBeliso MA, O'Shea JP, Harris C, et al. The relationship between trunk strength measures and lumbar disc deformation during stoop type lifting. Med Sci Sports Exerc 2003;35:(supplement) S134 (abstract).
83. Micheli LJ, Hall JE, Miller ME. Use of modified Boston back brace for back injuries in athletes. Am J Sports Med 1980;8:351–356.
84. Kothari NA. Imaging of musculoskeletal infections. Radiol Clin North Am 2001;39:653–671.
85. Frank G. Musculoskeletal infections in children. Pediatr Clin North Am 2005;52:1083–1106.
86. Thompson GH. The spine. In: Behrman RE, Kliegman RM, Jenson HB, eds. Behrman. Nelson Textbook of Pediatrics. 17th ed. Philadelphia: W.B. Saunders; 2004:2280–2288.
87. Mahboubi S, Morris MC. Imaging of spinal infections in children. Radiol Clin North Am 2001;39:215–222.
88. Fernandez M, Carrol C, Baker C. Discitis and vertebral osteomyelitis in children: an 18-year review. Pediatrics 2000;105:1299–1304.
89. Lampe RM. Osteomyelitis and suppurative arthritis. In: Behrman RE, Kliegman RM, Jenson HB, eds. Behrman. Nelson Textbook of Pediatrics. 17th ed. Philadelphia: W.B. Saunders; 2004:2297–2302.
90. Sassmannshausen G, Smith BG. Back pain in the young athlete. Clin Sports Med 2002;21:121–132.
91. Kaplan SL. Osteomyelitis in children. Infect Dis Clin North Am 2005; 19:787–797.
92. Leeson MC, Makley JR, Carter JR. Metastatic skeletal disease in the pediatric population. J Pediatr Orthop 1985;5:261–267.
93. Neff JR. Sarcomas of bone. In: Abeloff MD, Armitage JO, Niederhuber JE, et al., eds. Clinical Oncology. 3rd ed. Philadelphia: Churchill Livingston; 2004: 2471–2572.
94. Eismont FJ, Kitchel SH. Thoracolumbar spine. In: Delee JC, Drez DD, eds. DeLee and Drez's Orthopaedic Sports Medicine. 2nd ed. Philadelphia: W.B. Saunders; 2003:1525–1576.
95. Micheli LJ, Mintzer CM. Overuse injuries of the spine. In: Harries M, Williams C, Stanish WD, et al., eds. Oxford Textbook of Sport Medicine. 2nd ed. New York: Oxford University Press; 1998:709–720.

6
Thoracoabdominal Injuries

Hamish Kerr, Christine Curtis, and Pierre d'Hemecourt

Intrathoracic and Intraabdominal Injuries

A soccer player sustains trauma to his abdomen in a collision with an opponent. The player is taken out of the game, only to return within 2 min feeling little ill effect. He is noted to be coughing, but is able to continue. After the game he is complaining of left upper quadrant abdominal pain. The athletic trainer relates that the player has had a recent upper respiratory tract infection.

Did the player sustain a splenic rupture because of underlying splenomegaly, caused by infectious mononucleosis, or is this an abdominal wall hematoma or muscle strain? Alternatively, could the coughing be indicative of an intrathoracic injury, such as a pneumothorax?

This scene illustrates the difficulties involved in diagnosing injuries to the chest and abdomen. Unless there is a low threshold to pursue investigation, athletes may suffer serious consequences. Injuries to the chest and abdomen are often more subtle in presentation than other injuries, such as an acute ligament rupture. Injuries are uncommon and catastrophic events can occur if an intraabdominal or intrathoracic injury is unrecognized. Awareness of the organs that can be injured, and how injuries may present, is the best defense against missing potentially life-threatening thoracic and abdominal trauma (1).

Anatomy

The thorax contains the heart, the great vessels, and the lungs. The lungs are surrounded by two layers of pleurae protected by the ribs and the thoracic musculature. The diaphragm divides the thoracic and peritoneal cavities with a variable position in respiration (2). The expulsive motion of the diaphragm can raise the right crus to the level of the 4th anterior costal cartilage. Importantly, the abdominal contents may be raised well into the chest and exposed to chest wall trauma.

The peritoneal cavity contains solid organs, such as the liver, spleen, and pancreas, plus hollow viscous organs, including the stomach and the small and large intestine. Also in this area are the lower ribs, the abdominal wall musculature, vascular structures, the bladder, and retroperitoneal organs and spaces.

Clinical Evaluation

Thoracic Injury

Athletes with a thoracic injury may present with chest wall pain and, often, shortness of breath. Inspection for ecchymosis can also be helpful with intrathoracic injuries incurred in sport. Pulmonary auscultation is essential for assessment for lung pathology. Cardiac auscultation may be indicated for myocardial contusion or arrythmias. Further examination may include palpation for tenderness over a suspected rib fracture.

Abdominal Injury

Athletes can present with an immediate onset of pain or a more insidious onset (1). Athletes who have a history of an appropriate mechanism, such as a rapid deceleration or high-energy impact, who have continuous, persisting abdominal pain should be examined.

Physical exam should begin with the measurement of vital signs, which may be normal or reflect a state of shock. Inspection for ecchymosis and tenderness on abdominal palpation helps detect the potentially affected organ. Abdominal wall muscular contusion can be difficult to distinguish from intraabdominal injury. Contusions are usually only tender over the area of sustained injury, and pain may be evident with contraction of the underlying muscle. Conversely, intraabdominal injuries may elicit tenderness from various angles of palpation.

50% of athletes with a significant abdominal trauma have a negative initial exam, so re-examination can be crucial. One estimate is that 20% of patients with an acute hemoperitoneum have an initial benign abdominal exam (3).

Liver or spleen injuries can bleed, causing intraabdominal irritation and pain. Pain is often mild, without palpable tenderness. Injuries to hollow viscera and the pancreas cause peritonitis, often resulting in severe pain. Initially, this is localized to the site of injury. Peritoneal signs, such as referred tenderness and loss of bowel sounds, are found with progression of intraabdominal injury. Auscultation for bowel sounds can be misleading, as the presence of bowel sounds does not exclude injury. Walking or coughing can also precipitate pain. Retroperitoneal injuries may occur without peritoneal signs when there is minor trauma. Hematuria is often the only clinical manifestation of renal trauma.

Coexisting Injuries

It has been well recognized that lower chest wall trauma places the upper abdominal organs at risk for injury. Most commonly, a blow to the lower left chest wall can result in an injury to the spleen (1). Conversely, several case reports exist in the literature of abdominal impact resulting in an intrathoracic injury, such as a pneumothorax. One such report by Roberts (4) described an ice hockey player who was checked into the boards and sustained an impact over his left lower ribs. Initial concern for a splenic injury proved unfounded and he was allowed to return to the game. However, he was too uncomfortable to continue and assessment afterwards revealed a 15% pneumothorax on chest x-ray. Hence, pulmonary injury from abdominal trauma can occur without disruption of the diaphragm. Diaphragm rupture is uncommon, but is usually left sided (70–90%), as the liver appears to protect the right side.

Diagnostic Assessment

Laboratory investigations, including serial determination of hematocrit, diagnostic imaging, and diagnostic peritoneal lavage (DPL), can be performed in a hospital setting. DPL has become less commonly performed with the increased availability of computed tomography (CT). A chest x-ray is usually indicated. An erect view is helpful to exclude air under the diaphragm, suggesting bowel perforation. Abdominal CT scan after blunt trauma has 67% sensitivity in its ability to predict the need for surgery in a pediatric population (5). The negative predictive value was 98.7% in the same study. A combination of clinical exam and CT scan did not miss any significant injuries. Serial examination may be performed in a hospital setting. CT scan alone may miss clinically significant injuries.

Treatment

Field treatment for shock, before and during transfer to a trauma center, is essential when shock is detected. Intravenous access with a large-bore cannula should be established at two sites with rapid infusion of 0.9% saline, rather than dextrose-containing fluids.

Current surgical goals are for organ salvage and repair, rather than removal of injured intraabdominal organs. Indications for removal revolve around uncontrolled bleeding, particularly when associated with coagulopathy. In such circumstances, the risks of surgery are outweighed by the benefit of achieving hemostatic control, with a low likelihood of control being achieved any other way. Once stabilized, discharge with home observation is often practical. However, caution is required regarding delayed rupture of the spleen at 7–10 d.

Thoracic Injuries

Thoracic injuries generally result from rapid deceleration or high-energy impact, which occur most frequently in high-speed, high-energy contact and high-altitude sports, such as bicycling, skiing, football, hockey, and boxing (6). Statistically, adolescents have more penetrating thoracic trauma, with the mortality risk rising to 17% (7). The evolution of "extreme sports" may increase the potential for high-energy impacts, with lack of appropriate safety precautions and remoteness from immediate medical attention. In one study, 6.1% of injured snowboarders sustained chest trauma, whereas only 2.7% of skiers had similar injuries (8).

Lung Injuries

Pneumothorax

This is the most common intrathoracic injury after blunt thoracic trauma (9). Among all children who sustain high-energy thoracic trauma, approximately one third will develop a pneumothorax (10). Pneumothorax has been reported in several sports, including soccer and weightlifting (11–14). Tension pneumothorax occurs in 1–2% of patients with a spontaneous pneumothorax (15).

Pneumothorax results from the loss of air from the lung into the pleural space. If the loss of air into the pleural space continues, tension will result with concomitant shift of the mediastinum away from the side of the pneumothorax. Such a tension pneumothorax requires immediate decompression with, at minimum, a needle into the chest cavity and, optimally, by a tube thoracostomy. If this is not done, the continued pressure and mediastinal shift will lead to respiratory compromise by inhibition of airflow into the good lung and to cardiac compromise by a reduction in venous return to the heart.

Pneumothorax, whether simple or tension, can occur spontaneously from rupture of a bleb, from a sudden compressive force to the chest with a resulting rupture of the lung parenchyma, or from a displaced rib fracture that penetrates the lung. Both simple and tension pneumothoracies are associated with tachypnea, dyspnea, and sudden chest pain, though a simple pneumothorax may be subtle. A simple pneumothorax may present with a small shift of the mediastinal structures to the side of the pneumothorax, whereas tension pneumothorax is associated with a shift to the opposite side. Physical examination may also demonstrate decreased breath sounds

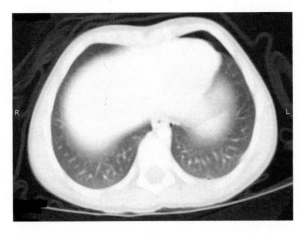

FIGURE 6.1. Left pneumothorax. Courtesy of David Mooney, MD, Children's Hospital, Boston, MA.

on auscultation and hyperresonance by percussion on the side of the lesion. Tension pneumothorax is also associated with tachycardia, neck vein distension, and hypotension.

The diagnosis is confirmed by chest x-ray, but as noted previously, tension pneumothorax should not await chest X-ray for treatment. Figure 6.1 illustrates a CT of a left pneumothorax.

Tube thoracostomy and suction at −20 cm H_2O is all that is required for the treatment of most pneumothoraces. The athlete can resume normal activity within a few days of discharge or as other injuries allow. Occasionally, a small, simple pneumothorax of 20% or less can be treated without tube thoracostomy if the patient is asymptomatic and has no other injuries. This approach requires careful observation and repeat chest x-ray to document stability. Return to normal activities should be delayed until the pneumothorax has completely resolved.

Pulmonary Contusion

This is a "bruise" of the lung associated with hemorrhage and edema into the lung parenchyma (6). It can result from a sudden deceleration in which the lung strikes the chest wall, from a concussive blow to the chest that compresses the lung, or from a displaced rib fracture (9). Children appear prone to this injury in the absence of a rib fracture because of the compressive nature of the rib cage (10). As a result, the force of impact is transmitted to the lungs, rather than being absorbed by the ribs, which do not fracture.

Patients present with cough, hemoptysis, and dyspnea. Exam shows diminished breath sounds, crackles, or both. Chest x-ray findings vary from fluffy, patchy infiltrates to consolidation. It is diagnostic in 85–97% of patients (16,17). Fluid intake should be minimized if possible, to reduce pulmonary edema. Supportive ventilation is necessary in severe instances. Pulmonary contusion after athletic injury is usually self-limited, without long-term sequelae. Once resolved, an athlete can resume training, but should do so gradually, because exercise tolerance and pulmonary reserve will be reduced.

Hemothorax

Hemothorax may result from injury to the lung parenchyma or any of the intrathoracic vessels that may be lacerated by a traumatic rib fracture. Clinically relevant hemothoraces occur in 14% of children sustaining blunt-force chest injury (10). Blood in the thorax is often asymptomatic, unless the volume is large. In this instance, hemothorax can present similarly to tension pneumothorax, with decreased breath sounds and hypotension. Dullness to percussion is noted over the area of pooled blood. Treatment involves supporting ventilation and circulation with intravenous fluids, and then placing a chest tube once transferred to an appropriate setting.

Cardiac Injuries

Commotio Cordis

Commotio cordis is a cause of sudden death resulting from blunt, nonpenetrating, and usually innocent-appearing chest blows, resulting in cardiac arrhythmias (18–22). A series of 128 cases consecutively entered into the U.S. Commotio Cordis Registry had a median age of 14 yr (23). Narrow and underdeveloped chest cages may make younger athletes more susceptible to commotio cordis. 81% of the 107 commotio cordis events recorded in the registry were part of competitive sport and involved a blunt precordial blow from a projectile propelled against a stationary chest wall. Projectiles were most commonly baseballs, although softballs, hockey pucks, and lacrosse balls were also involved. All had a hard solid core, except one event involving a soccer ball.

The uncommon occurrence of commotio cordis is largely explained by its mechanism, which requires the exquisite confluence of several determinants. This includes a direct blow over the heart (18), with a precise timing to the vulnerable phase of repolarization just before the T wave peak (24–26). 84% of people died as a consequence of the commotio cordis event (23). Of the survivors, 19 out of 21 had resuscitative measures instituted for cardiac arrest; the other 2 survivors were judged likely to be examples of aborted commotio cordis. Data from the initial electrocardiogram conducted after the collapse in 82 cases included 33 with ventricular fibrillation,

3 with ventricular tachycardia, 3 with bradyarrythmias, 2 with idioventricular rhythm, 1 with complete heart block, and 40 with asystole, which was unlikely to be the initial rhythm after impact (23).

Chest barriers and safety balls may reduce risk, but protection is not absolute from commotio cordis and the equipment may provide a false sense of security. Prompt cardiopulmonary resuscitation or defibrillation is a major determinant of surviving a commotio cordis event.

Myocardial Contusion

A cardiac "bruise" results from a direct blow to the chest or from a rapid deceleration of the heart, causing it to strike the rib–sternum complex. It can occur in contact sports, but is more common in high-speed events. Significant cardiac events are rare after blunt trauma in young patients. Presentation is typically with collapse after a blow to the chest. Assessment should begin with airway, breathing, and circulation (ABCs). The initial electrocardiogram (EKG) is a better indicator of potential cardiac problems than are more sensitive tests, such as troponin or creatine kinase. Cardiac enzymes and echocardiography results are not related to outcome (27).

Most dysrhythmias from cardiac trauma occur in the first 24 h after injury. Barring EKG abnormalities, which require immediate intervention, patients with a significant mechanism for myocardial injury should be monitored for 24 h. Although this may not require an intensive care setting, the cardiac rhythm should be monitored, as well as hemodynamic parameters including blood pressure, pulse rate, and neck vein distension. Abnormalities in these parameters may signal a more lethal cardiac injury, such as pericardial effusion, valvular injury, or cardiac tamponade. In the absence of EKG or hemodynamic abnormalities for 24 h, the individual can resume normal activities as other injuries allow (6).

Chest Wall Injuries

Rib Fractures

Rib fractures are considered the most common serious injury of the chest wall (28,29). Children are less vulnerable to rib fractures than adults because of the increased elasticity and flexibility of their thoracic cage (30,31). The most commonly fractured ribs in any age group are the 4th to 9th ribs from direct impact (28).

A fracture of the rib may signal significant injury and should increase clinical suspicion of other injuries, such as intrathoracic and intraabdominal injuries. Fractures of the first four ribs or the last two ribs, multiple fractures, and flail segments are less benign than other fractures and may result in injury to surrounding structures (29). Acute direct impact fractures of the 1st and 2nd rib are associated with neck trauma and vascular injuries, as well as pneumothorax, lung laceration, and hemothorax. However, direct external trauma is a rare cause of first rib fractures because of the protection of the shoulder girdle (28). Direct impact fractures of the lower two ribs may damage the kidneys, liver, or spleen. Splenic trauma has been reported in up to 20% of left lower rib fractures and acute liver trauma in up to 10% of right lower rib fractures (28).

First rib fractures may occur from indirect trauma, and have been reported in tennis players, surfers, windsurfers, rowers, jive dancers, and basketball players (32–37). These occur with hyperabduction of the arm and falling on an outstretched arm, as well as sudden muscle contraction (32,38–41). The fracture occurs at the first rib by the opposing forces of muscle contraction. The anterior scalene muscle produces bending forces at the subclavian sulcus, which is the usual fracture site. This groove endures great stress from the downward tensile forces of the intercostals and serratus anterior musculature inferiorly and the upward forces of the scalene muscles. Floating lower rib fractures may also occur with indirect trauma (29). They are caused by avulsion of the attachments of the external oblique muscles and latissimus dorsi muscles with sudden contraction (29). These types of fractures have been reported in baseball players and batters (28,42).

The diagnosis of rib fractures is often indicated by a traumatic event. The pain may initially be diffuse and gradually localize over the affected rib. Direct palpation, deep inspiration, coughing, and twisting or flexion to the side may exacerbate the pain. Palpation of the 1st rib may be difficult. There may be tenderness medial to the superior angle of the scapula, at the root of the neck, supraclavicular triangle, or deep in the axilla. There may be subcutaneous emphysema with pleural injury.

A chest x-ray may establish the diagnosis and exclude other diagnoses, such as a pneumothorax or hemothorax. Rib fractures are often not seen on routine radiographs and often require rib views for accurate diagnosis (28).

The majority of rib fractures heal with rest. The goal of therapy for uncomplicated rib fractures is pain relief, improvement of ventilation, prevention of worsening injury, and a safe return to sport. Pain is usually controlled with oral analgesics. Ice may also be used. Local intercostal nerve blocks are sometimes required if the patient's respiratory status is impaired (6). Deep breathing should be encouraged to prevent atelectasis. Taping is controversial and may lead to increased splinting, pulmonary complications, and atelectasis. Activities should be modified until symptoms resolve. Training should be resumed gradually. Return to play should only be considered in patients whose symptoms resolve and who have minimal pain with palpation.

Rib Stress Fractures

There are more reports of stress fractures of the first rib than any other single rib (43). This has been reported in overhead activities such as baseball, basketball, tennis, and weightlifting (44–49), as well as surfers and jive dancers (48,50) (Figure 6.2).

In a study of 44 patients with a diagnosis of upper extremity or rib stress fractures, Sinha and Kaeding found that lower rib stress fractures predominated in patients who engaged in swinging activities such as golf and tennis

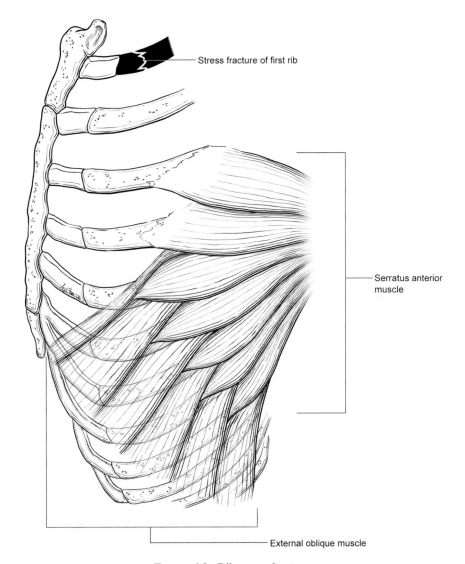

Stress fracture of first rib

Serratus anterior muscle

External oblique muscle

FIGURE 6.2. Rib stress fracture.

(51). Etiological factors associated with these sorts of fractures include technique problems, training errors, equipment problems, and lack of flexibility and strength (52,53).

Stress fractures of the fourth and fifth ribs have also been reported in rowers (54). In a 14-mo period, 12% of a national rowing team were diagnosed with rib stress fractures (55). Gaffney reported a rower with a serratus anterior avulsion from rowing, attesting to the large forces exerted by this muscle (56). Stress fractures in the ribs in rowers are postulated to be caused by excessive action of the serratus anterior muscle (56).

An athlete with a rib stress fracture typically presents with an insidious onset of pain, which is frequently reported in the posterior thorax at the spinal border of the scapula. In a study by Lord et al., plain radiographs revealed stress fractures in 16 cases of 19 rib fractures performed 2 wk after the injury (57). However, plain radiographs may initially be negative with stress fractures. Diagnosis typically requires a triple-phase bone scan. CT scans and MRI may also be useful for accurate diagnosis. Rest from sport is suggested for a period of 4–6 wk. The athlete may undertake light training, including cardiovascular training.

Delayed union and nonunion are the most common complications of first rib stress fractures in throwing athletes. Gurtler et al. described one baseball pitcher in whom it took 9 mo to radiographically heal, despite avoidance of pitching (58). A transaxillary resection to the level of the transverse process may be used to treat a painful nonunion (59).

Rib Tip Syndrome

Rib tip syndrome, or slipping rib syndrome, was defined by Scott and Scott as pain in the lower chest or abdomen, a tender spot on the lower costal margin, and reproduction of pain by pressing that spot (60). The condition typically involves the eighth, ninth, and tenth ribs. These ribs are attached to each other by fibrous tissue. If these fibrous connections are weakened or ruptured by trauma, the ribs can slip and impinge on the intercostal nerve, producing pain. Rib tip syndrome is usually unilateral; however it may be bilateral (60–62). This condition particularly affects running, vigorous arm exercise, arm abduction, and swimming (43). It frequently occurs in contact sports such as football, ice hockey, wrestling, lacrosse, and rugby (28).

Pain is localized to the upper abdomen, epigastrium, or inferior costal regions. Some patients report a slipping movement of the ribs or a popping sensation. Athletes in tennis, cricket, and throwing sports have reported a sudden onset of localized pain, described as sharp, stabbing, or dull, at the costal margin, when side flexing and hyper extending away from this side. In one study, 46% of patients reported the pain as a minor nuisance, whereas another 41% reported pain as moderately severe (60). The remaining 11% reported pain as interfering with activities (60). Symptoms can be reproduced upon clinical examination by hooking the fingers under the inferior rib and pulling anteriorly, referred to as the "hooking maneuver" (63). A positive test reproduces the patient's pain and results in a click. Direct tenderness over the cartilage is another frequent finding. Diagnostic imaging is not helpful, although it may exclude other conditions.

Conservative management includes strapping the ribs, avoidance of aggravating motions, and manipulative techniques. Eastwood was able to manage the condition by manipulating the costovertebral joint (64). Some patients have reported favorable outcomes with single or multiple local anesthetic nerve blocks (65,66). Corticosteroids added to an injection may be beneficial. In recalcitrant cases, surgical intervention may be necessary.

Costosternal Syndromes (Costochondritis)

A variety of diagnostic terms have been used in this group of syndromes, including costochondritis, costosternal syndrome, and anterior chest wall syndrome. Costochondritis is a common cause of atraumatic chest pain in children and adolescents. This condition may account for 9–22% of cases of pediatric chest pain (67). It occurs in contact sports such as football and wrestling. The sites most typically involved are the fourth, fifth, and sixth ribs. Costochondritis may be preceded by exercise or an upper respiratory infection, and it may persist for several months. Morning stiffness and an increased sedimentation rate have suggested inflammation in some patients.

Diagnosis of costochondritis is based on a history of chest pain. Anterior chest wall tenderness may be localized to one or more costochondral junctions. Horizontal arm flexion maneuvers have also been found to be useful in diagnosis.

Most patients recover spontaneously from the condition. Antiinflammatory agents, ice, muscle relaxants, and injection of lidocaine (with or without corticosteroid) have been used in selected cases. Symptoms typically resolve in 9–12 wk, but may recur. Padding is recommended upon the athlete's return to play.

Sternal Fractures

Sternal stress fractures have been reported in golfers, weight lifters, and wrestlers (43). Isolated sternal fractures from direct impact do not pose significant risk to the athlete. Studies have shown the mortality associated with sternal fractures to be less than 1% (68,69). Sternal fractures are frequently seen in association with deceleration injuries and/or direct blows to the chest.

Injuries to the sternum have traditionally led to a search for associated cardiac, great vessel, and pulmonary injuries caused by the anatomic proximity of these structures. Associated morbidity with these injuries is low. Nevertheless, it is important that one carefully assess the pediatric patient who presents with symptoms of a sternal fracture for other potentially associated injuries. These include pneumothorax and cardiopulmonary stress.

Sternal fractures are often seen on lateral sternal x-rays. Because most of these fractures are oriented transversely, they can be missed with anterior–posterior (AP) radiographs. In cases in which a fracture is questionable, CT scans may be helpful. If intrathoracic trauma is suspected, an EKG and chest x-rays should be ordered.

Scapular Fractures

Scapular fractures represent less than 1% of all skeletal injuries and 5% of shoulder fractures (70,71). Fractures of the scapula are rare in athletes, with the majority of reported cases occurring in football players (70–72). Injuries occur during tackling, when the shoulder is in abduction and the scapula is pulled away from the chest wall and is unable to dissipate direct force.

There are eight types of scapular fractures. They are classified by anatomic location: body, glenoid rim, glenoid fossa, anatomic and surgical neck, acromion, spine, and coracoid process. The majority of scapular fractures are body fractures (73). Approximately 10% of fractures occur in the acromion, coracoid, and spine (73).

A scapular fracture may present with symptoms that are similar to a rotator cuff injury. Cain and Hamilton reported that rotator cuff injuries were initially suspected in half of football players who were diagnosed with scapular fractures (70). Clinical examination reveals weakness to abduction and external rotation of the shoulder. Pain and weakness in the shoulder region is exacerbated with movement. Localized tenderness, swelling, and hematoma formation over the fracture site may also be present.

Scapula fractures are often not seen on standard scapula x-rays (AP, lateral, and axillary views). In one study, 43 out of 100 of scapular fractures were missed on initial radiographs (74). Therefore, CT or MRI may be necessary.

Treatment of scapular fractures is usually conservative and involves rest from sport(s) and physical therapy. The application of ice is recommended for the first 48 h. A sling may also be used for immobilization. Early pendulum exercises, increasing passive range of motion exercises and relative immobilization for 2–4 wk usually allows for complete healing. In severe cases, surgical fixation should be considered.

Abdominal Injuries

Ten percent of all abdominal injuries have been reported to result from sports-related trauma (75). Football (76,77), rugby (78), soccer (79–81), and wrestling (82) are the most common contact sports for abdominal trauma.

TABLE 6.1. Sport-related abdominal trauma.

Intraabdominal pathology	Abdominal wall contusions	Splenic ruptures	Ruptured jejunum	Pancreatic injury	Renal injuries
No. of patients	11	4	1	1	7

(*Source:* Ref. 75. Reprinted with permission from Elsevier.)

Noncontact sports, such as downhill skiing (83–86), water skiing (87), and horseback riding (76,88), result in high-speed deceleration mechanisms and may result in very serious injuries.

A retrospective cohort study of Swedish children by Bergqvist et al. (76,89), involving 348 injuries over 30 yr, revealed 7.1% of abdominal trauma was sport related (Table 6.1). Sports involved were ice hockey (8 cases), skiing (6 cases), soccer (5 cases), pole vaulting (1 case), and gymnastics (1 case).

The same study contrasted recreational cycling with organized sport and found 12% of abdominal trauma in children was related to this pastime. In addition to the pathologies detailed in Table 6.1, there were liver injuries, a mesenteric rupture, muscle lacerations, a stomach rupture, and colon injuries with cycling. Ballham (90) showed that bicycle injuries had a higher injury severity index than other sports. Pediatric bicycle injury data from Puranik (91) of 211 children under 15 yr old revealed 9% had internal organ injuries. The handlebar imprint can sometimes be seen along the upper edge of the abdomen (Figure 6.3) (92). Bicycles (93–95), and other types of sports-related vehicular use may result in the same patterns of abdominal injury that are seen in automobile accidents.

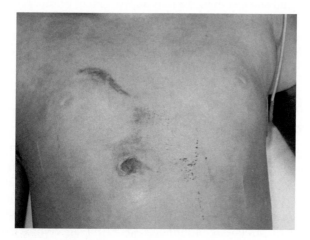

FIGURE 6.3. Duodenal injury from a bicycle fall. Courtesy of David Mooney MD, Children's Hospital, Boston, MA.

Splenic Injury

Injuries to the spleen can result from a direct force to the abdomen, especially the left upper quadrant; from a sudden deceleration when the hilum is torn; or by displacement of lower left rib fractures. Any of these mechanisms are possible in high-speed or contact sports.

The mechanism of splenic injury was explored in a study of downhill skiers (96). In high-velocity or high-impact collisions, e.g. with a tree, a chairlift pole, or a snow fence, multiple trauma was always present (fractures or damage to multiple organs). Skiers were unable to move at the scene and splenectomy resulted in 5 out of 6 cases (83%). With low-velocity or low-impact collisions, often just a single organ was involved. Such injuries resulted from falls on ski trails, on moguls, or on tree stumps or rocks. Presentation in these cases was often delayed for hours while the individual continued skiing. Splenectomy was necessary in 5 of 12 cases (42%).

Machida et al. (97) found a significantly higher abdominal injury rate in snowboarders compared to skiers. Injuries to the kidney, liver, and spleen were seen in both. In snowboarders, riding mistakes after jumping and subsequent falls were responsible for 31.6% of the abdominal traumas. Skiers were more likely to have a collision as the mechanism for their abdominal injury.

Physical exam is neither sensitive nor specific for splenic injury. Therefore, patients with an appropriate mechanism or pain should undergo CT scan. The most important determinant of nonoperative management of splenic rupture is hemodynamic stability, including hematocrit. Nonoperative management of splenic injuries consists of careful hemodynamic monitoring, frequent physical and laboratory examination, and, most importantly, strict bed rest. Given a stable course, a CT scan should be repeated after 5–7 d and should show stabilization or improvement of the injury. Rest and avoidance of contact sports is recommended for up to 4 mo after injury. This is determined largely by the severity of the injury seen on CT and its resolution. Nonoperative splenic management seems to be more successful in children (90%) than in adults (70%) (98).

Epstein-Barr Virus, Infectious Mononucleosis, and Splenomegaly

By age 30, 90% of the population has been exposed to the Epstein-Barr virus, which causes infectious mononucleosis (99). This may frequently be unrecognized, particularly in children. From 1–3% of college students are affected each year (100). The peak incidence is in 15–24 yr-olds.

A recent study using physical exam alone reported splenomegaly in 8% of patients with infectious mononucleosis (101). In comparison, a study utilizing ultrasonography demonstrated that 100% of patients with infectious mononucleosis had an enlarged spleen; physical examination detected the abnormality in less than 20% of the same cases (102). These studies indicate that physical exam alone is an insensitive tool to diagnose splenomegaly in the setting of infectious mononucleosis.

Infectious mononucleosis causes the splenic architecture to become distorted, making the spleen susceptible to rupture from any increased abdominal pressure, even from sneezing or coughing. Splenic rupture in infectious mononucleosis occurs in 0.1–0.2% of cases, with the highest estimate being 0.5% (103). The timing of this complication is predictable, being noted in the first 3 wk of the illness. Splenic rupture is unusual beyond 3 wk from the onset of symptoms (headache, sore throat, and fever). The prodromal period is not considered when determining the onset of the illness.

Splenic rupture is associated with abdominal pain, left shoulder pain (Kehr's sign), or periscapular pain. Left upper quadrant abdominal tenderness may or may not be accompanied by peritoneal signs, such as generalized tenderness, guarding, and rebound tenderness. Indicators of hypovolemia, such as tachycardia and hypotension, are worrisome signs. This complication fortunately is often not fatal. Splenectomy is necessary in some instances, although nonoperative management is often successful (104). Treatment should be individualized. There is no evidence to suggest corticosteroids reduce spleen size or shorten the duration of the illness (105).

The appropriate time to allow an athlete with infectious mononucleosis to resume his or her activity is determined by the duration of symptoms, as well as the presence of splenomegaly and risk of splenic rupture. There is concern that contact trauma may precipitate splenic rupture. In a 1976 survey of college team physicians, the respondents identified 22 cases of splenic rupture. At the time of the trauma, 41% of these were diagnosed with infectious mononucleosis. Seventeen of the student athletes were participating in football (106). Most splenic ruptures in the setting of infectious mononucleosis, however, are spontaneous, not the result of contact.

Return-to-play recommendations in the literature have been varied (107). To protect the enlarged spleen, which should probably be assumed to be present in all cases (105), all strenuous activity should be avoided for the first 21 d. At this point the athlete may start a graded aerobic program, avoiding contact, if the athlete is asymptomatic, afebrile, and does not have a palpable spleen. At 4 wk, if the signs are equivocal or the athlete is at a high risk for collision, an imaging study such as an ultrasound should be considered (108). It should also be noted that normal spleen size has been directly correlated with athlete size; hence, a large athlete with an appropriately sized spleen may be mistakenly diagnosed with splenomegaly if the splenic volume/body mass is not considered (109).

Hepatic Injury

With the evolution of CT scanning, recognition of minor liver injuries has been enhanced. Although the spleen was previously asserted to be the most

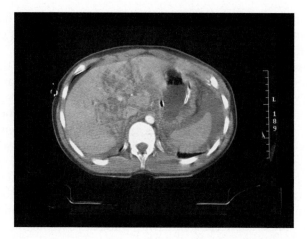

FIGURE 6.4. Hepatic injury. Courtesy of David Mooney MD, Children's Hospital, Boston, MA.

commonly injured intraabdominal organ, the incidence of liver injuries may be similar (110). This is not surprising considering the large size, soft substance, and unprotected position of the liver. Injury can result from a direct blow, especially to the right upper quadrant; a sudden deceleration; or by displacement of right lower rib fractures. Hepatomegaly results in an increased risk of injury, not only because of the increased size, but also because an enlarged liver is softer than normal. Therefore, hepatomegaly is a contraindication to high-speed or contact sports.

The mechanism of injury, especially for lower rib fractures, is much more important than the physical exam to suggest a possible liver injury. Right upper quadrant abdominal tenderness, an abrasion/contusion over the right upper abdomen, right shoulder pain, or hemodynamic instability may be present. A CT scan is warranted with any appropriate mechanism. The typical appearance of a liver laceration is illustrated in Figure 6.4. Unstable patients should have an immediate laparotomy. However, even high-grade injuries can be managed nonoperatively despite an imposing CT appearance, if the patient is hemodynamically stable.

Renal Injury

The kidney is the most commonly injured intraabdominal organ in some sports, such as rugby. Renal injuries may be relatively asymptomatic, even with repeated blows, such as in boxers, or they may result in renal contusions causing microscopic or gross hematuria. Occult hematuria without radiographic evidence of injury is extremely common in several sports. It is present in 25% of boxers (111), college football players (112), and dis-

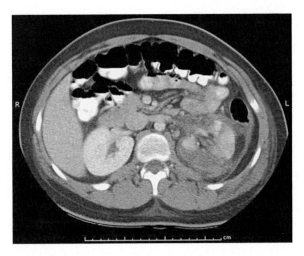

FIGURE 6.5. Left kidney injury. Courtesy of David Mooney MD, Children's Hospital, Boston, MA.

tance runners (113). Kidney trauma from a direct blow is particularly common in football and rugby. 25% of renal injuries and 40% of renal pedicle injuries do not demonstrate hematuria (114). An injury to the kidney is shown by CT in Figure 6.5.

Gross hematuria should be evaluated in the hospital. Nonoperative management is appropriate as long as the athlete is not in shock, there is no expanding hematoma, and no free extravasation of urine by intravenous contrast CT. Complete healing is essential before return to sports. Most renal injuries heal within 6–8 wk. Microscopic hematuria may persist for 3–4 wk after injury.

Younger patients require special attention, as renal injury is more common than splenic or hepatic injury. Up to 30% of renal trauma in children is related to sport. This may be caused by a proportionally larger kidney size or a lack of musculoskeletal protection (5).

Pancreas

The pancreas is injured in 1–2% of abdominal trauma. A forceful blow to the upper abdomen is the most common mechanism of injury (78,81). For instance, a bicycle fall where the handlebar twists and "spears" the child may be the presenting history (1,92). As with other internal organs, there are often minimal physical signs. Patients can develop nausea, vomiting, and abdominal pain up to 48 h later. Typically, the pain radiates to the back. CT is the most useful imaging modality.

Bowel Injury

Bowel injury is infrequent and most commonly occurs as a result of a forceful blow to a small area over the small intestine. Physical findings may be limited. An erect chest x-ray may reveal air beneath the diaphragm, although CT is the most sensitive diagnostic imaging.

Groin Pain and Injuries

This is one of the more difficult problems to diagnose in athletes, especially if chronic. Soccer, hockey, hurdling, and skiing are sports where groin injuries are especially common (115). The etiology is most commonly soft tissue injury, contusion or hematoma, and muscle–tendon strain. However, consideration of inguinal hernia, bursitis, and nerve entrapment is warranted.

Additionally, there is evidence evolving in the literature regarding the sportsman's hernia (116). This is a tear in the transversalis fascia in the posterior inguinal floor that Hackney (117) describes as an "incipient direct inguinal hernia." The mechanism of injury is aggressive abduction in specific athletic situations, such as cutting maneuvers. Sportsman's hernias are particularly common in sports such as soccer and hockey, where athletes frequently change direction at high speed (117–119). The sportsman's hernia is resistant to conservative therapy and will recur after a period of rest. The key physical exam finding is tenderness at the pubic tubercle. This injury does not show up on imaging. Surgical repair of the inguinal floor will return approximately 90% of patients to full activity without pain (116).

Prevention

Thoracoabdominal trauma is uncommon in pediatric athletes. Certain injuries may be preventable. Sport-specific safety equipment should be worn to minimize the risk of injury. For instance, chest barriers and safety balls in baseball have decreased the risk of commotio cordis (18). An automated external defibrillator (AED) should be present at venues.

Conditioning is also important. Appropriate core strength, including the entire trunk, will maximize protection in contact sports and minimize overuse stress in noncontact sports. Attention to proper sports technique, can also minimize the possibility of overuse.

Return to Play Guidelines

Onsite return to play decisions should be based on pain resolution, unless a minor abdominal wall injury is considered likely. Vital signs should be normal and peritoneal signs absent. Further, players should be able to exercise without an increase in symptoms.

Athletes who have sustained a solid organ contusion require a normal CT scan 2–3 wk before being allowed to return to practice. Lacerations and subcapsular hematomas require longer periods of recovery because of the greater architectural damage sustained; hence, a prolonged period of healing is necessary. If an organ has to be removed, full tissue postoperative healing takes 6–24 wk. Strenuous activity should therefore be postponed for 6–8 wk and contact sports for 12–24 wk, although advice varies by surgeon.

Rib injuries should be considered on a case-by-case basis, but return to sport is usually possible in 4–8 wk. Tullos and Erwin described a baseball pitcher who was asymptomatic with a first rib injury at 3 wk and was able to return to pitching with a pain-free nonunion (42). The athlete with a sternal fracture can return to play when he/she can compete in a pain-free manner. If the patient engages in contact sports a flank jacket or other similar device can be used to protect the injury.

Clinical Pearls

- It is essential, when assessing an athlete who has sustained trauma to the thorax or abdomen, to maintain a high level of suspicion for internal injury.
- There may be no external sign initially, and serial physical examinations are crucial.
- If a significant injury is suspected, the athlete should be transferred to a setting where CT imaging and advanced medical care is available.
- Rib fractures may be traumatic from direct impact or secondary to acute muscle contraction. They may also occur as a stress injury.
- Fractures of the first 4 ribs or the last 2 ribs, multiple fractures, and flail segments may result in injury to surrounding structures.
- Scapular fractures are unusual in sports and are often missed initially.

References

1. Diamond DL. Sports-related abdominal trauma. Clin Sports Med 1989;8(1): 91–99.
2. Gray H. Anatomy of the Human Body. Philadelphia: Lea & Febiger; 1918: 1396.
3. Roberts WO. GI trauma in sports. ACSM Team Physician Course Lecture, 2002.
4. Roberts JA. Viral illnesses and sports performance. Sports Med 1986;3(4): 296–303.
5. Sievers EM, Murray JA, Chen D, Velmahos GC, Demetriades D, Berne TV. Abdominal computed tomography scan in pediatric blunt abdominal trauma. Am Surg 1999;65(10):968–971.

6. Amaral JF. Thoracoabdominal injuries in the athlete. Clin Sports Med 1997; 16(4):739–753.

7. Bliss D, Silen M. Pediatric thoracic trauma. Crit Care Med 2002;30(11); S409–S415.

8. Machida T, Hanazaki K, Ishizaka K, et al. Snowboarding injuries to the chest: Comparison with skiing injuries. J Trauma Inj Infect Crit Care 1999;46:1062–1065.

9. Richardson JD, Miller FB. Injury to the lung and pleura. In Feliciano DV, Moore EE, Mattox KL, eds. Trauma. 3rd ed. Stamford, CT: Appleton & Lange; 1996:387–407.

10. Nakayama DK, Rammenofsky ML, Rowe MI. Chest injuries in children. Ann Surg 1989;210:770–775.

11. Sadat-Ali M, Al-Arfaj AL, Mohanna M. Pneumothorax due to soccer injury [letter]. Br J Sports Med 1986;20(2):91.

12. Simoneaux SF, Murphy BJ, Tehranzadeh J. Spontaneous pneumothorax in a weight lifter: a case report. Am J Sports Med 1990;18(6):647–648.

13. Volk CP, McFarland EG, Horsmon G. Pneumothorax: on-field recognition. Phys Sportsmed 1995;23(10):43–46.

14. Partridge RA, Coley A, Bowie R, Woolard RH. Sports-related pneumothorax. Ann Emerg Med 1997;30(4):539–541.

15. Erickson S, Rich B. Pulmonary and chest wall emergencies. Phys Sportsmed 1995 23:95–104.

16. Wagner RB, Crawford WO, Schimpf PP, Jamieson PM, Rao KC. Quantitation and pattern of parenchymal lung injury in blunt chest trauma: Diagnostic and therapeutic implications. J Comput Tomogr 1988;12:270–281.

17. Bonadio WA, Hellmich T. Post-traumatic pulmonary contusion in children. Ann Emerg Med 1989;18:1050–1052.

18. Maron BJ, Poliac L, Kaplan JA, Mueller FO. Blunt impact to the chest leading to sudden death from cardiac arrest during sports activities. N Engl J Med 1995;333:337–342.

19. Curfman GD. Fatal impact: concussion of the heart [editorial]. N Engl J Med 1998;338:1841–1843.

20. Estes NAM, III. Sudden death in young athletes [editorial]. N Engl J Med 1995;333:380–381.

21. Abrunzo TJ. Commotio cordis: the single, most common cause of traumatic death in youth baseball. AJDC 1991;145:1279–1282.

22. Kaplan JA, Karofsky PS, Volturo GA. Commotio cordis in two amateur ice hockey players despite the use of commercial chest protectors: case reports. J Trauma 1993;34:151–153.

23. Link MS, Maron BJ, VanderBrink BA, et al. Impact directly over the cardiac silhouette is necessary to produce ventricular fibrillation in an experimental model of commotio cordis. J Am Coll Cardiol 2001;37:649–654.

24. Link MS, Wang PJ, Pandian NG, et al. An experimental model of sudden death due to low-energy chest-wall impact (commotio cordis). N Engl J Med 1998;338:1805–1811.

25. Link MS, Wang PJ, VanderBrink BA, et al. Selective activation of the K_{ATP}^{+} channel is a mechanism by which sudden death is produced by low energy chest-wall impact (commotio cordis). Circulation 1999;100:413–418.

26. Link MS, Maron BJ, Wang PJ, VanderBrink BA, Zhu W, Estes NAM, III. Upper and lower energy limits of vulnerability to sudden death with chest wall impact (commotio cordis) J Am Coll Cardiol 2003;41(1):99–104.
27. Ivatury RR. Injury to the heart. In: Feliciano DV, Moore EE, Mattox KL, eds. Trauma. 3rd ed. Stamford, CT: Appleton & Lange; 1996:409–440.
28. Chang CJ, Graves DW. Athletic injuries of the thorax and abdomen. In: Mellion MB, Walsh MW, Madden C, et al. Team Physicians Handbook. 3rd ed. Philadelphia: Hanley & Belfus; 2001:441–458.
29. Miles JW, Barrett GR. Rib fractures in athletes. Sports Med 1991;12(1): 66–69.
30. Kirsch MM. Injuries to the chest wall. In: Blunt Chest Trauma. Boston, MA: Little, Brown, and Company; 1977.
31. Cogbill TH, Landercasper J. Injury to the chest wall. In: Feliciano DV, Moore EE, Mattox KL, eds. Trauma. 3rd ed. Stamford, CT: Appleton & Lange; 1996:525–550.
32. Bailey P. Surfer's rib: isolated first rib fracture secondary to indirect trauma. Ann Emerg Med 1985;141:346–349.
33. Brooke, R. Jive fracture of the first rib. J Bone Joint Surg 1959;41B: 370–371.
34. Gurler R, Pavlov H, Torg JS. Stress fracture of the ipsilateral first rib in a pitcher. 1985;13:277–279.
35. Lankenner PA Jr, Micheli LJ. Stress fracture of the first rib. A case report. J Bone Joint Surg Am 1985;67(1):159–160.
36. Pereira J. Stress fracture of a rib. Br J Sports Med 1985;(1):26.
37. Saccherti AD, Beswick DR, Morse SD. Rebound rib: stress induced first rib fractures. Ann Emerg Med 1983;12:177–179.
38. Albers JE, Rath RK, Glaser RS, Poddar PK. Severity of intrathoracic injuries associated with first rib fractures. Ann Thorac Surg 1982;33(6): 614–618.
39. Blichert-Toft M. Fatigue fracture of the first rib. Acta Chir Scand 1969; 135:675–678.
40. Breslin FJ. Fractures of the first rib unassociated with fractures of other ribs. Am J Surg 1937;35:384–389.
41. Lorentzen Je, Movin M. Fracture of the first rib. Acta Orthopaedica Scanda 1976;47:632–634.
42. Tullos HS, Erwin WD, Woods GW, et al. Unusual lesions of the pitching arm. Clin Orthop 1972;88:169–182.
43. Gregory PL, Biswas AC, Batt ME. Musculoskeletal problems of the chest wall in athletes. Sports Med 2002;32(4):235–250.
44. Colosimo AJ, Byrne E, Heidt RS Jr, Carlonas RL, Wyatt H. Acute traumatic first-rib fracture in the contact athlete: a case report. Am J Sports Med. 2004;32(5):1310–1312. Epub 2004 May 18.
45. Jenkins SA. Spontaneous fractures of both first ribs. J Bone Joint Surg 1952; 34B:9–13.
46. Lorentzen JE, Movin M. Fracture of the first rib. Acta Orthop Scand 1976;47(6): 632–634.
47. Aitken AP, Lincoln RE. Fracture of the first rib due to muscle pull. N Engl J Med 1939;220:1063–1064.

48. Brooke R. Jive Fracture of the first rib. J Bone Joint Surg Br 1959; 41B:370–371.
49. Leung HY, Stirling AJ. Stress fracture of the first rib without associated injuries. Injury 1991;22(6):483–484.
50. Bailey P. Surfer's rib: isolated first rib fracture secondary to indirect trauma. Ann Emerg Med 1985;14(4):346–349.
51. Sinha AK, Kaeding CC, Wadley GM. Upper extremity stress fractures in athletes: clinical features of 44 cases. Clin J Sports Med 1999;9(4):199–202.
52. Holden DL, Jackson DW. Stress fracture of the ribs in female rowers. Am J Sports Med 1985;13(5):342–348.
53. Lin HC, Chou CS, Hsu TC. Stress fractures of the ribs in amateur golf players. Zhonghua Yi Xue Za Zhi (Taipei). 1994;54(1):33–37.
54. Karlson KA. Rib stress fractures in elite rowers. A case series and proposed mechanism. Am J Sports Med 1998;26(4):516–519.
55. Christensen E, Kanstrup IL. Increased risk of stress fractures in the ribs of elite rowers. Scand J Med Sci Sports 1997;7(1):49–52.
56. Gaffney KM. Avulsion injury of the serratus anterior: a case history. Clin J Sports Med 1997;7(2):134–136.
57. Lord MJ, Ha KI, Song KS. Stress fractures of the ribs in golfers. Am J Sports Med 1996;24(1):118–122.
58. Gurtler R, Pavlov H, Torg JS. Stress fracture of the ipsilateral first rib in a pitcher. Am J Sports Med 1985;13(4):277–279.
59. Proffer DS, Patton JJ, Jackson DW. Nonunion of a first rib fracture in a gymnast. Am J Sports Med 1991;19(2):198–201.
60. Scott EM, Scott BB. Painful rib syndrome: A review of 76 cases. Gut 1993;34(7):1006–1008.
61. Wright JT. Clicking rib. Lancet 1973 I: (7809):935.
62. Parry W, Breckenridege I, Khalil YF. Bilateral clicking ribs. Thorax 1989; 44(1):72–73.
63. Heinz GJ, Zavala DC. Slipping rib syndrome. JAMA 1977;237(8):794–795.
64. Eastwood NB. Slipping-rib syndrome. Lancet 1980;1898:219–220.
65. Spence EK, Rosato EF. The slipping rib syndrome. Arch Surg 1983;118(11): 1330–1332.
66. Arroyo JF, Vine R, Reynaud C, Michel JP. Slipping rib syndrome: don't be fooled. Geriatrics 1995;50(3):46–49.
67. Selbst SM. Chest pain in children. Am Fam Physician. 1990;41(1):179–186.
68. Potaris K, Gakidis J, Mihos P, et al. Management of sternal fractures: 239 cases. Asian Cardiovasc Thorac Ann 2002;10:145–149.
69. Athanassiadi K, Gerazounis M, Moustardas M, Metaxas E. Sternal fractures: Retrospective analysis of 100 cases. World J Surg 2002;(10):1243–1246.
70. Cain TE, Hamilton WP. Scapular fractures in professional football players. Am J Sports Med 1992;20(3):363–365.
71. McBryde JP. Scapular fracture in a high school football player. Phys Sportsmed 1997;25(10):64–68.
72. Brown MA, Sikka RS, Cuanche CA, Fischer DA. Bilateral fractures of the scapula in a professional football player. Am J Sports Med 2004;32: 237–242.
73. Miller M, Ada J. Injuries to the shoulder girdle. Skeletal Trauma. 1992;2:1291–1301.

74. Harris RD, Harris JH Jr. The prevalence and significance of missed scapular fractures in blunt chest trauma. AM J Roentgenol 1988;151(4):747–750.
75. Bergqvist D, Hedelin H, Karlsson G, Lindblad B, Matzsch T. Abdominal trauma during thirty yrs: Analysis of a large case series. Injury 1981;13:93–99.
76. Bergqvist D, Hedelin H, Karlsson G, Lindblad B, and Matzsch T. Abdominal injury from sporting activities. Br J Sports Med 1982;16:76–79.
77. Murphy CP, Drez D. Jejunal rupture in a football player. Am J Sports Med 1987;15:184–185.
78. Harrison JD, Branicki FJ, Makin GS. Pancreatic injury in association football. Injury 1985;16:232.
79. Johnson WR, Harris P. Isolated gallbladder injury secondary to blunt abdominal trauma: Case report. Aust NZ J Surg 1982;52:495–496.
80. Maehlum S, Daljord OA. Football injuries in Oslo: A one year study. Br J Sports Med 1986;18:186–190.
81. Speakman M, Reece-Smith H. Gastric and pancreatic rupture due to a sports injury [letter]. Br J Surg 1983;70:190.
82. Wilton P, Fulco J, O'Leary J, Lee JT. Body slam in no sham. N Engl J Med 1985;313:188–189.
83. Blankstein A, Salai M, Israeli A, Ganel A, Horoszowski H, Farine I. Ski injuries in 1976–1982: Ybrig region, Switzerland. Int J Sports Med 1985;6:298–300.
84. Hildreth TA, Cass AS, Khan AU. Skiing injuries to the urinary tract. Minn Med 1979;62:155–156.
85. Jurkovich GJ, Pearce JH, Cleveland HC. Thoracic and abdominal injuries in skiers: The role of air evacuation. J Trauma 1983;23:844–848.
86. Scharplatz D, Thurleman K, Enderlin P. Thoracoabdominal trauma in ski accidents. Injury 1979;10:86–91.
87. Kleiman AH. Renal trauma in sports. West J Surg Obstet Gynecol 1961;69:331–340.
88. Pounder DJ. "The grave yawns for the horseman." Equestrian deaths in South Australia 1973–1983. Med J Aust 1984;141:632–635.
89. Bergqvist D, Hedelin H, Lindblad B, and Matzsch T. Abdominal injuries in children: an analysis of 348 cases. Injury 1985;16(4):217–220.
90. Ballham A, Absoud EM, Kotecha MB, Bodiwala GG. A study of bicycle accidents. Injury 1985;16(6):405–408.
91. Puranik S, Long J, Coffman S. Profile of pediatric bicycle injuries. S Med Journal 1998;91(11):1033–1037.
92. Erez I, Lazar L, Gutermacher M, and Katz S. Abdominal injuries caused by bicycle handlebars. Eur J Surg 2001;167(5):331–333.
93. Friede AM, Azzara CV, Gallagher SS, Guyer B. The epidemiology of injuries to bicycle riders. Pediatr Clin North Am 1985;32:141–151.
94. Kiburz D, Jacobs R, Reckling F. Bicycling accidents and injuries among adult cyclists. Am J Sports Med 1986;14:416–419.
95. Sparnon AL, Ford WDA. Bicycle handlebar injuries in children. J Pediatr Surg 1986;21:118–119.
96. Sartorelli KH, Pilcher DB, Rogers FB. Patterns of splenic injuries seen in skiers. Injury 1995;26(1):43–46.
97. Machida T, Hanazaki K, Ishizaka K, et al. Snowboarding injuries of the abdomen: comparison with skiing injuries. Injury 1999;30(1):47–49.

98. Esposito JT, Gamelli RL. Injury to the spleen. In Feliciano DV, Moore EE, Mattox KL, eds. Trauma. 3 ed. Stamford, CT; Appleton & Lange; 1996:525–550.

99. Kaye KM, Kieff E. Epstein-Barr virus infection and infectious mononucleosis. In: Gorbach SL, Bartlett JG, Blacklow NR, eds. Infectious Diseases. Philadelphia: W.B.Saunders; 1992:1646–1654.

100. Brodsky AL, Heath CW Jr. Infectious mononucleosis epidemiological patterns at United States colleges and universities. Am J Epidemiol 1972;96:87–93.

101. Rea TD, Russo JE, Katon W, Ashley RL, Buchwald DS. Prospective study of the natural history of infectious mononucleosis caused by Epstein-Barr virus. J Am Board Fam Pract 2001;14:234–242.

102. Dommerby H, Stangerup SE, Stangerup M, Hancke S. Hepatosplenomegaly in infectious mononucleosis, assessed by ultrasonic scanning. J Laryngol Otol 1986;100:573–579.

103. Maki DG, Reich RM. Infectious mononucleosis in the athlete: diagnosis, complications, and management. Am J Sports Med 1982;10:162–173.

104. Askari MM, Begos DG. Spontaneous splenic rupture in infectious mononucleosis: a review. Yale J Biol Med 1997;70:175–182.

105. Kinderknecht JJ. Infectious mononucleosis and the spleen. Curr Sports Med Rep 2002;1:116–120.

106. Frelinger DP. The ruptured spleen in college athletes: a preliminary report. J Am Coll Health Assoc 1978;26:217.

107. Burroughs KE. Athletes resuming activity after infectious mononucleosis. Arch Fam Med 2000;9:1122–1123.

108. Waninger KN, Harcke HT. Determination of safe return to play for athletes recovering from infectious mononucleosis. A literature review. Clin J Sport Med 2005;15(6):410–416.

109. Spielmann AL, DeLong DM, Kliewer MA. Sonographic Evaluation of Spleen size in tall healthy athletes. Am J Roentgenol 2005;184:45–49.

110. Pachter HL, Liang HG, Hofstetter SR. Liver and biliary tract trauma. In: Feliciano DV, Moore EE, Mattox KL, eds. Trauma. 3rd ed. Stamford, CT: Appleton & Lange; 1996:487–523.

111. Kleiman AH. Renal trauma in sports. West J Surg Obstet Gynecol 1961;69:331–340.

112. Boone AW, Haltiwanger E, Chambers RL. Football hematuria. JAMA 1955;158:1516–1517.

113. Alyea EP, Parish HH. Renal response to exercise. JAMA 1958;167:807–813.

114. Peterson NE. Genitourinary trauma. In: Feliciano DV, Moore EE, Mattox KL, eds. Trauma. 3rd ed. Stamford, CT: Appleton & Lange; 1996:661–693.

115. Renstrom PA. Tendon and muscle injuries in the groin area. Clin Sports Med 1992;20:640–643.

116. Joesting DR. Diagnosis and treatment of sportsman's hernia. Curr Sports Med Rep 2002;1(2):121–124.

117. Hackney RG. The sports hernia: a cause of groin pain. Br J Sports Med 1993;27:58–62.

118. Gilmore OJ. Gilmore's groin. Sportsmed Soft Tissue Trauma 1992;3:12–14

119. Fricker PA. Management of groin pain in athletes. Br J Sports Med 1997;31:97–101.

7
Adolescent Shoulder Injuries

John A. Guido, Jr., and Treg Brown

Injury to the adolescent shoulder poses a unique challenge to the sports medicine team. To determine best practice patterns, the team must utilize an evidenced-based approach. These young athletes sustain injuries caused by both acute, traumatic events and chronic overuse patterns. These injuries affect both osseous and soft-tissue structures. Some of the injuries encountered are unique to this age group.

With growing numbers of adolescents participating in sports and increasing pressure to perform, shoulder injuries in this young age group have steadily risen. Acute injuries resulting from a fall or collision are seen in all sports, but are particularly prevalent in collision, contact, and extreme sports, such as football, hockey, gymnastics, and skateboarding. Year-round competition and sports-specific training have further contributed to the rise in overuse injuries seen in this young patient population. Participation in sports such as baseball, softball, tennis, and swimming create potential repetitive overuse injuries of the shoulder. Forty to eighty percent of swimmers and 50–95% of baseball players demonstrate signs and symptoms of shoulder dysfunction (1). The incidence of shoulder pain in youth baseball pitchers has a frequency of 32%, and nearly one third of 298 pitchers reported shoulder symptoms over the course of two seasons (2).

The current body of scientific literature regarding the athletic adolescent shoulder is limited. Therefore, extrapolation of research findings on the adult overhead athlete will be necessary. As physicians continue to improve and refine the diagnosis and surgical intervention for the athletic shoulder, physical therapists and athletic trainers have been challenged to develop creative rehabilitation programs to care for these athletes. Understanding the epidemiology, functional anatomy, basic science, normal and abnormal biomechanics, pathophysiology, and a variety of therapeutic approaches are vital to achieving success when working with the adolescent athletic shoulder.

Functional Anatomy

Adolescent athletes are faced with a triumvirate of predisposing factors for shoulder injury. Open physeal plates, joint laxity, and underdeveloped musculature are three unique aspects of the developing body (3). When combined with trauma or the stresses of overhead activity, these factors can result in a host of shoulder injuries unique to the skeletally immature athlete. To better recognize these injuries, an understanding of normal development is paramount. As embryologic development ends, shoulder anatomy progresses such that the shoulder is fully developed and the structures are identical to the adult shoulder. Skeletal maturation may continue well into the second decade of life, and it is during this time that the stress of overhead activity will remodel the humerus. Ossification of the humeral head is accomplished by three centers: one for the humeral head and one for each tuberosity (4). This area accounts for approximately 80% of the growth of the upper extremity. The epiphyseal plates at these sites are weaker than the surrounding ligaments, so adolescents are more likely to sustain avulsion fractures when more mature athletes would sustain tendon or ligament injuries (5). Normal skeletal development continues through adolescence, culminating in proximal humeral physeal closure in girls by 14–16 yr of age and in boys by 16–21 yr of age.

As development occurs, the type III collagen is progressively converted to the more stable and "soluble" type I collagen found in adults. The increased level of type III collagen in the young athlete explains why young people with shoulder instability are more prone to recurrent instability compared with older people (6). The developing shoulder also undergoes considerable adaptation from the stress of sports. As the shoulder continues to develop, the head is inclined and retroverted relative to the shaft. Osseous and soft tissue changes have been shown to occur both radiographically and by simple range of motion comparisons of the dominant and nondominant shoulders. The normal angle of humeral retroversion in the adult population varies markedly, but has been found to be increased in the dominant shoulder of baseball pitchers (7–10). This variability should be kept in mind when evaluating the young overhead athlete.

The superior biceps–labrum complex is a structure of significant importance to the overhead athlete. The superior portion of the labrum inserts directly onto the biceps tendon, and the biceps tendon inserts on the supraglenoid tubercle (11). Huber and Putz describe the superior and inferior portions of the labrum and the surrounding glenohumeral ligaments and tendons as a periarticular fiber system (PAFS), forming a basket of fibers around the neck of the scapula and constituting a functional unit (Figure 7.1) (12). Morphologically, the fibers of the upper portion of the PAFS are indistinguishable from those of tendons (10). Clinically, tendons are designed to handle tensile forces. Therefore, the superior portion of the PAFS may be adapted to handle the tensile forces of deceleration as

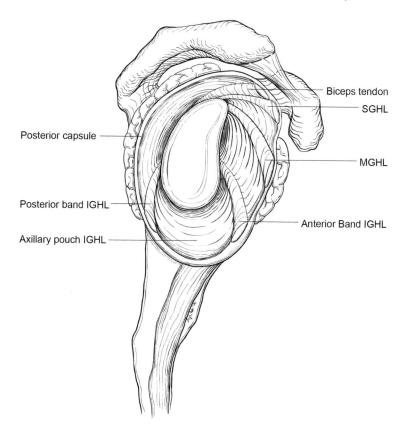

Biceps tendon

SGHL

Posterior capsule

MGHL

Posterior band IGHL

Anterior Band IGHL

Axillary pouch IGHL

FIGURE 7.1. Schematic of glenoid fossa, labrum, biceps tendon, and glenohumeral ligaments.

opposed to the shear stress that occurs in maximum external rotation (over-head sports).

The shoulder joint capsule, in combination with the labrum, reinforces the glenohumeral joint. The shoulder capsule has three primary bands or thickenings, termed the glenohumeral ligaments (superior, middle, and inferior). These "tissues" and the glenohumeral ligaments in particular, provide static stability to the glenohumeral joint, allowing it to reach extreme angles of mobility, while preventing subluxation or dislocation. The inferior glenohumeral ligament (IGHL) supports the humeral head much like a hammock, with the bands reciprocally tightening as the humeral head is rotated in the abducted position (13). It is the primary restraint to AP translation in the abducted, externally rotated position (13,14). The superior glenohumeral ligament and rotator interval provide stability against inferior and posterior forces with the arm adducted. AP translation is restricted by the middle glenohumeral ligament in the abducted arm. The posterior capsule limits posterior translation when the arm is forward flexed, internally rotated, and adducted. Joint concavity provided by the glenoid socket and accentuated by the labrum provides further stability.

The rotator cuff is the "workhorse" of the shoulder. As in the adult, the adolescent rotator cuff has three main functions: glenohumeral stabilization, rotation of the humerus, and assisting with elevation of the upper extremity. The rotator cuff consists of the subcapularis, supraspinatus, infraspinatus, and teres minor muscles and their tendons. The subscapularis inserts onto the lesser tuberosity, whereas the remaining tendons insert onto the greater tuberosity. Optimal performance of these dynamic stabilizers requires proper functioning of the deltoid and periscapular stabilizers (trapezius, levator scapulae, serratus anterior, and rhomboids).

Clinical Evaluation

History

A thorough history and physical exam is critical to effectively diagnose shoulder injuries. A physician must take a detailed history from the athlete regarding the events surrounding the injury, whether traumatic or atraumatic. This should include, but is not limited to, the following: date of onset of symptoms; the mechanism of injury; the location of the pain; the presence of any mechanical or instability symptoms; previous injuries or surgeries; and previous and immediate management of the injury. Questions pertinent to the overhead athlete include: practice and competition level, number of repetitions, and where in the "overhead motion" pain occurs.

Physical Examination

Physical examination consists of observation, range of motion, strength, palpation, and special tests, which should confirm the working hypothesis determined from the history. Exposure of the entire shoulder region is mandatory. The shoulder and periscapular region should be inspected and compared to the contralateral shoulder for any signs of asymmetry, atrophy, discoloration, or deformity. Palpation of key bony and soft tissue structures should be performed in a systematic fashion. These structures should include the sternoclavicular (SC) and acromioclavicular (AC) joints, clavicle, acromion, scapula, greater tuberosity, deltoid, and proximal bicep tendon.

Range of Motion

Range of motion should be assessed in all planes, and any deficits or painful arcs-of-motion should be noted. Both active and passive ranges of motion should be evaluated. The supine position will better enable the clinician to stabilize the scapula, and thereby better assess true glenohumeral motion. The examination may be modified to a sport-specific injury if the history warrants. External and internal rotation measurements have been utilized as an indirect measure of the status of a thrower's shoulder (Figure 7.2). Meister et al. examined the differences in range of motion in an adolescent male baseball population (8–16 yr of age) to determine developmental changes (15). Range of motion differed significantly between the 8-yr-old and 16-yr-old groups. Differences between the dominant and nondominant shoulders grew larger as the age of the group increased. Interestingly, total shoulder motion decreased as the athletes aged, indicating decreased soft tissue laxity. Differences in range of motion in the throwing shoulder occur with differing levels of competition (Table 7.1). Werner et al. documented similar, but increased, shoulder ranges of motion in adolescent windmill softball pitchers (16). This was felt to be caused by the increased generalized ligamentous laxity found in females.

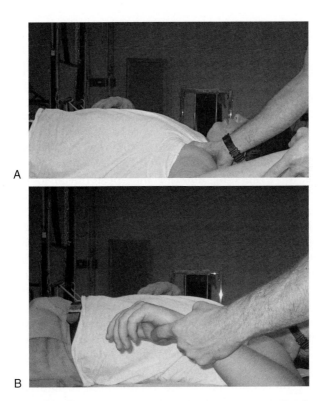

FIGURE 7.2. **(A)** Passive external rotation range of motion of the glenohumeral joint in the supine position with scapular stabilization. **(B)** Passive internal rotation range of motion of the glenohumeral joint in the supine position with scapular stabilization.

TABLE 7.1. Comparison of external and internal rotation range of motion in three levels of baseball competition.

Level	Passive ER/IR	Max ER°
Pro	121–137°/62°	184°
College	107–160°/48°	158°
Youth	120–148°/44°	163°

Maximum external rotation data from our lab during the actual pitching motion.

Strength Testing

Strength testing should be performed with the athlete seated facing the examiner. Resistance is then provided to assess supraspinatus strength (thumb down abduction in the plane of the scapula), infraspinatus (external rotation with the arm adducted), and deltoid (abduction with the arm at the side). Grade of strength and any associated pain with these tests should be noted.

Special Tests

A thorough ligamentous stability examination will often require examining the patient in the supine position if any guarding or apprehension is present. Several "special" tests are utilized to discern the presence of any instability. Anterior instability is by far the most frequent type of instability pattern encountered, and it may easily be assessed performing a standard apprehension relocation maneuver (Figure 7.3). This is a useful test and easily mastered in a brief period. The load and shift maneuver is also useful for evaluating anterior and posterior instability patterns (Figure 7.4). This exam requires complete relaxation of the patient and the findings should always be compared to the contralateral shoulder. A useful grading system for this examination is as follows: grade 0 = no translation, grade 1 = translation up to the glenoid rim, grade 2 = translation onto the rim (subluxation), grade 3 = translation over the rim (dislocation). The O'Brien's test has been described as a useful adjunct in the diagnosis of superior labral (SLAP) injuries that are often found in conjunction with a variety of instability patterns (Figure 7.5). Unfortunately, false positives are common, often representing the presence of an AC injury, bicep tendinitis, or posterior instability. The sulcus test may be performed either seated or supine and, again, requires complete relaxation of the patient (Figure 7.6). This test evaluates for the presence of inferior laxity and rotator interval injuries. The exam should be performed with the arm in the neutral position and repeated in full external rotation (ER). If the sulcus sign remains positive with the arm in full external rotation of the glenohumeral joint, a rotator interval injury should be suspected; however, bilateral sulcus signs are

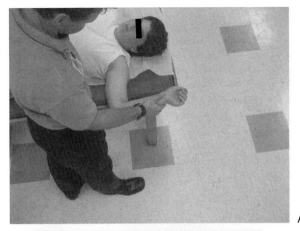

A

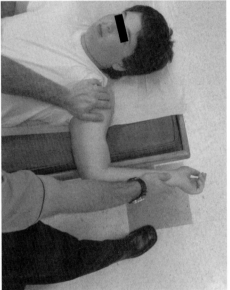

B

FIGURE 7.3. **(A)** Anterior apprehension test for anterior instability. Patient's gleno-humeral joint is passively moved into external rotation until guarding is demon-strated (+) or capsular end feel is reached (−). **(B)** Relocation test for anterior instability. After a (+) apprehension test, a posteriorly directed force is applied to center the humeral head in the glenoid fossa, and apprehension disappears with a concomitant increase in passive external rotation range of motion.

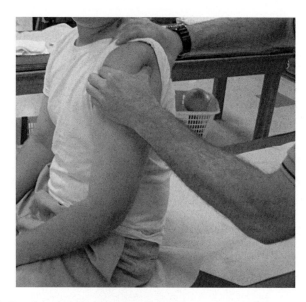

FIGURE 7.4. Load and shift maneuver is also useful for evaluating anterior and posterior instability patterns. Gentle force is applied to the humeral head to center it on the glenoid fossa, and an anteriorly or posteriorly directed force is applied to determine instability.

often indicators of generalized ligamentous laxity. All patients suspected of having generalized laxity should be inspected for hyperextension of the elbows and metacarpal-phalangeal joints, and hyper-flexion of the first carpometacarpal/wrist joint.

Impingement tests are performed to evaluate the rotator cuff and sub-acromial bursae. These tests are performed with the athlete seated. The classic Neer impingement sign and Hawkins sign are good indicators of subacromial inflammation, and they should be correlated with appropriate strength testing to better evaluate for rotator cuff pathology. An "impingement test" (subacromial injection of local anesthetic) may be performed when there is a question regarding the source of the patient's pain. Intraarticular injuries (biceps and capsulolabral injuries) will not be relieved with a subacromial injection.

The AC and SC joints should be palpated, and areas of tenderness should be noted. If an AC injury is suspected, a painful cross-arm adduction maneuver will help confirm pathology at this site. If an injury to this area remains in question, pain relief after a selective injection of local anesthetic into the AC joint may confirm the diagnosis.

Scapulothoracic Region

The scapulothoracic region should also be closely inspected. Injuries to this area are particularly prevalent in the overhead athlete. Winging and

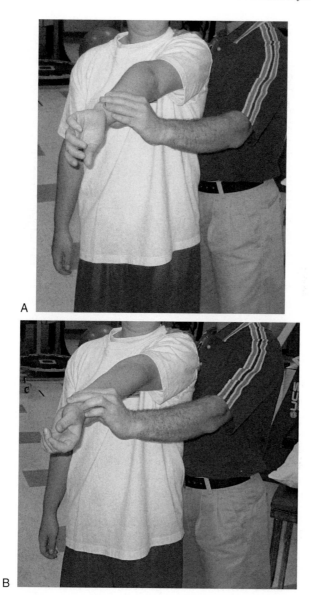

FIGURE 7.5. **(A and B)** The O'Brien's test has been described as a useful adjunct in the diagnosis of superior labral (SLAP) injuries that are often found in conjunction with a variety of instability patterns.

scapular dyskinesia should be sought. Unfortunately, direct observation of scapula position and orientation has proven elusive in the overhead athletic population. Myers et al., studying an adult population, demonstrated significantly increased upward rotation, internal rotation (IR), and retraction

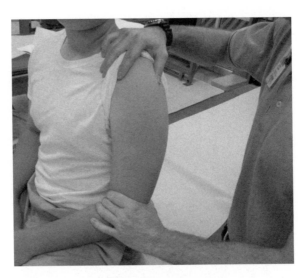

FIGURE 7.6. The sulcus test, used to determine multidirectional instability, may be performed either seated or supine and, again, requires complete relaxation of the patient.

of the scapula during humeral elevation (17). They concluded that throwing athletes have a different resting scapular position and orientation than their nonthrowing counterparts. At what point during development these adaptive changes occurs has not been determined. However, it is important to note that differing scapular positions between dominant and nondominant shoulders in the overhead adolescent athlete may be a normal adaptation. These changes should be distinguished from Sprengel's deformity, a rare congenital malformation of the scapula.

Diagnostic Imaging

The physical examination may warrant further evaluation with routine radiographs, computed tomography (CT) scan, bone scan, or magnetic resonance imaging (MRI). Although arthroscopy remains the "gold standard" for diagnosing rotator cuff and labral injuries, MRI has become increasingly useful in the detection of these injuries. An initial report of 95% accuracy in the detection of labral injuries using MRI has not been duplicated by other studies (18,19). Arthrography using MRI is currently the recommended diagnostic study of choice for imaging SLAP lesions. MRI without contrast can be useful for detecting suspected rotator cuff tears; however, the physician should be aware of recent studies showing apparent partial- and full-thickness rotator cuff tears and labral injuries in asymptomatic overhead athletes (20,21). Ultimately, it is up to the physician and the radiologist to determine the usefulness of diagnostic testing and to correlate this with the clinical presentation.

Acute Shoulder Injuries

Adolescent macrotraumatic injuries can occur during collision and contact sports, most notably from a fall on an outstretched hand or from direct contact with the ground, enclosure, or another player. Such force can result in a glenohumeral subluxation, dislocation, acromioclavicular separation, or a variety of fractures. Because of the developmental and structural differences between the young athlete and adults, the diagnosis and management of these injuries can differ.

Acromioclavicular and Sternoclavicular Separations and Dislocations

AC and SC separations are rare in the young athlete. Injuries to these joints typically occur from a direct blow to the superior aspect of the shoulder or a direct lateral blow with the arm adducted. The corresponding physes for these joints fuse late, with the medial clavicular physis remaining open until 24–25 yr of age (22). Therefore, injuries to this area in children 15 yr of age and younger are usually physeal fractures or pseudodislocations that are difficult to distinguish from the common adult AC separation.

AC joint injuries should be evaluated with AP views of both AC joints for comparison and an axillary view to determine the presence of any anterior or posterior positioning or intraarticular involvement. True AC separations have been classified as grades I–VI (23). Grade I and II injuries are essentially nondisplaced injuries. Grade III injuries will demonstrate displacement of 25–100% on radiographs. These injuries should be distinguished from grade V separations, which result in significant superior displacement in excess of 100%. Grade IV and VI injures are rare and displace posteriorly and inferiorly, respectively.

Grade I and II AC separations are treated nonoperatively. The player should be given a sling for comfort and will likely be unable to participate in contact sports for 2–3 wk. When all motion and strength have returned and pain has diminished they may be allowed to return to play as tolerated. Management of grade III separations remains controversial, but most authors continue to recommend nonoperative management in most cases. Injuries to the dominant arm in overhead athletes or weightlifters are exceptions, and will likely benefit from early repair. Grade IV–VI require anatomic repair or distal clavicle excision and stabilization using one of many techniques described in the literature.

Medial physeal fractures can mimic adult SC dislocations and are more frequent than medial shaft fractures. Sternoclavicular separations are usually anterior and respond to nonoperative measures. Attempts to reduce anterior SC joint dislocations typically fail; however, these injuries tend to respond to initial activity modification and gradually return to activities as pain allows. Posterior dislocations are rare, but can result in dysphagia, dysphonia, and pulmonary and neurovascular compromise. Closed reduction may be successful. Open reduction should be reserved for open injuries and injuries with significant displacement or compromise of the neighboring vital structures. Once reduced, these injuries tend to be quite stable, and range of motion may begin after 2–3 wk. Distinguishing between anterior and posterior dislocations can be quite difficult using routine radiographs; therefore, CT scans are routinely recommended to evaluate this injury. Physeal fractures of either the AC or SC joint should be treated with a sling for 2–3 wk, followed by gradual progression of physiotherapy. Return to play can be expected in 4–6 wk.

Clavicle Fractures

Fractures of the clavicle are one of the most common fractures seen in this age group. The healing capacity of the skeletally immature athlete allows for considerable displacement and deformity to occur with little to no residual sequelae. Nonoperative treatment involves a sling for 3–4 wk and pendulum exercises at 2–3 wk. As the athlete reaches skeletal maturity, the healing capacity diminishes and consideration may be given for surgical fixation of fractures with significant shortening or displacement, which may cause an increased risk of nonunion and residual dysfunction (24). Open fractures or fractures causing tenting of the skin are absolute indications for surgery. Return to play for these injuries requires clinical union of the fracture site and pain-free, normal range of motion.

Proximal Humerus Fractures

Fractures of the proximal humerus in the skeletally immature athlete usually occur at the physes. These fractures may be missed on routine AP views; therefore, a standard trauma series consisting of AP, scapula Y, and axillary lateral views should be obtained when evaluating any patient with a suspected shoulder injury. Salter–Harris type II fractures are most commonly seen (Figure 7.7 A–C). These fractures have tremendous remodeling capability and are typically treated nonoperatively in a sling and swathe. Proximal humerus fractures with associated lytic areas likely represent a simple bone cyst that should be evaluated further. Unstable or significantly displaced fractures require closed reduction and percutaneous pinning. If a closed reduction is not possible, then open reduction should be performed as soft tissue interposition of the biceps tendon in the fracture site has likely occurred. A sling and swathe for 3–4 wk and early range of motion will result in return to play as early as 8 wk.

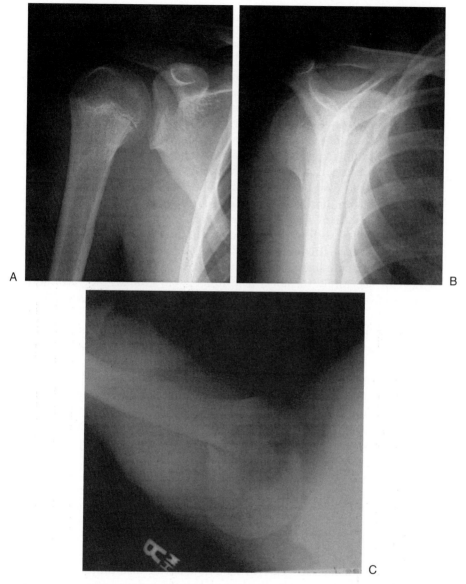

FIGURE 7.7. A 12-yr-old basketball player with severe pain after a fall onto an outstretched arm. **(A)** AP radiograph and **(B)** Scapula Y views are nondiagnostic for injury. **(C)** Axillary lateral view shows obvious Salter–Harris fracture of the surgical neck.

Glenohumeral Dislocation

Glenohumeral instability encompasses a wide spectrum of shoulder disorders. A discussion of glenohumeral instability requires proper classification by the physician, distinguishing between an actual dislocation, a subluxating episode, or subtle microinstability. The instability pattern must then be characterized as anterior, posterior, or multidirectional in nature. Finally, the etiology of the instability should be defined as traumatic or atraumatic. Patients with an atraumatic etiology should then be further classified as exhibiting involuntary versus voluntary instability. Only after the shoulder disorder is properly classified will the physician be able to accurately diagnose and treat the young athlete.

Shoulder dislocations and subluxations are common in the older adolescent athlete, and their frequency approaches that of adults. The extreme degree of mobility seen in the glenohumeral joint is likely to blame. Furthermore, the elastic nature of the immature, capsuloligamentous structures can exacerbate the problem. On the contrary, athletes younger than 10–12 yr of age rarely sustain a true dislocation; instead, they are more likely to have a fracture at the weaker, open proximal humeral physis (25).

Traumatic instability typically develops after a fall or injury with the arm in an abducted and externally rotated position. Anterior instability is the most common pattern. Traumatic injuries may result in tears or plastic deformation of the capsuloligamentous structures and/or labrum. The anterior–inferior glenohumeral ligament and labrum are the most commonly injured structures, and are termed Bankart lesions. Numerous investigators have studied these injuries and have noted the high recurrence rate for anterior shoulder instability in this age group. Marans et al. reported the results of 21 adolescent patients with traumatic anterior shoulder dislocations and reported a recurrence rate of 100% (26). Deitch et al. retrospectively evaluated the outcome in 32 patients between the ages of 11–18 yr with radiographically documented anterior shoulder dislocations. All patients were immobilized from 1–8 wk, and 24 of them received supervised physical therapy. Nonetheless, instability recurred in 75% of patients (27).

Athletes sustaining an acute, traumatic anterior dislocation will often hold the affected extremity in an abducted and externally rotated position. A prominence in the anterior joint region and hollow space in the posterior subacromial area are often present. The axillary nerve may be injured, and it should be thoroughly evaluated before initiation of any treatment. Radiographs should be obtained for anyone suspected of having a dislocation or subluxating event. These studies should include the standard shoulder trauma series mentioned previously, and they should be performed before any reduction. This is particularly important in the skeletally immature child who is more likely to have a physeal fracture that clinically mimics a dislocation. Postreduction radiographs should always be obtained to confirm an adequate reduction. If the diagnosis remains in doubt, a magnetic resonance arthrogram (MRA) can be quite useful to detect capsulolabral injuries, occult glenoid fractures (bony Bankart lesions), and posterior or anterior humeral head impaction fractures (Hill-Sach's and reverse Hill-Sach's lesions).

Posterior dislocations are seen far less frequently than anterior dislocations. There is no available data to determine the exact incidence of this injury in the adolescent population; posterior dislocations in the child are limited to case reports only (28).

Posterior shoulder instability most frequently occurs in a position of forward flexion above 100 degrees, with the shoulder in mild internal rotation and slight adduction. This position is commonly achieved in weight training, hockey, and blocking in football. These injuries may also follow a direct blow to the anterior aspect of the shoulder as occurs with contact sports. Posterior dislocations are more difficult to diagnose on clinical exam. The arm is usually held across the body in full internal rotation and adduction. These patients will have pain with any attempts at motion and have an inability to externally rotate.

The treatment for athletes sustaining an acute, first-time anterior and posterior glenohumeral dislocation varies considerably amongst surgeons, and it continues to evolve. In general, first-time "dislocators" are initially placed in a sling, for comfort, and are counseled regarding the natural history of this injury and high incidence of recurrent dislocations in this young, athletic population. Conservative management is directed toward restoring full range of motion and strength through a supervised physical therapy program. Emphasis is placed on rotator cuff and periscapular strengthening. Overhead athletes should progress through an interval throwing program before returning to play (27).

In collision and contact athletes with anterior instability involving their dominant arm, and for those athletes with recurrent anterior or posterior instability, surgical stabilization is a consideration. Treatment is tailored to each athlete, with some midseason athletes being allowed to return to play upon regaining full motion and strength, with the plan to proceed with surgery upon completion of the season. Early surgical repair should be reserved for collision, contact, and throwing athletes sustaining an acute anterior dislocation in the dominant shoulder (28).

This treatment approach reflects the findings of numerous recent studies demonstrating significantly reduced redislocation rates with operative stabilization when compared to nonoperative measures. Lawton et al. performed a retrospective review of 70 shoulders in 66 patients, aged 16 and younger, with shoulder instability (29). At a 2-yr follow-up, those individuals treated with conservative management including physical therapy had a 60% success rate, whereas 40% went on to have surgery. In the surgical group, 90% felt they were performing at the same or higher levels of competition and work. Bottoni et al. also recommended surgical stabilization for their series of young patients with acute, traumatic, first-time anterior shoulder dislocations (30). They noted that of the 12 patients treated nonoperatively, 9 went on to have recurrent instability (75%), whereas only 1 out of 9 treated operatively (11%) recurred. These studies emphasize the inherent pitfalls of conservative management for these injuries (31). The majority of these injuries may be corrected through an arthroscopic approach. However an "open" approach should be considered for those contact athletes with bony Bankart lesions and/or large impaction fractures (Hill-Sach's deformities) of the humeral head.

After surgery, the patient is placed in a sling and swathe for 3–4 wk. Physical therapy for passive range of motion is begun the first week after surgery, and is slowly progressed until full motion is achieved by 12 wk. Strengthening is begun on the second visit and steadily progressed over the ensuing 12 wk, at which point more sport-specific activities are emphasized. Progressive weight training continues, and the athlete is allowed to return to collision or contact sports after a minimum of 4 mo if all goals have been met. Overhead athletes, and pitchers in particular, may require 6–9 mo to return to play. There have recently been encouraging reports of decreased recurrence rates treating first time dislocators in an external rotation sling (32). Although this technique is promising for initial nonsurgical management, more studies are warranted.

SLAP Lesions

Injuries to the biceps–superior labrum complex can occur from a variety of occurrences, including falls on an outstretched arm, traction pulls from lifting, a direct blow to the shoulder, and overuse (33–35). These injuries have been termed "SLAP" lesions, describing their "superior labral anterior–posterior" location. Tennis, volleyball, baseball, and windmill softball pitchers are all at risk of developing a SLAP injury over time. These injuries are rare in the young athlete, but their incidence increases as late adolescence arrives.

Athletes with a SLAP injury will often complain of pain in either the anterior or posterior aspect of the shoulder, usually during the later cocking and early acceleration phases of throwing (36,37). They occasionally describe a "clicking" or "catching" sensation, and the O'Brien sign is often positive. Posterior capsule contracture is the most common cause for shoulder pain in the young overhead athlete, and it can accompany labral injuries. Internal rotation should therefore be assessed and compared to the contralateral shoulder. Plain radiographs are typically normal. If the clinician strongly suspects the presence of a labral injury, a MR arthrogram of the shoulder may be useful. Connell et al., utilizing conventional MRI and using arthroscopy as the gold standard, concluded that MRI had a sensitivity of 98%, specificity of 89%, and an accuracy of 95% for detection of superior labral tears (18). However, this level of accuracy has been difficult to reproduce by other clinicians (15). To further confuse the issue, Connor et al. and Miniaci et al., analyzing the MRI results of asymptomatic overhead athletes (baseball and tennis players), noted findings consistent with partial- or full-thickness rotator cuff tears and abnormalities of the labrum (20,21).

Initial treatment for SLAP injuries should mimic the treatment outlined for acute shoulder dislocations. An initial course of relative rest and early physical therapy is indicated (38). Patients sustaining a SLAP lesion secondary to a compressive injury, such as a fall onto an outstretched arm, should avoid closed chain exercises to minimize compression and shear stresses to the healing labrum. Patients with a peel-back mechanism should avoid excessive external rotation while the lesion is healing. However, they may need stretching of a tight posterior capsule (13). To stretch a tight posterior capsule, the scapula should be stabilized and the shoulder should be internally rotated.

There are seven key exercises we utilize in the early stages of shoulder rehabilitation for the scapula and rotator cuff musculature: seated press ups, push up plus, rows, scaption, side-lying external rotation, prone shoulder extension with external rotation, and prone horizontal abduction with external rotation (39–41). When painless range of motion and full strength are achieved, the athlete is progressed to a "reentry to sport" program, documenting the number of throws, swimming yards, or tennis strokes and the athlete's response to these sessions. Pain before and during activity necessitates a return to rehabilitative activities, whereas pain after activity that resolves in a few hours with cryotherapy, allows the athlete to continue through the program. Athletes that have failed a 4–6-mo course of conservative treatment may require diagnostic arthroscopy. Partial, stable tears of the superior labrum should be debrided, whereas complete, unstable tears are repaired. Early, supervised physical therapy is critical for these athletes and should parallel the nonoperative rehabilitation program. A return to overhead sports is prohibited for a minimum of 4–6mo postoperatively.

Rotator Cuff Injury

The incidence of complete rotator cuff tears in the adolescent population has been reported to be as low as 0.8–1.0% of patients of all ages diagnosed with a cuff tear (42,43). This low rate is attributed to the absence of degenerative changes in the tendon, as is often present in the elderly. Perhaps more importantly, the tensile strength of the young, healthy tendon is greater than bone. This explains the still infrequent, but more common, finding of an avulsion fracture of the greater or lesser tuberosity after a traumatic injury (44). Because of the physiology of the young shoulder, pitchers may also develop a "Little Leaguer's shoulder" rather than an isolated cuff tear (45). Young pitchers will occasionally sustain an overuse rotator cuff tear; however, the injury is typically preceded by a more traumatic event (46,47).

Physical exam will reveal pain with impingement testing and weakness of the rotator cuff, most commonly the supraspinatus tendon. Tenderness over the greater or lesser tuberosity may also be present. The patient should also be evaluated for a concomitant labral injury. Routine radiographs, including AP, scapula Y, and axillary lateral views, should be obtained. MRI is reserved for those athletes with persistent, atypical pain or weakness after a fall, or those failing a protracted course of conservative treatment. It is quite useful for diagnosing supraspinatus and infraspinatus tears; however, accurate diagnosis of small subscapularis tears remains problematic.

Rotator cuff strains and small, partial-thickness tears should initially be treated conservatively. This treatment should include a physical therapy program focusing on rotator cuff and scapular strengthening, as previously mentioned. The athlete should be restricted from overhead sporting activities. An initial course of nonsteroidal antiinflammatory medication may be helpful. Restoration of a swimmer or thrower's range of motion, rotator cuff and scapular strength and endurance, and an elimination of pain are achieved before a return to overhead activities.

Surgical intervention is reserved for those patients who have failed a 6-mo course of conservative treatment or those athletes with MRI confirmation of a full-thickness rotator cuff tear. Surgery should begin with a thorough examination under anesthesia, followed by diagnostic arthroscopy. Partial-thickness tears estimated to be <30–40% in thickness at the time of arthroscopy may be debrided, whereas larger tears should be repaired. In the rare event that a complete rotator cuff tear is encountered in an adolescent, it should be repaired. If no rotator cuff tear is seen at the time of arthroscopy, a secondary impingement syndrome because of underlying instability is likely. In this setting, a selective arthroscopic capsulorrhaphy and subacromial bursectomy is performed, as described below. A selective capsular plication technique is recommended to address the instability; thermal capsulorrhaphy should be avoided in this young age group.

Chronic Overuse Shoulder Injuries

Little Leaguer's Shoulder

Little Leaguer's shoulder describes a clinical entity characterized by pain with throwing, in conjunction with radiographic evidence of widening of the proximal humeral physis (Figure 7.8). This condition is typically the result of overuse in the overhead athlete, particularly pitchers. These athletes will often have mild shoulder pain for several months that increases

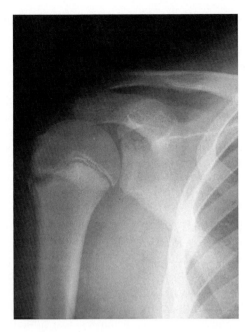

FIGURE 7.8. Radiograph of Little Leaguer's shoulder. A 13-yr-old Little League pitcher with onset of pain after routine pitch late in season. Note widening of the physis, with fragmentation along the lateral aspect.

dramatically while pitching in a game (48). They will have tenderness over the proximal humerus and may have associated swelling. Pain and weakness are noted with resisted abduction and external rotation. Radiographs of the contralateral shoulder are useful to confirm subtle physeal widening. If the diagnosis remains questionable, a bone scan may be useful for revealing increased, asymmetric uptake in the involved proximal humerus.

The development of Little Leaguer's shoulder appears to result from the extreme, repetitive force placed across the proximal humeral physis in these young athletes. Mair et al. found that the increased external rotation and shear stress arising from the throwing motion causes adaptive changes to the proximal humeral epiphysis (49). Furthermore, Sabick et al. used a biomechanical study to demonstrate how shear stress arising from the high torque in late cocking is large enough to lead to deformation of the weak proximal humeral epiphyseal cartilage, causing either humeral retrotorsion or proximal humeral epiphysiolysis over time (5).

Treatment is nonsurgical and includes rest and gentle range of motion. As the pain resolves, a light rotator cuff strengthening program is begun. Pitching is not allowed for a minimum of 6–8 wk, or until all pain has resolved. A supervised throwing program is begun, and improper pitching mechanics are corrected. If any symptoms return, the throwing program is discontinued for an additional month.

Long-term consequences are rare; however, premature physeal closure with resultant humeral length discrepancy or deformity and physeal fractures have occurred (50). Proximal humeral epiphysiolysis or osteochondrosis of the proximal epiphysis should be sought in the skeletally immature pitcher. This condition is distinguishable by the radiographic signs of avascular necrosis or fragmentation of the proximal epiphysis in the presence of a normal-appearing physeal plate (45). This condition is rare and has a less predictable outcome.

Glenohumeral Instability

Glenohumeral subluxation often follows a single traumatic event (recurrent traumatic instability), but may also occur as a result of overuse in the overhead athlete (atraumatic, microinstability). Young athletes with generalized laxity and no history of trauma will frequently demonstrate multidirectional instability (atraumatic MDI). Overhead athletes with multidirectional instability will commonly complain of soreness, fatigue, decreased velocity, and a decline in accuracy. Capsulolabral tears are not as commonly seen in this subgroup of athletes, and their symptoms tend to be a product of rotator cuff imbalance, overuse, and improper technique. These athletes usually present with complaints caused by secondary impingement resulting from their instability. They will occasionally relate a subluxating episode and, less frequently, have a true dislocating event (29). Athletes experiencing subluxating events will complain of pain and "slipping" or "popping" of their shoulder. Occasionally they will describe a "dead arm" sensation after a particular throw. This sensation is brief in duration and usually precludes further pitching that day.

Athletes with recurrent subluxations or multidirectional instability (MDI) should initially be treated with 4–16wk of activity modification, specifically avoiding overhead throwing activities. A supervised physical therapy program focusing on rotator cuff and periscapular strengthening is begun immediately. Strengthening of the trunk and lower extremities is often neglected, and should be addressed. Pitchers should be evaluated for a posterior capsular contracture, and an appropriate stretching program should be begun if present. As symptoms subside, a return to play program should be utilized that will ensure a slow, progressive, and safe return to functional activities. If the patient is an overhead athlete, their technique should be evaluated and corrections made before a return to their respective sport. Athletes who do not respond to this treatment regimen may warrant a selective capsulorrhaphy, addressing only the capsuloligamentous structures contributing to the instability pattern. Capsular suture plication is recommended, as thermal capsulorrhaphy has demonstrated an unacceptably high rate of recurrence in this patient group (51). Furthermore, reports of severe chondrolysis after thermal capsulorrhaphy are particularly concerning for this young age group (52,53). Superior labral tears (SLAP lesions) may also occur in this patient group, and should be repaired if encountered at the time of surgery. The postoperative regimen for these athletes is similar to that described for glenohumeral dislocations, with the exception of return to play typically requiring 6–9 mo in the multidirectional instability group.

SLAP Lesions

Several theories have been proposed to explain the etiology of overuse-related SLAP injuries. Adolescent athletes demonstrate a significant amount of joint laxity, which may manifest as increased external rotation, particularly in throwing athletes (15). Studies have shown the highest strain rate on the superior labrum to occur during the late cocking position (maximum external rotation) (54,55). Overhead athletes with increased external rotation in the presence of subtle instability have been found to be at risk of developing a biceps–labral complex tear (56–59). Biomechanically, when a pitcher over rotates (excessive ER) or horizontally abducts his shoulder in early and late cocking, shear stress develops that can damage the superior biceps–labral complex. In addition, pitchers with less than a 180-degree arc of internal/external rotation are particularly at risk for SLAP injury. Poor mechanics combined with capsular laxity, underdeveloped musculature, or fatigue (overuse) adversely affects the dynamic stability, leading to shoulder injuries and SLAP lesions in particular (57,60).

Overuse SLAP lesions may not be entirely caused by overhead forces. Windmill softball players also are at increased risk of developing this injury despite using an underhand windmill technique. These athletes typically present with hyperlaxity or even MDI. Most notable in females, windmill softball pitchers have been found to develop distraction forces across the glenohumeral joint that are 94% of body weight (16). This distraction force occurs as the momentum created by the windmill motion results in the arm being pulled away from the body immediately after ball release. This mechanism of injury was demonstrated by Bey et al. through the creation of unstable SLAP lesions in 7 out of 8 cadaveric shoulders when combining traction and inferior subluxation, as occurs during a typical windmill pitch (61). This mechanism of injury should be remembered when examining the young softball pitcher with persistent shoulder pain.

Internal Impingement

Throwing a baseball, softball, or football can cause shoulder dysfunction caused by the high rotational velocities and torques generated at the glenohumeral joint. Other sports, such as volleyball, tennis, and swimming, have unique biomechanics, but similar injury patterns. However, internal impingement is one overuse injury that tends to affect a disproportionate number of baseball pitchers. The exact etiology of this injury is debated, but it may represent a combination of injuries, including superior labral tears, rotator cuff injury, posterior capsule contracture, and anterior instability (62). These athletes complain of pain while throwing and note a decrease in control and speed with their pitches. They will also occasionally complain of a "dead arm" sensation (5). On physical exam they will have a positive apprehension relocation test, pain with resisted external rotation, and a positive O'Brien sign. Internal rotation is often limited, and should be compared to the contralateral shoulder. Once again, pitchers with less than a 180-degree arc of internal/external rotation are particularly at risk for SLAP injury. If the diagnosis remains in question, a MRA may be helpful in detecting a SLAP lesion and/or rotator cuff injury.

Conservative management follows those principles discussed for anterior instability and SLAP lesions. Once the overhead athlete regains painless full range of motion and rotator cuff strength, they may progress through an interval throwing program. Once completed, the athlete undergoes biomechanical analysis. Recommendations should be made providing specific drills to correct biomechanical issues. The athlete must complete all aspects of the conservative management program before return to competition.

Absolute indications for operative treatment include MRI evidence of an unstable SLAP lesion or full-thickness rotator cuff tear. Relative indications include failure of 4–6 mo of conservative treatment as outlined. SLAP injuries are surgically treated as discussed in SLAP injuries. Partial-thickness rotator cuff tears <20–30% in thickness are debrided, and larger tears are repaired. These athletes often display subtle anterior instability, which will require a selective anterior–inferior capsulorrhaphy, if present (63). The postoperative course is similar to that described for SLAP lesions and anterior instability. The basic principles of therapy are directed toward achieving full range of motion, full strength, no swelling, and no pain. This will create a foundation for the athlete to begin a functional exercise progression. Sports-specific activities and interval throwing programs will then enable the athlete to return to their preinjury level of function, often requiring 6 mo or longer for the overhead athlete.

"Secondary" Impingement Syndrome

The adolescent shoulder may be more susceptible to overuse injuries than the adult shoulder. Smaller muscle mass, decreased muscular endurance, and increased tissue laxity may lead to microtraumatic injuries. The overhead athlete is particularly susceptible to this mechanism of injury. These athletes often participate in daily practices or games and may play on more than one team during the course of the year—a perfect recipe for overuse injuries. Characteristically, overuse injuries are manifested as "secondary" impingement in the subacromial space. Here, contact between the superior humeral head and inferior surface of the acromion process can inflame the bursa, rotator cuff, and bicep tendon. This abnormal contact occurs when the static and dynamic stabilizers are no longer able to properly balance the glenohumeral joint. Glenohumeral instability is the most common cause for this imbalance. Athletes demonstrating generalized joint laxity are particularly susceptible and will often develop MDI that is frequently mistaken for pure "outlet" impingement. These athletes appear to primarily have a rotator cuff injury when in reality, their rotator cuff symptoms are a result of underlying instability. If the laxity and subsequent instability are not recognized and addressed, the rotator cuff is placed at a disadvantage by performing activities related to overhead motion, while concomitantly maintaining congruency of the glenohumeral joint (60). As the instability continues, more demands are placed on the rotator cuff, resulting in inflammation with possible progression to an undersurface tear over time.

The young athlete will nearly always describe a history of repetitive overhead throwing, serving, or swimming. If such a history is not offered, it should be pursued with questions pertaining to number of practices and competitions per week, the duration of sport-specific training, number of teams they participate on, and number of pitches, serves, or laps performed leading up to or immediately preceding the injury. Patients will complain of anterolateral shoulder pain that increases with overhead activities. On exam they demonstrate pain with provocative impingement testing, although significant weakness is not typically found (50). The apprehension and relocation exam is usually abnormal, prompting further evaluation with load and shift testing. A positive sulcus sign is also helpful for detecting underlying MDI. Standard radiographic studies are typically normal. Patients that have not responded to an appropriate conservative treatment program or are suspected of having a rotator cuff tear may require MRI evaluation. Increased signal in the subacromial space and distal supraspinatus tendon is not uncommon, and may represent tendonitis and impingement; however, false positives in the overhead athlete are common.

Rotator cuff impingement in the young adolescent will typically respond to 4–16 wk of conservative therapy. Many of the athletes have underlying instability of the glenohumeral joint, and therefore the treatment program is identical to that discussed in the instability section. A gradual re-entry to sport program is initiated, documenting the number of throws, swimming yards, or tennis strokes and the athlete's response to these sessions. Pain before and during activity necessitates a return to rehabilitative activities, whereas pain after activity that resolves in a few hours and with cryotherapy, allows the athlete to continue through the program. A baseball or softball player that is asymptomatic while batting, but develops pain during throwing will often respond to conservative management. When following an appropriately designed conservative rehabilitation program, these athletes may demonstrate improvements with as few as 4–6 treatments.

Surgery is considered only after the patient has shown no improvement after a minimum of 6 mo of conservative treatment. Surgery entails an exam under anesthesia, followed by a diagnostic arthroscopy. Tears of the labrum and rotator cuff are treated as previously described. In the presence of a relatively normal arthroscopic exam, but clinical instability, a selective capsulorrhaphy is performed addressing only the area of instability. A suture plication technique is preferred and thermal capsulorrhaphy avoided in the skeletally immature athlete. A subacromial bursectomy is often helpful, but an acromioplasty is not indicated in this age group.

Prevention

Returning the injured overhead athlete to their preinjury level of competition can be difficult at times. Unfortunately, numerous studies focusing on the normal mechanics in baseball and windmill softball pitching found the shoulder to undergo potentially damaging forces on every pitch (5,16,64). It is therefore critical to prevent injury from occurring, rather than treat it after the fact. Numerous studies have thus been conducted to determine effective measures to prevent injuries in the overhead athlete. Lyman et al. found young pitchers had a lower incidence of injury when they were limited to throwing no more than 75 pitches per game and 600 pitches per season (2). Curveballs and sliders were associated with higher incidence of injury and should be discouraged in children under 14–15 yr of age. In addition, they felt young pitchers should be removed from the game if demonstrating any signs of fatigue, and should not be allowed to participate in more than one league at a time (2). Proper pitching mechanics should be taught early and year-round conditioning encouraged, with emphasis also placed on core strengthening and posterior capsule stretching for pitchers in particular (64).

There are several critical instants during overhead throwing motions, and some are shared by baseball, football, and softball. Balance point, occurring at the end of the wind-up phase, is unique to baseball pitching. If the pitcher does not achieve a solid balance point, the legs and trunk will not be in sync with the upper extremity, placing greater stress on the shoulder and elbow to achieve ball velocity. Keeping the hand on top of the ball during the early cocking phase and restricting the arm from moving behind the body in late cocking minimizes the stress placed on the anterior capsule and is a characteristic shared by all three sports. Taking an adequate stride length is also important. This ensures that the legs and trunk are in sync with the arm and the athlete can take advantage of the explosiveness of the body to impart force to the ball with the least amount of stress to the shoulder. This underscores the importance of lower extremity and core strengthening in the adolescent overhead athlete.

Return to Play Guidelines

Adolescent athletes must achieve certain clinical or impairment goals before completing a functional exercise progression. This includes achieving full range of motion at the shoulder, and thrower's range of motion in the overhead athlete. They must demonstrate full strength throughout the rotator cuff, scapula, and prime movers of the shoulder girdle, as well as core and lower extremity strength and power. Pain and effusion must be eliminated. The functional exercise progression consists of sports-specific activities and practice drills that will mimic the stresses the athlete will encounter in competition. For the overhead athlete, an interval throwing program, or long toss program, must be completed for position players, and an additional mound interval-throwing program must be completed for pitchers. The athlete must also demonstrate appropriate mechanics for their respective sport to minimize the risk of reinjury and to enable them to achieve peak performance. Achievement of all the impairment goals and completion of the interval throwing program will ensure that the athlete can return to full competition as quickly and safely as possible, with a minimal risk for reinjury.

Clinical Pearls

- There are numerous conditions that can affect the adolescent athlete's shoulder.
- Overuse injuries occur more frequently than acute, traumatic injuries. Most of these injuries can be prevented.
- When an injury does occur, early recognition and conservative care will allow a safe return to sport in the majority of cases. Conservative treatment revolves around a well-structured and supervised physical therapy program for many of these injuries.
- Sport-specific return-to-play programs enable a safe and efficient return to competition and a long, healthy career.
- When surgical intervention is needed, recent advances in surgical techniques allow the majority of procedures to be performed arthroscopically.
- The sports medicine specialist is in a unique position to educate coaches, parents, and athletes on preparation, prevention, training, and participation to minimize the risk of shoulder injury.

References

1. Lephart SM, Kocher MS. The role of exercise in the prevention of shoulder disorders. In: Matsen FA, Fu FH, Hawkins RJ, eds. The Shoulder: A Balance of Mobility and Stability. Rosemont, IL: American Academy of Orthopedic Surgeons; 1993;597–620.

2. Lyman S, Fleisig GS, Waterbor JW, et al. Longitudinal study of shoulder and elbow pain in youth baseball pitchers. Med Sci Sports Exerc. 2001;Nov 33(1):1803–1810.
3. Hutchinson MR, Ireland ML. Overuse and throwing injuries in the skeletally immature athlete. Instr Course Lect 2003;52:25–36.
4. Clark WA. Anatomy. In: Kelley MJ, Clark WA eds. Orthopedic Therapy of the Shoulder. Philadelphia: J.B. Lippincott Co; 1995.
5. Sabick MB, Kim YK, Torry MR, et al. Biomechanics of the shoulder in youth baseball pitchers: Implications for the development of proximal humeral epiphysiolysis and humeral retrotorsion. Am J Sports Med 2005; Nov 33(11):1716–1722. Epub 2005 Aug.
6. Walton J. Paxinos A, Tzannes A, et al. The unstable shoulder in the adolescent athlete. Am J Sport Med 2002;30(5):758–767.
7. Robertson DD, Yuan J, Bigliani LU, et al. Three-dimensional analysis of the proximal part of the humerus: Relevance to arthroplasty. J Bone Joint Surg-Am 2000; Nov 82-A(11):1594–1602.
8. Pearl ML. Proximal humeral anatomy in shoulder arthroplasty: Implications for prosthetic design and surgical technique. J Shoulder Elbow Surg 2005; Jan-Feb 14(1 Suppl S):99S–104S.
9. Sarrafian SK. Gross and functional anatomy of the shoulder. Clin Orthop 1983;173:11.
10. Regan FM, Meister K, Horodyski MB, et al. Humeral retroversion and its relationship to glenohumeral rotation in the shoulder of college baseball players. Am J Sports Med 2002;May-June 30(3):354–360.
11. Cooper DE, Arnoczky SP, O'Brien SJ, et al. Anatomy, histology and vascularity of the glenoid labrum. J Bone Joint Surg 1992;74-A(1):46–52.
12. Huber WP, Putz RV. Periarticular fiber system of the shoulder joint. Arthroscopy 1997;December 13(6):680–691.
13. O'Brien SJ, Neves MC, Arnoczky SP, et al. The anatomy and histology of the inferior glenohumeral ligament complex of the shoulder. Am J Sports Med 1990;18(5):449–456.
14. Cole BJ, Warner JJP. Anatomy, biomechanics, and pathophysiology of glenohumeral instability. In: Iannotti JP, Williams GR, eds. Disorders of the Shoulder: Diagnosis and Management. New York: Lippincott, Williams & Wilkins; 1999:207–232.
15. Meister K, Day T, Horodyski M, et al. Rotational motion changes in the glenohumeral joint of the adolescent/Little League baseball player. Am J Sports Med 2005; May 33(5):693–698.
16. Werner SL, Guido JA, McNeice RP, et al. Biomechanics of youth windmill softball pitching. Am J Sports Med. 2005;33(4):552–560.
17. Meyers JB, Laudner KG, Pasquale MR, et al. Scapular position and orientation in throwing athletes. Am J Sports Med. 2005;33(2):263–271.
18. Connell DA, Potter HG, Wickiewicz TL, et al. Noncontrast magnetic resonance imaging of superior labral lesions: 102 cases confirmed at arthroscopic surgery. Am J Sports Med 1999;27(2):208–213.
19. Bencardino JT, Beltran J, Rosenberg ZS, et al. Superior labrum anterior-posterior lesions: Diagnosis with MR arthrography of the shoulder. Radiology 2000;214:267–271.

20. Connor PM, Banks DM, Tyson AB, et al. MRI of the asymptomatic shoulder of overhead athletes: A 5-year follow up study. Am J Sports Med 1993;31(5):724–727.
21. Miniaci A, Mascia AT, Salonen DC, et al. MRI of the shoulder in asymptomatic professional baseball pitchers. Am J Sports Med 2002;30(1):66–73.
22. Gray H. Anatomy of the Human Body. Philadelphia: Lea & Febiger; 1985.
23. Dameron TB, Rockwood CA. Fractures and Dislocations of the shoulder. In: Rockwood CA, Wilkins KE, King RE, eds. Fractures in Children. Philadelphia: J.B. Lippincott; 1984:624–653.
24. Nowak J, Holgersson M, Larsson S. Can we predict sequelae following fractures of the clavicle based on initial findings? A prospective study with 9–10 years follow-up. In: Program and Abstracts of the American Shoulder and Elbow Surgeons 18th Open Meeting; 2002 Feb 16; Dallas, TX.
25. Wagner KT Jr, Lyde ED. Adolescent traumatic dislocations of the shoulder with open epiphyses. J Pediatr Orthop 1983;3:61–62.
26. Marans HJ, Angel KR, Schemitsch EH, et al. The fate of traumatic anterior dislocation of the shoulder in children. JBJS 1992;74A:1242–1244.
27. Dietch J, Mehlman CT, Foad SL, et al. Traumatic anterior shoulder dislocations in adolescents. Am J Sports Med 2003;Sept-Oct 31(5):758–763.
28. Foster WS, Ford TB, Drez D. Isolated posterior shoulder dislocation in a child. Am J Sports Med 1985;13:198–200.
29. Lawton RL, Choudhury S, Mansat P, et al. Pediatric shoulder instability: Presentation, findings, treatment, outcomes. J Pediatr Orthop 2002;Jan–Feb 22(1):52–61.
30. Bottoni CR, Wilckens JH, DeBerardino TM, et al. A prospective, randomized evaluation of arthroscopic stabilization versus nonoperative treatment in patients with acute, traumatic, first-time shoulder dislocations. Am J Sports Med 2002;Jul-Aug 30(4):576–580.
31. Postacchini F, Gumina S, Cinotti G. Anterior shoulder dislocation in adolescents. J Should Elbow Surg 2000;9:470–474.
32. Itoi E, Hatakeyama Y, Kido T, et al. A new method of immobilization after traumatic anterior dislocation of the shoulder. A preliminary study. JSES 2003: 12:413–415.
33. Snyder SJ, Banas MP, Karzel RP. An analysis of 140 injuries to the superior glenoid labrum. J Shoulder Elbow Surg 1995;Jul-Aug 4(4):243–248.
34. Maffet MW, Gartsman GM, Moseley B. Superior labrum-biceps tendon complex lesions of the shoulder. Am J Sports Med 1995; Jan-Feb 23(1):93–98.
35. Snyder SJ, Karzel RP, DelPizzo W, et al. SLAP lesions of the shoulder. Arthroscopy. 1990;6(4):274–279.
36. Meister K. Injuries to the shoulder in the throwing athlete. Part Two: Evaluation/Treatment. Am J Sports Med 2000;28(4):587–601.
37. Altchek DW, Warren RF, Wickiewicz TL, et al. Arthroscopic labral debridement: A three-year follow up study. Am J Sports Med 1992;20(6):702–706.
38. Wilk KE, Reinhold MM, Dugas JR, et al. Current concepts in the recognition and treatment of superior labral (SLAP) lesions. J Orthop Sports Phys Ther 2005;35(5):273–291.
39. Moseley JB, Jobe FW, Pinks M, et al. EMG analysis of the scapular muscles during a shoulder rehabilitation program. Am J Sports Med 1992;20(2):128–134.

40. Blackburn TA, McLeod WD, White B, et al. EMG analysis of posterior rotator cuff exercises. J Athl Train 1990;25(1):41–45.

41. Reinhold MM, Wilk KE, Fleisig GS, et al. Electromyographic analysis of the rotator cuff and deltoid musculature during common shoulder external rotation exercises. J Orthop Sports Phys Ther 2004;Jul 34(7):385–394.

42. Itoi E, Tabata S. Rotator cuff tears in the adolescent. Orthopaedics 1993; 16:78–81.

43. Norwood LA, Barrack R, Jacobson KE. Clinical presentation of complete tears of the rotator cuff. J Bone Joint Surg 1989;71A:499–505.

44. Meister K, Andrews JR. Classification and treatment of rotator cuff injuries in the overhand athlete. J Orthop Sports Phys Ther 1993; Aug 18(2): 413–421.

45. Ireland ML, Satterwhite YE. Shoulder Injuries in Baseball. Andrews JR, Zarins B, Wilk KE, eds. Philadelphia: Lippincott-Raven; 1998:271–281.

46. Sugalski MT, Hyman JE, Ahmad CS. Avulsion fracture of the lesser tuberosity in an adolescent baseball pitcher: A case report. Am J Sports Med 2004; Apr–May 32(3):793–796.

47. Tarkin IS, Morganti CM, Zillmer DA, et al. Rotator cuff tears in adolescent athletes. Am J Sports Med 2005;Apr 33(4):596–601.

48. Carson WG, Gasser SI. Little leaguer's shoulder: A report of 23 cases. Am J Sports Med 1998;26(4):575–580.

49. Mair SD, Uhl TL, Robbe RG, et al. Physeal changes and range-of-motion differences in the dominant shoulders of skeletally immature baseball players. J Should Elbow Surg 2004;Sept-Oct 13(5):487–491.

50. Chen FS, Diaz VA, Loebenberg M, et al. Shoulder and Elbow Injuries in the Skeletally Immature Athlete. J Am Acad Orthop Surg 2005;13(3):172–185.

51. Montgomery SC, Miller MD. What's new in sport medicine. J Bone Joint Surg 87A;3;March 2005:686–692.

52. Levine WN, Bigliani LU, Ahmad CS. Thermal capsulorrhaphy. Orthopedics August 2004;27(4):823–826.

53. Levine WN, Clark AM Jr., D'Alessandro DF, Yamaguchi K. Chondrolysis following arthroscopic thermal capsulorrhaphy to treat shoulder instability: A report of two cases. JBJS 2005;87-A(3):616–621.

54. Shepard MF, Dugas JR, Zeng N, et al. Differences in the ultimate strength of the biceps anchor and the generation of type II superior labral anterior to posterior lesions in a cadaveric model. Am J Sports Med 2004;32(5): 1197–1201.

55. Pradhan RL, Itoi E, Hatakeyama Y, et al. Superior labral strain during the throwing motion: A cadaveric study. Am J Sports Med 2001;29(4):488–492.

56. Mihata T, YeonSoo L, McGarry MH, et al. Excessive humeral external rotation results in increased shoulder laxity. Am J Sports Med 2004;32(5): 1278–1285.

57. Burkhart SS, Morgan CD, Kibler WB. The disabled throwing shoulder: Spectrum of pathology. Part I: Pathoanatomy and biomechanics. Arthroscopy 2003; 19(4);404–420.

58. Walch G, Boileau J, Noel E, et al. Impingement of the deep surface of the supraspinatus tendon on the posterior superior glenoid rim: An arthroscopic study. J Shoulder Elbow Surg. 1992;1:238–243.

59. Jobe FW, Giangarra CE, Kvitne RS, et al. Anterior capsulolabral reconstruction of the shoulder in athletes in overhand sports. Am J Sports Med 1991;Sept-Oct 19(5):428–434.
60. Fleisig GS, Andrews JR, Dillman CJ, Escamilla RF. Kinetics of baseball pitching with implications about injury mechanisms. Am J Sports Med 1995;23(2):233–239.
61. Bey MJ, Elders GJ, Huston LJ, et al. The mechanism of creation of superior labrum, anterior, and posterior lesions in a dynamic biomechanical model of the shoulder: The role of inferior subluxation. J Shoulder Elbow Surg 1998;7(4):397–401.
62. Jobe CM. The rotator cuff, part II: Superior glenoid impingement. Orthop Clinic North Am 1997;April 28(2):137–143.
63. Levitz CL, Dugas J, Andrews JR. The use of arthroscopic thermal casulorrhaphy to treat internal impingement in baseball players. Arthroscopy: The Journal of Arthroscopic and Related Surgery. 2001;17(6):573–577.
64. Fleisig GS, Barrentine SW, Zheng N, et al. Kinematic and kinetic comparison of baseball pitching among various levels of development. J Biomech 1999;Dec 32(12):1371–1375.

8
Elbow and Forearm Injuries

Anthony Luke, Margaret Lee, and Marc Safran

The elbow and forearm create a fascinating joint complex. It is a highly congruous joint that provides a wide range of motion required for functions such as sports. The adolescent athlete has the added dimensions of growth and development, which can affect forces around the joint, as well as motor function, and can be the source of multiple potential problems (1). The elbow has a complex maturation process, developing from multiple ossification centers, which can complicate the diagnosis and treatment of injuries. As a growing individual is able to perform with greater speed, strength, and endurance, the loading forces, torques, and risk of injury increase (2,3).

Injuries to the elbow and forearm can result from overuse or acute trauma. Throwing sports, such as baseball (4), lead to frequent elbow problems. Overuse elbow injuries are also commonly seen in athletes who use the upper extremities and are involved in repetitive training, such as gymnastics (5,6) weight lifting, tennis (1,7), and golf (8). Trauma, typically a fall on the outstretched arm, can result in fractures and dislocation. Fractures in the upper extremity in children most frequently involve the radius and ulna, followed by hand and carpal bones, and then the distal humerus (9).

The literature on management of elbow problems is extremely limited in clinical studies, especially for the adolescent athlete. The majority of elbow research includes cadaveric studies, case reports and series in adults, or kinematic and epidemiologic studies in youth pitchers, who are often preadolescent. Treatment of most sport-related elbow injuries for the adolescent athlete is based on expert experience and opinion often expressed in review papers and textbooks.

Anatomy

Bony Anatomy

The elbow joint is made up of the articulations between the humerus, ulna, and radius. The forearm is composed of the radius and ulna with its proximal and distal articulations, as well as its overlying muscles and soft tissue structures. The distal humerus has two major articulating surfaces: the trochlea, which articulates with the coronoid and olecranon of the ulna, and the capitellum, which opposes the radial head. The elbow joint can be divided into the following three articulations: a) the radiocapitellar joint, b) the ulnohumeral joint, and c) the proximal radioulnar joint. The ulnohumeral joint allows flexion and extension, whereas the radiocapitellar and radioulnar joints allow supination and pronation of the forearm, with the radius pivoting around the ulna. The bony hinge of the elbow provides osseous stability with its greatest contribution below 20 degrees and greater than 120 degrees of flexion; between these ranges, the ligaments and capsule are the primary motion restraints (10). Children often demonstrate hyperextensibility of the elbow associated with capsular and ligamentous laxity (11,12).

Ossification Centers

The development of the elbow from multiple ossification centers makes the elbow vulnerable to fracture and apophyseal injuries. The growth plates are areas of vulnerability from traction or shearing forces. The ossification centers follow a predictable order of formation, which can help assess bony maturity, based on their appearances on x-ray. They appear in the following order: the capitellum (age 1–2), the Radial head (age 3), the Internal (medial) epicondyle (age 5), the Trochlea (age 7), the Olecranon (age 9), and the External (lateral) epicondyle (age 10 in girls and 11 in boys) (mnemonic "CRITOE") (Figure 8.1) (13). Eighty percent of the growth of the humerus occurs at the proximal end. Therefore, there is less potential for remodeling at the elbow if fractures should occur there. (12)

Ligament Complexes

On the medial aspect of the elbow, the ulnar collateral ligament (UCL) complex is composed of three ligaments: anterior oblique, posterior oblique, and transverse (Figure 8.2). The anterior oblique ligament is functionally divided into anterior and posterior bands. The anterior band is responsible for most of the stability of the elbow and is most prone to injury with acute or repetitive valgus strain.

On the radial side of the elbow, the lateral collateral ligament (LCL) complex is composed of the radial collateral ligament (RCL), the lateral ulnar collateral ligament (LUCL), the accessory lateral collateral ligament (ALCL), and the annular ligament (AL), which wraps around the radial head (14). The LCL complex is the main ligament responsible for withstanding varus and external rotatory stress in the elbow. The LUCL has been shown to help control posterolateral rotatory motion around the elbow (15). Injuries involving the LCL at the humeral insertion, primarily involving the LUCL and the RCL, produce maximal rotatory instability (16,17).

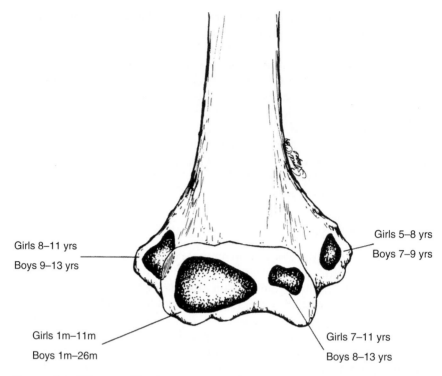

Girls 8–11 yrs
Boys 9–13 yrs

Girls 5–8 yrs
Boys 7–9 yrs

Girls 1m–11m
Boys 1m–26m

Girls 7–11 yrs
Boys 8–13 yrs

FIGURE 8.1. Elbow ossification centers and their roentgenographic appearance according to age. (Reprinted from: Bradley JP. Upper extremity: elbow injuries in children and adolescents. In: Stanitski CL, DeLee JC, Drez D Jr, eds. Pediatric and Adolescent Sports Medicine. Vol 3. Philadelphia: WB Saunders; 1994:244. With permission from Elsevier.)

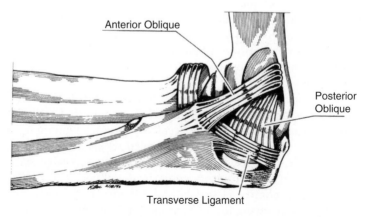

Anterior Oblique

Posterior Oblique

Transverse Ligament

FIGURE 8.2. The ulnar collateral ligament complex. (From Safran MR. Elbow Injuries in Athletes: A Review. Clin Orthop 1995;310:260. With permission.)

Muscle Tendon Units

Muscles that cross the elbow contribute a compressive joint reaction force. The joint reactive forces of the anterior and posterior muscles (biceps, brachialis, brachioradialis, and triceps) provide stability to the joint by compressing the congruous joint (18). The lateral elbow is also statically and dynamically stabilized by the extensor and supinator muscles (19). The common extensor muscle group inserts onto the lateral epicondyle and is composed of the extensor carpi radialis brevis, extensor digitorum, extensor digiti minimi, extensor carpi ulnaris extensor pollicis, and the supinator. The supinator, abductor pollicis longus, extensor pollicis longus and brevis, and extensor indicis muscles originate from the ulna and radius to compose the deep extensors of the forearm. The flexor-pronator group provides some dynamic stability to the medial elbow, but its role is minor (17). The common flexor group includes the pronator teres, flexor carpi radialis, palmaris longus, and flexor carpi ulnaris. The flexor digitorum superficialis and profundus, flexor pollicis longus, and pronator quadratus make up the deeper muscles of the forearm.

Neurovascular Structures

The ulnar nerve is the neurologic structure most commonly injured in sports because of its superficial course. The ulnar nerve passes behind the medial epicondyle and lies over the ulnar collateral ligament. It is anterior to the medial triceps and fairly mobile, allowing it to slide out of the cubital tunnel in some patients. The median nerve travels with the brachial artery under the ligament of Struthers in the medial arm, into the antecubital fossa medial to the biceps, and then under the bicipital aponeurosis and pronator teres (20). The radial nerve passes from the posterolateral arm towards the anterior aspect of the elbow at the level of the distal third of the humerus. It divides into the superficial radial nerve and the posterior interosseus nerve, which is the deep branch. The posterior interosseus nerve supplies the extensor muscles of the forearm and runs in close proximity to the radial neck and under the supinator, passing the arcade of Frohse, where it can occasionally become compressed. (20)

After the age of 5, the capitellum is supplied by only one or two blood vessels, which act as end arteries. Anastomoses interconnecting the metaphysis, epiphysis, and diaphysis of the humerus form by the age of 19, when the growth plate has closed, to bring blood supply to the capitellum (21–23). It has been suggested that repetitive valgus stress on the elbow during a period when the capitellum has its most vulnerable blood supply, such as from repetitive throwing or gymnastic maneuvers, can cause microtrauma to these vessels, which may lead to osteochondroses (24).

Clinical Evaluation

History

In the evaluation of an upper extremity injury in an athlete, it is important to obtain information about the patient's age, hand dominance, side of involvement, position played, duration, and nature of symptoms. Most athletes will complain of pain, instability, or lack of function. In throwers, this may be described as not being able to throw the ball as far or as accurately, or in other sports like tennis or volleyball, not hit the ball as hard. Loss of range of motion is common in children with acute or overuse injuries, and it may be caused by pain, capsular contracture, effusion, or internal joint derangement. Mechanical symptoms such as catching or locking suggest an intraarticular pathology, such as a loose body, chondral injury, or osteochondritis dissecans. Patients may complain of instability of the elbow with hard throwing or pushing up with the arms from a seated position. If neurologic symptoms are reported, such as paresthesias or weakness, the distribution of symptoms may indicate whether the injury is more central involving the neck or brachial plexus, or if a peripheral nerve is affected.

The mechanisms of injury, as well as activities that exacerbate and alleviate the symptoms, are useful for narrowing the differential diagnosis. A fall on the outstretched hand usually has different consequences and pathologies than an atraumatic problem with gradual onset from repetitive overuse. Instability of the elbow most often occurs with hard throwing or weight-bearing loading such as push-ups or gymnastic maneuvers. For patients who are throwers, the style of throwing, mechanics, types, and volume of throws/pitches, velocity, accuracy, and any training errors should be noted (7). One should determine which phase of throwing produces symptoms. Pain during cocking and late acceleration suggests ulnar-sided pathology caused by valgus stress, whereas pain during deceleration and follow-through are suspicious for posterior impingement and stress injuries (10). The location of symptoms can also help focus the examiner towards the most probable diagnosis (25). For example, posterior pain typically occurs during hyperextension.

Physical Examination

Observation, Palpation, and Range of Motion (Look, Feel, Move)

The elbow should be examined for deformity, areas of ecchymosis, and swelling. Patients with a fracture or dislocation will usually present with significant tenderness, swelling, and deformity. The sulci on either side of the olecranon should be observed for intraarticular effusion. The carrying angle can be observed in the relaxed, extended, position.

Several superficial landmarks can be palpated for tenderness, including the lateral and medial epicondyles, the olecranon, the radial head, the capitellum, the distal biceps insertion into the radial tubercle, and the ulnar nerve. The ulnar collateral ligament, which lies under the flexor carpi ulnaris, can also be palpated for tenderness. The ulnar nerve can be palpated in the posterior aspect of the medial epicondyle area during flexion and extension of the elbow to determine if the nerve subluxes or dislocates.

Range of motion can be checked with active and passive assessments of elbow flexion, extension, and forearm supination and pronation. Average motion includes flexion from 0 degrees to 145 ± 10 degrees, with pronation and supination at about 80 and 85 degrees, respectively (26). Lack of extension can suggest an internal derangement or chronic flexion contracture.

Stress Tests

The UCL is best tested with the elbow in approximately 70 degrees of flexion. There are several stress maneuvers to test the functional integrity of the UCL, including the valgus stress test, the milking maneuver, and the moving valgus stress test.

Valgus stress testing can be performed with the elbow flexed to approximately 30 degrees. Though the test has often been described with the forearm in pronation, cadaveric studies suggest that the valgus laxity of the elbow is most pronounced with the forearm in neutral rotation (Figure 8.3) (18).

The "Milking Maneuver" can be performed with the arm in more flexion, ideally at 70 degrees, with the valgus force applied by supporting the elbow and tractioning the thumb, similar to milking a cow (Figure 8.4). This

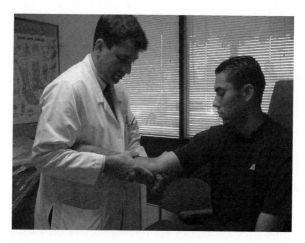

FIGURE 8.3. Valgus stress test. (The patient's wrist and hand are fixed, and a valgus stress is applied with the patient's elbow at 30 degrees.)

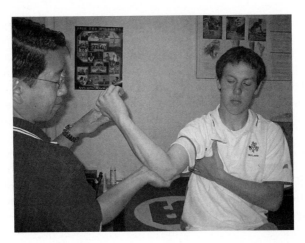

FIGURE 8.4. The "Milking Maneuver" is performed with the arm at 70 degrees, with the valgus force applied by supporting the elbow and tractioning the thumb, similar to milking a cow.

position recreates the valgus throwing position and helps hold the shoulder in external rotation, thereby reducing the effect of shoulder rotation on the assessment of the UCL (27).

The "Moving Valgus Stress test" is described by O'Driscoll et al. (Figure 8.5) (28). With the shoulder abducted to 90 degrees, the examiner maintains a valgus force to the elbow until the shoulder is fully externally rotated then quickly extends the elbow from full flexion to approximately 30 degrees, similar to the acceleration phase of throwing. In a positive test, the athlete describes the reproduction of pain at the UCL that the patient experiences with activities, which typically occurs maximally between 120 and 70 degrees of flexion, as the elbow is extended. The test has been suggested to be 100% sensitive and 75% specific with a small sample of patients (28).

Varus stress testing is performed by flexing the elbow to 30 degrees with the forearm in full pronation and applying a varus force to the lateral elbow. Pain or laxity indicates a positive test, although varus laxity is exceedingly rare (29). The lateral pivot-shift apprehension test is the most sensitive test for reproducing posterolateral instability of the elbow (Figure 8.6). This test allows for the radial head to sublux posterolaterally as the elbow rotates around the axis of the UCL with the applied forces (30).

Provocative tests

The valgus extension overload test involves quickly placing the athlete's elbow in maximal extension with the forearm pronated (10). Valgus stress in hyperextension that accentuates the pain suggests posterior impingement of the olecranon in the olecranon fossa.

Resisted muscle testing is useful for identifying underlying tendinopathies. Pain over the lateral epicondyle is often demonstrated with resisted forearm supination, wrist extension, or third-digit extension with elbow in full extension, if the common extensor tendon is injured. Passive wrist palmarflexion while the elbow is extended may also reproduce symptoms of lateral epicondylosis. Conversely, resisted wrist palmarflexion or pronation and passive wrist dorsiflexion/extension while the elbow is in extension can reproduce pain if the common flexor tendons are affected.

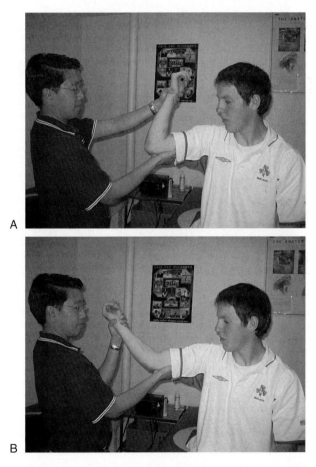

FIGURE 8.5. Moving valgus stress test. **(A)** With the patient sitting with the shoulder abducted to 90 degrees, the examiner applies a valgus force to the elbow until the shoulder is fully externally rotated. **(B)** While maintaining the valgus torque, the examiner quickly extends the elbow to approximately 30 degrees. A positive test reproduces pain at the UCL, typically occurring maximally between 120 degrees and 70 degrees of flexion.

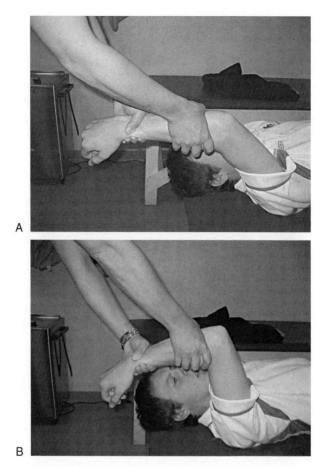

FIGURE 8.6. Pivot shift. **(A)** With the athlete lying supine with the arm overhead, the elbow is supinated and a valgus and axial force is applied to the elbow. The athlete may complain of pain or apprehension. **(B)** Starting in extension, the elbow is flexed with a reduction "clunk" occurring typically at 40 degrees to 70 degrees of flexion.

Looking Beyond the Elbow

Physical examination should include evaluation of the cervical spine, bilateral shoulders, elbows, and wrists (31), as well as motor strength testing and neurologic sensation. Patients with ulnar nerve symptoms may exhibit a positive Tinel's sign over the cubital fossa, as well as subluxation of the ulnar nerve with flexion of the elbow.

A thorough examination should also include an assessment of the kinetic chain. A coordinated sequence of joint movement and muscle contracture is necessary to produce an efficient functional task such as pitching. For example, key events before release of the ball include generation of momentum through the lower extremities and trunk, elbow elevation and extension, internal rotation of the shoulder, and pronation of the elbow. "Dropping the elbow," which positions the elbow below the shoulder, increases the tensile loads on the elbow ligaments (32). This can happen in a young pitcher because of poor technique or fatigue. Specifically, assessments of core trunk stability, one-leg stance, and squat testing for weakness, scapular dyskinesis, and glenohumeral internal rotation deficit (GIRD) are suggested in throwing athletes (33). The elbow simply may be the weakest link in the chain, and thus more susceptible to injury.

Imaging

Standard radiographs of the elbow include anterior–posterior (AP), lateral, and one or two oblique views of the elbow. Radiographs of the contralateral elbow are sometimes helpful for comparison in young patients. Though comparison films are commonly ordered, two studies found that opposite side elbow films did not improve diagnostic accuracy (34,35) and do not need to be routinely obtained. A posterior fat pad sign has been reported to be predictive of an occult, intracapsular fracture (supracondylar, radial head, olecranon) in as high as 76% of children with otherwise normal radiographs, though previous reports ranged from 6 to 29% (36). The capitellum should not be posterior to the anterior humeral line, as this suggests a supracondylar extension fracture with displacement of the capitellum posteriorly (13). Stress radiographs performed manually or by gravity can be obtained to demonstrate ligamentous insufficiency in the UCL; however, they can be misleading (18).

Other imaging modalities may be required for the elbow. A computed tomography (CT) scan is still ideal for fractures and bone definition. Bone scan is useful to detect stress injuries of the olecranon or medial apophysis. In the setting of osteochondritis dissecans, bone scans are useful to determine bony activity and assess healing potential. However, magnetic resonance imaging (MRI) is being used more frequently for identifying stress and occult fractures without radiation (37). MR arthrogram has a high sensitivity for complete and partial tears of the UCL in adults (95% and 86% respectively) (38). MRI is still the gold standard for soft tissue pathology, although diagnostic ultrasound has been increasing in utility for soft tissue injuries as well as fractures (39,40).

Acute/Traumatic Elbow Injuries

Elbow Dislocation

During a fall on the outstretched hand, an axial force is applied to the elbow. When other stresses, such as a hyperextension, valgus, or a valgus/external rotation mechanism, are added to the axial load, the elbow may dislocate. These additional forces can lead to posterior dislocation, disruption of the anterior ulnar collateral ligament, or posterolateral instability respectively (41). In younger children, aged 5–10, the anatomy of the distal humerus is predisposed to fracture in the supracondylar region, because the area of bone is very thin between the olecranon fossa posteriorly, the coronoid fossa anteriorly, and the medial and lateral columns of the distal humerus (42). Extension fractures, which cause the distal fragment to displace posteriorly, occur 97.5% of the time, whereas flexion fractures occur much less frequently (2.5%) (43). Elbow dislocations in children younger than 13 yr of age are relatively uncommon, with an incidence of 3–6% of all elbow injuries (44).

The peak incidence of elbow dislocation is between 13–14 yr of age, when the physes begin to close (45). Boys are affected more than girls (7:3), and the injury usually involves the nondominant arm (60%). The most common dislocation is posterior, with posterolateral displacement of the proximal radius and ulna articulation from the humerus and an intact radioulnar articulation (46). In posterior elbow dislocations, the mechanism of injury is usually a fall backward with the arm in abduction and extension. Over one half of posterior elbow dislocations will have an associated fracture, with fractures of the medial epicondyle being the most common (12,44). Anterior elbow dislocation is rare, and divergent elbow dislocation is extremely rare. A direct blow to the posterior aspect of the flexed elbow leads to anterior elbow dislocations. Divergent elbow dislocation signifies a posterior elbow dislocation with disruption of the radioulnar articulation leading to lateral displacement of the radial head and medial displacement of the proximal ulna. Divergent elbow dislocations are caused by high-energy trauma.

A child with a posterior elbow dislocation presents with obvious elbow swelling, deformity, and forearm shortening. The patient frequently holds his or her elbow in a semiflexed position and refuses to move the elbow secondary to pain. Routine radiographs are usually diagnostic and must be examined carefully for associated fractures.

Nonoperative treatment by closed reduction should be performed promptly after adequate pain control and muscle relaxation is established. A careful neurovascular exam must be done before and after reduction, paying special attention to the median nerve and brachial artery. After reduction, a posterior splint is used to immobilize the elbow at 90 degrees of flexion for 2 wk. Active range of motion is then started as early as 2 wk to minimize the risk of fixed contracture, although stable reductions may be accompanied by earlier range of motion as pain subsides. Indications for surgical treatment include an inability to obtain a closed reduction, an open dislocation, or a displaced osteochondral fracture. Fractures need to be immobilized for 4–6 wk (46).

The most serious neurologic complication is damage to the median nerve directly by the dislocation or by entrapment within the joint. Approximately 10% of patients experience neuropraxia of the median or ulnar nerve, which usually resolves within 6–8 mo (42). Late complications include loss of motion, myositis ossificans, recurrent dislocations, radioulnar synostosis, and cubitus recurvatum (46). Initiating early mobilization 2 wk after injury can help minimize loss of motion, which is a common complication. Recurrent instability in elbow dislocations without associated fracture is rare.

Posterolateral Rotatory Instability

Posterolateral rotatory instability (PLRI) is a common form of recurrent instability in the elbow. With a fall on the outstretched hand and internal rotation of the body, a valgus and supination moment can occur, causing the posterolateral movement as the elbow subluxes or dislocates. Athletes usually present complaining of recurrent painful clicking, snapping, and/or locking of the elbow after a dislocation, trauma, or elbow surgery (30). The injury is associated with tearing of the LCL complex, particularly the LUCL, with recurrent episodes of instability caused by the ulna and radius rotating posteriorly as a unit (47). The posterolateral pivot-shift apprehension test is the most sensitive test for reproducing the patient's symptoms (Figure 8.6) (30). Radiographs may demonstrate a small flake fracture of the coronoid process, which suggests a shear fracture from an elbow subluxation or dislocation (30). Stress radiographs with the arm supinated and slightly flexed with the lateral elbow against the x-ray cassette may demonstrate the rotatory instability. MRI can be helpful in identifying LCL injuries directly. It can also be useful to identify osteochondral injury to the capitellum, which may result in problems for a young athlete (48). In one series, 8 out of 44 patients requiring surgical reconstruction, usually after a dislocation, were under 18 yr of age (47). The LUCL can be repaired if the LCL has been directly avulsed from the lateral epicondyle, and any associated osteochondral defects should be addressed during surgery (48). Otherwise, reconstruction of the LUCL is performed for chronic ligament insufficiency (47).

Forearm fractures

Forearm fractures can occur in young athletes after angular loading with rotational displacement. A Monteggia fracture is a fracture of the ulna with a dislocation of the radial head caused by rupture of the proximal radioulnar ligaments. These are frequently missed, and all patients who present with an ulnar fracture should have their elbow assessed clinically and radiographically to avoid missing the concomitant instability of the radial head. In younger patients, the ulnar fracture usually involves the coronoid process or is just distal to it (49). Nightstick fractures are transverse fractures of the ulna from direct trauma. Galeazzi fractures involve a fracture of the distal radius with a disruption of the distal radioulnar joint, although this usually presents in preadolescent athletes.

The athlete will typically present with pain, swelling, and deformity over the fracture site, although a mildly displaced fracture may not be obvious. A careful neurovascular assessment must be performed to rule out complications of forearm fractures, including nerve injury and compartment syndrome. If an athlete complains of both elbow and wrist pain with an isolated ulna fracture, a dislocated radial head should be ruled out. Those with a distal radius fracture should be assessed for pain at the wrist to rule out distal radioulnar joint injury.

X-rays of the forearm should be assessed for alignment. Specifically, on a true lateral, a line drawn along the anterior aspect of the humerus (anterior humeral line) should pass through the anterior third of the capitellum. Similarly, a line drawn through the head of the radius (radiocapitellar line) should intersect the capitellum (49).

Although treatment of forearm fractures in adults is operative, pediatric forearm fractures are usually treated conservatively (50). Uncomplicated forearm fractures can be immobilized with a short arm cast. If reduction is necessary, gentle longitudinal traction and the opposite force from the mechanism of injury are typically applied. The radial head usually dislocates laterally or anteriorly in young athletes, and can be reduced with flexion, supination, and direct pressure (49). When acceptable reduction has been achieved, a sugar-tong splint can be applied around the fractured forearm to avoid the risk of developing compartment syndrome from bleeding. Once the acute swelling has ceased, treatment involves a long-arm cast, initially at approximately 110 degrees, to avoid rotation of the forearm, rather than using a short-arm cast. The forearm is casted in the neutral position, rather than in supination or pronation (51). Molding of the cast may be needed.

Open fractures, unstable fractures, and severely malaligned fractures require surgical attention. Advantages of open reduction with internal fixation are more stable and anatomic healing and the ability to start earlier range of motion, for example, in treating isolated lateral condyle fractures. If the angulation of the fracture is more than 10 degrees, it may require operative fixation to enable healing. Some angulation may be accepted, especially if there is growth remaining; however, rotational deformities have much less capacity for remodeling (51). Also, proximal radial and ulnar fractures have less potential for remodeling because the distal growth plates are responsible for over three quarters of the longitudinal growth of each bone (50). In Monteggia fractures, the ulnar fracture alignment should be restored for proper healing; the radioulnar joint congruency is usually addressed once the ulna is realigned.(49) Long-term complications after a Monteggia fracture include persistent valgus instability, cubitus valgus, elbow stiffness, and arthritis. A poorly treated Galeazzi fracture may result in chronic wrist pain, limited motion, and arthritis from ulnocarpal impaction. Plates used to repair a forearm fracture are best left in place, especially if the individual is involved in a contact sport (51).

Medial Epicondyle Avulsion

The medial epicondyle can avulse after acute valgus stress and/or sudden contraction of the flexor–pronator group. Medial humeral epicondyle fractures account for 12% of all elbow fractures that occur in children (52,53), Woods and Tullos have classified medial epicondyle avulsions into types 1, 2, and 3 (54). Type 1 fractures are described as large avulsions involving the whole epicondyle and affect athletes under age 14. These avulsions do not result in elbow instability. Type 2 injuries involve avulsion of the epicondyle and the anterior band of the UCL. Type 3 injuries are fragments smaller than the epicondyle and usually occur in the adolescent athlete.

Nonoperative treatment typically involves casting for 2–3 wk at 90 degrees, followed by protected motion with a hinge brace for at least 6 wk. Current recommendations for surgical treatment include fragment displacement greater than 2 mm, valgus instability greater than 3 mm, entrapment of the fragment in the joint, and ulnar nerve dysfunction (55). Displacement of the fragment into the joint usually occurs when the elbow also dislocates. Surgical treatment of adolescent athletes, consisting of open reduction internal fixation (ORIF) and early range of motion after 4 d with a brace ($n = 8$), has been successful with full return to sports and no valgus stress instability (45,56). Josefsson and Nilsson have reported on long-term follow-up of conservatively treated patients with medial epicondyle fractures. They found that 31 out of 35 healed with fibrous nonunion with good function and range of motion (45). Similarly, in a long-term retrospective study from Italy, 42 patients with medial epicondyle fractures with displacement between 5 and 15 mm, which occurred between 8 and 15 yr of age, were followed for an average of 34 yr after injury (52). They reported that 16 out of 19 patients who were treated conservatively with casting at 90 degrees for 4 wk demonstrated good results and function, which was similar to ORIF and better than excision.

Chronic / Atraumatic Injuries

"Little League Elbow"

"Little leaguer's elbow" is a term that has been misrepresented throughout the literature, as it has been applied to medial apophysitis, osteochondritis dissecans (OCD), Panner's disease, and any other elbow pain in a young thrower. The use of this term should be avoided and the specific diagnosis should be used. Classically, Little Leaguer's elbow is a medial apophyseal injury that affects young baseball players, usually pitchers, around 9–12 yr of age (57). A study done in 1965 showed abnormal changes in the radiographic appearance of the elbows of 80 California Little League pitchers aged 9–14 yr, with 39 elbows (49%) reported to demonstrate medial epicondylar apophyseal fragmentation (58). Hutchinson and Wynn reported that 4–12% of young baseball pitchers had a mild flexion contracture, and that 3–37% had a valgus deformity (1). Excessive, repetitive throwing at an early age is felt to be the cause of these changes. As the adolescent throwing athlete matures, the forces generated by the upper extremity can lead to overuse injuries. During the cocking and acceleration phases of throwing, the ulnar collateral ligament sustains high-tension valgus stress, whereas a compressive force is applied over the radial head and capitellum (1). Medial epicondyle apophysitis or avulsion, radial head hypertrophy, or avascular changes in the capitellum (osteochondritis dissecans) are adaptational or pathological changes that occur in the immature elbow (1,4).

Osteochondritis Dissecans of the Capitellum

Osteochondritis dissecans is a progressive form of osteochondrosis of the capitellum involving focal injury to subchondral bone. leading to a loss of structural support for the overlying articular cartilage (22). OCD typically affects the dominant extremity of adolescents and young adults with onset of symptoms between 11 and 16 yr of age. Most cases are seen in high-level athletes who experience repetitive valgus stress and lateral compression across the elbow (overhead-throwing athletes, gymnasts, weight lifters) (21,31,59,60). The lesion only affects a portion of the capitellum. Loose bodies and articular surface deformation can develop (61).

The etiology of OCD is unclear. Most authors believe that repetitive microtrauma in the setting of a tenuous blood supply is the primary mechanism of injury (12,62,63). Genetic factors, trauma, and ischemia have also been proposed (59,60,64). The histopathology of OCD is consistent with findings of subchondral bone osteonecrosis (22,62).

Patients typically present with a gradual onset of lateral elbow pain and flexion contracture in the affected arm, more often the dominant one. The pain is intermittent, aggravated by activity, and relieved by rest. Elbow swelling may develop, as well as locking, popping, and catching of the elbow as loose bodies form. On physical exam, there may be tenderness to palpation and crepitus over the radiocapitellar joint. Loss of 10–20 degrees of extension is common, and mild loss of flexion and forearm rotation may also be seen (21,31,62).

Characteristic plain film findings of elbow OCD include a focal area of radiolucency and rarefaction in the subchondral bone in the anterior aspect of the capitellum (Figure 8.7). Early OCD can appear as flattening of the capitellum without fragmentation, typically in children around

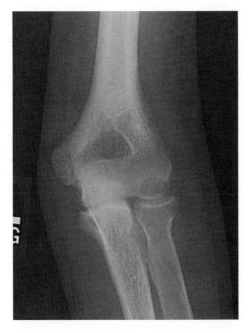

FIGURE 8.7. Osteochondritis dissecans of the capitellum in a 15-yr-old baseball pitcher.

11 yr of age (65). More advanced and/or older lesions become fragmented (65), may have a sclerotic border, or demonstrate loose bodies on radiographs.

The preferred method in the evaluation of OCD lesions is MRI because it is both sensitive and specific (61). It demonstrates the extent of the OCD lesion more accurately, and it also identifies loose bodies that may not be seen on plain film, as well as the integrity of the articular cartilage overlying the area of bony rarefaction, helping dictate treatment. CT scans can also help define bony anatomy and identify loose bodies. Bone scintigraphy is very sensitive for identifying osteoblastic activity or increased vascularity at the site of an OCD lesion; however, it is nonspecific and is less useful in diagnosis (31). Ultrasonography can also facilitate the assessment of capitellar lesions (66). Although there is no universal classification system, Baumgarten et al. have proposed an arthroscopic classification of OCD lesions (Table 8.1).

The prognosis of OCD of the capitellum and the choice of conservative or surgical management depend on the patient's age and the severity of the original lesion (31), as determined by symptoms, size of the lesion, and stage of the lesion; specifically, the integrity of the cartilage surface. To provide the best outcome, early detection and appropriate treatment are

TABLE 8.1. Classification of osteochondritis lesions of the elbow.

Grade	Arthroscopic findings	Treatment
Grade 1	Smooth but soft, ballottable articular cartilage.	If symptomatic, undergo drilling.
Grade 2	Fibrillations or fissuring of the articular cartilage.	Lesions not responding to nonoperative treatment should undergo removal of all affected cartilage back to a "stable" rim and then abrasion chondroplasty of the underlying bone.
Grade 3	Exposed bone with a fixed osteochondral fragment.	Removal of the osteochondral fragment and abrasion chondroplasty.
Grade 4	Loose but undisplaced fragment.	Removal of the osteochondral fragment and abrasion chondroplasty.
Grade 5	Displaced fragment with resultant loose bodies.	Abrasion chondroplasty of the exposed crater with diligent search of the remaining elbow joint for loose bodies, which should be removed. Any associated osteophyte or synovitis in other elbow compartments should be removed. An early ROM and strengthening program should begin ASAP postoperatively.

Source: Adapted from Baumgarten TE, Andrews JR, Satterwhite YE. The arthroscopic classification and treatment of osteochondritis dissecans of the capitellum. Amer J Sports Med 26(4):520–523. Reprinted by permission of Sage Publications, Inc.

imperative. Small, nondisplaced lesions in younger athletes with intact articular cartilage on MRI are best managed conservatively with rest, ice, and NSAIDs, particularly if the bone scan demonstrates increased bony activity. Serial plain films should be obtained to follow resolution of disease. Unfortunately, many may not heal (12,67). Prevention through activity modification and education is an important and effective management strategy (21). Proper education of athletes, parents, and coaches about this problem is crucial, as development of a loose body from continued sports participation can lead to permanent symptoms and disability.

The prognosis for more advanced lesions and older athletes, particularly when the articular cartilage is not intact, the bone scan is cold, or if loose bodies are present, is less favorable. Even after 6mo of rest, 13 out of 24 athletes still had pain during activities (68). Indications for surgical treatment include persistent symptoms despite conservative management, symptomatic loose bodies, articular cartilage fracture, or displacement of the osteochondral lesion. The surgeon must assess the size, stability, and viability of the fragment and decide whether to remove the fragment or attempt to surgically reattach it. Most fragments cannot be reattached, and therefore are excised, followed by local debridement. Although symptoms usually improve, approximately half of all patients will continue to have chronic pain or limited range of motion, and many athletes are unable to return to their prior levels of competition (63,69,70). Arthroscopic abrasion chondroplasty or subchondral drilling may be performed to encourage healing (31,62,70,71). In advanced stage OCD, a case series of osteochondral autograft transplantation to repair the defect using bone cartilage plugs from nonweightbearing areas of the knee has been described, with subjective improvements postoperatively, although persistent irregularities were still demonstrated over the articular cartilage on MRI. Sixteen out of eighteen subjects were able to return to throwing activities by 2 yr (72).

Panner's Disease

Panner's disease is an osteochondrosis of the capitellum. Age, pain onset, and the radiographic appearance of the lesion help differentiate between Panner's disease and OCD (61). It is a self-limiting, benign process that involves the entire ossification center and commonly occurs in children between the ages of 4–10 yr old (73). The dominant extremity is usually involved.

Children typically complain of several weeks of a vague, dull, aching pain over the lateral elbow of the dominant extremity that is exacerbated by activity and relieved by rest (21,22,31,62). On physical exam, there is usually a 10–20-degree loss of extension and maximal palpation tenderness over the radiocapitellar joint. Edema and effusion are rare (22). Typical radiographic findings in Panner's disease include demineralization of the capitellum with poorly defined cortical margins, fissuring, and/or fragmentation of the entire capitellum (74). Abnormal development of the radial head may also be observed. CT is occasionally helpful to further define bony pathology. MRI is very sensitive and useful in the early detection of Panner's disease (21,23). Follow-up plain films show healing with consolidation, but persistent flattening of the capitellum may occur.

Treatment is conservative and involves rest, activity modification, avoidance of valgus stress, maintenance of range of motion, ice, and nonsteriodal antiinflammatory drugs (NSAIDs). A prolonged period of healing of up to 3 yr is common. Long-term clinical and radiographic results are excellent. In most patients, there is no long-term sequelae or residual deformity (31).

Medial Apophysitis

Repetitive valgus overload can lead to microtrauma in the apophysis of the medial epicondyle. Athletes will present with medial elbow pain or decreased throwing velocity. They may present with or without flexion elbow contracture. Where adults would suffer from UCL injury, physeal injuries occur in young overhead or throwing athletes. Radiographs may show some widening of the medial apophysis or fragmentation of the epicondyle. These changes can best be delineated by comparing with contralateral elbow radiographs. Bone scan and MRI will demonstrate changes over the medial apophysis representing stress injury or possible stress fracture. Treatment usually involves relative rest from valgus loading activities such as throwing. Antiinflammatories and ice are commonly used, though long-term evidence of benefit is not available. Nondisplaced stress injuries to the medial epicondyle respond well to conservative treatment, with no functional deficits (4).

Ulnar Collateral Ligament Injury

Ulnar collateral ligament injuries of the elbow are less common in the adolescent athlete (75). When the growth plate is no longer the weakest link, repetitive valgus stress can produce tensile forces on the medial elbow, leading to microtrauma of the UCL. Factors leading to overuse include velocity, power, and the repetitious nature of the throwing motion (7,76). Pain during the acceleration phase of throwing, pain at ball release during delivery, or pain at point of impact when hitting a baseball are the common complaints (77). Because of the chronic nature of UCL instability, patients may also present with symptoms of ulnar nerve irritation or loose bodies (7). Patients typically have point tenderness 2 cm distal to the medial epicondyle. Ecchymosis may develop in the medial joint line 2–3 d after an acute injury. Valgus loading stress maneuvers can demonstrate any ligament insufficiency.

Plain radiographs are needed to evaluate for possible medial epicondyle fracture and/or instability. A relatively increased widening of 2 mm or more at the medial joint space compared with the unaffected elbow on valgus stress AP radiographs is considered pathologic (22). Arthrography is helpful with an acute injury, but has limited usefulness in chronic UCL insufficiency. In one study of 25 adult baseball players, CT scan with intraarticular contrast was 86% sensitive and 91% specific for acute and chronic injuries to the UCL (78). MRI can also be useful in identifying a torn UCL (78–80); however, some radiologists prefer an MR arthrogram.

Nonoperative treatment consists of rest, antiinflammatory medication, and ice. After the pain is controlled, physical therapy should be initiated. Approximately 6 wk after the initial injury, the elbow should be reevaluated (22). In a study of 31 throwing athletes with an average age of 18 yr who had a UCL injury, 42% were able to return to their previous level of play at an average of 24.5 wk (13–54 wk) of conservative management (81).

For patients who continue to have pain with activity after 3 mo or more of rest and rehabilitation, referral to an orthopedic surgeon should be considered (22). In some cases, surgical UCL reconstruction has been performed, preferentially using autologous grafts of the palmaris longus or gracilis (7). Petty, Fleisig, and Cain suggest that indications for surgical treatment are more complex in the adolescent than in the adult, because teens tend to display more significant signs and symptoms related to a given injury and they have better healing potential. For these reasons they feel that conservative management has a higher chance of being effective in the adolescent than the adult for UCL injuries (76).

Posterior Impingement, Olecranon Stress Injury, and Apophysitis

Many sports require the elbow to forcefully extend to generate force, or to lock out to provide stability, leading to valgus extension overload. During throwing, the olecranon is loaded and can impinge in the olecranon fossa when the elbow is extended during acceleration and follow through (1). This is accentuated in the face of valgus laxity of the elbow. To stabilize the elbow with many gymnastics maneuvers, the elbow is often locked in extension. The olecranon can develop stress injury from impacting the olecranon fossa or from eccentric triceps traction forces (82–84). If a growth plate is present, widening may occur leading to apophysitis. Rarely, the epiphysis can acutely displace (82). Wilson has recommended radiographing the elbow at 110 degrees of flexion with the arm lying on the cassette, and the beam angled 45 degrees towards the ulna to better demonstrate osteophytes in the posteromedial elbow, which are commonly seen with valgus extension overload (13,83). MRI is the best test to identify degenerative changes, apophysitis, or developing stress fracture. Initial treatment is directed toward symptom control, activity modification, and physical therapy. If symptoms persist despite rest, arthroscopic debridement can be considered (71).

Treatment

Initial Management

Traumatic injuries, including fracture and dislocation, are treated initially by protecting the arm in a splint until it can be assessed by a physician or an orthopedic surgeon. A posterior splint can, ideally, keep the elbow at 90 degrees with the hand supinated, which is the position of function for the elbow. Emergency attention is required if there is neurovascular compromise, a joint dislocation, an open fracture, or a severely displaced and unstable fracture. As a rule of thumb, intraarticular fractures that involve more than a 2-mm step-off or displacement may require surgical management (12). A hinged brace is useful to protect the elbow from valgus instability, while allowing flexion and extension range of motion.

Physical Therapy

Physical therapy for the elbow is often directed towards protected early range of motion. After even severe trauma such as a dislocation, rehabilitation can be started immediately in a hinged cast-brace with the elbow in full pronation (41). Priest and Weise concluded that elbow immobilization for as short a time as possible was beneficial to regaining range of motion after dislocations in gymnasts (5). A randomized control trial with 43 patients showed that physical therapy helped improve motion at 12 and 18wk postoperatively in supracondylar fractures; however, it was not shown to demonstrate differences in motion at 1 yr (84). This suggests that physical therapy of the elbow can restore good range earlier in young patients. Low-load, long-duration stretches are suggested to improve motion (85). If athletes have a persistent flexion contracture and no other internal derangement or instability, a dynamic splint may be used to help increase range of motion (86).

Sport-specific exercise can be introduced once an adequate healing period has passed after injury or surgery. Wilk et al. start an early range of motion program, including joint mobilizations, followed by strengthening exercises. Throwing programs are often introduced by 6wk after injury, with a gradual sequence of progressive exercises involving different distances, resistances, coordination, and proprioceptive exercises (87).

Surgery

Arthroscopic surgery in the elbow, in the hands of an experienced surgeon, has a safe and effective role in the treatment of selective pathologies. In a series from 1979 to 1995, 49 elbow arthroscopies were performed for osteochondritis dissecans (58%), arthrofibrosis and joint contracture (20%), synovitis (10%), acute trauma (10%), and posterior olecranon impingement syndrome (70). Based on a modified Andrews elbow scoring system, 85% of patients had a good or excellent result, with 90% of the children returning to sports without limitation. Although no complications were reported in the mentioned series, potential complications, including nerve injuries, flexion contracture, and infection, have been identified after elbow arthroscopy in an adult population (88).

In general, surgical assessment is required for functional ligamentous instability; cartilage defects and intraarticular lesions, including loose bodies and OCD; displaced fractures; and injuries resulting in malformation causing persistent dysfunction. As a rule of thumb, fractures that have less than 2mm of displacement are treated nonoperatively (53,89).

Prevention

To avoid traumatic and overuse elbow injuries, proper technique in a given sport should be emphasized. In a biomechanical study, Fleisig et al. analyzed the throwing mechanics of youth, high school, college, and professional pitchers (2). He found that the increases in joint forces and torques were most likely caused by increased strength and muscle mass in the higher level athlete. The greater shoulder and elbow angular velocities produced by high-level pitchers were most likely caused by the greater torques they generated during the arm cocking and acceleration phases. The valgus torque around the elbow is closely correlated with the throwing athlete's weight ($r = 0.79$) (3). The other kinetic factors that were associated with elbow torque are maximum shoulder abduction torque and maximum internal rotation torque (3). Younger pitchers often take a shorter stride and drop the elbow, leading to less velocity overall for the pitch. This may force the athlete to "use more arm" to improve the speed. Thus, it appears that the natural progression for successful pitching is to learn proper mechanics as early as possible, and build strength as the body matures (2).

Modifying training risk factors, especially the type and volume of activity, is useful. In a prospective, descriptive cohort study, Lyman et al. studied 472 pitchers ages 9–14 over 1 season in Alabama (90). Their study tools included pre- and postseason questionnaires, injury and performance interviews after each game, pitch count logs, and video analysis of pitching mechanics. They determined that there was an increase in elbow and shoulder injuries with cumulative pitch count over 600 pitches per season. Breaking pitches and high pitch counts were risk factors for injuries. The 13 and 14 yr old pitchers had 3 times the number of elbow injuries when throwing the slider (OR 3.49; $p < 0.01$) (90).

Training volume and activities are important to discuss with the athlete, parents, and coaches to identify if there are any training errors or areas that can be modified. Rules should be enforced by referees and coaches, to avoid reckless play and dangerous training practices. For gymnastics, Priest and Weise recommend employing spotters, using thicker mats, and educating young gymnasts in techniques of falling (5). For throwing sports, coaches should emphasize proper pitching mechanics to optimize power from the lower part of the body and to align the upper extremity properly to decrease valgus stress on the elbow.

Specific recommendations have been made for young baseball players. Experts recommend that adolescent baseball players should not throw more than 80 pitches a game, should not participate in more than 8 mo of competition per year, and should limit their total number of pitches in competition to 2,500 per year (91). Throwing breaking pitches should not be started until after 13 yr of age (91). At least 3 d of rest is recommended between outings to allow adequate recovery and to avoid fatigue. As recommendations continue to be refined, activity recommendations, including pitching, should be made based on physical maturity of the athlete rather than chronological age, because the onset of puberty varies widely, and strength and flexibility are based more on physical maturity rather than age (92) .

During the preparticipation physical exam, suggestions to improve strength and flexibility in joints in the kinetic chain may help prevent injuries. A GIRD from tightness of the posterior shoulder capsule can often cause shoulder problems in throwing athletes, which subsequently move down the chain to affect the elbow. High-school pitchers were also noted to have stronger internal rotators on the dominant versus the nondominant arm during isokinetic strength testing (93,94). In these overhead athletes, a proper conditioning program should target stretching the shoulder and elbow, including posterior shoulder capsule stretching, and strengthening of the rotator cuff and periscapular stabilizers.

Return to Play Guidelines

An athlete should have full, pain-free range of motion before returning to sports. The athlete should be returned gradually, with limited activities early on. After surgery, not all athletes will return to their sport, depending on the type and severity of injury. After ulnar collateral ligament surgery in high school baseball players, 20 out of 27 athletes returned to play after approximately 11 mo (76). Return to play with OCD and intraarticular lesions is difficult to determine. Radiographic healing is ideal, though not always possible. The athlete should be completely asymptomatic with all activity, especially if they are overhead athletes, before returning to play. After trauma to the elbow, such as dislocation or fracture, the athlete will most likely not resume upper extremity training for at least 3 mo, with full activities expected at approximately 6 mo. With most elbow soft tissue injuries and nonoperative problems, adolescent athletes recover well after an adequate period of healing.

Clinical Pearls

- Elbow pain in the adolescent athlete deserves careful attention.
- Reproducing the mechanisms that produce symptoms through physical exam maneuvers or by having them perform pushups or throwing will help identify the problem.
- Elbow tendinopathies can still occur from overtraining, but they are much less common in adolescents than adults.
- If the adolescent athlete has persistent, reproducible pain within the elbow, osteochondritis dissecans should be ruled out. MRI can be useful to help stage the OCD lesion to determine treatment.

- When there is a history of trauma and an effusion in the elbow, a dislocation or occult fracture, especially involving the radial head, should be suspected.
- In fractures of the radius and ulna, carefully examine the proximal and distal radioulnar joints to rule out complex fractures.
- With almost all elbow injuries, the athlete should begin protected motion early, at the latest by 3 wk, to avoid excessive stiffness.
- Forced range of motion after trauma is discouraged in physical therapy to avoid heterotopic ossification.
- Any apophyseal avulsion or fracture with more than 2 mm of displacement is more concerning and should be evaluated by an orthopedic surgeon familiar with elbow problems.
- Fortunately, there can be good healing potential and remodeling for elbow injuries in young patients with open growth plates.

References

1. Hutchinson MR, Wynn S. Biomechanics and development of the elbow in the young throwing athlete. Clin Sports Med 2004;23:531–544.
2. Fleisig GS, Barrentine SW, Zheng N, Escamilla RF, Andrews JR. Kinematic and kinetic comparison of baseball pitching among various levels of development. J Biomech 1999;32:1371–1375.
3. Sabick MB, Torry MR, Lawton RL, Hawkins RJ. Valgus torque in youth baseball pitchers: A biomechanical study. J Shoulder Elbow Surg 2004;13:349–355.
4. Gugenheim Jr, JJ, Stanley RF, Woods GW, Tullos HS. Little League survey: the Houston study. Am J Sports Med 1976;4:189–200.
5. Priest JD, Weise DJ. Elbow injury in women's gymnastics. Am J Sports Med 1981;9:288–295.
6. Snook GA. Injuries in women's gymnastics. A 5-year study. Am J Sports Med 1979;7:242–244.
7. Safran, M. Ulnar collateral ligament injury in the overhead athlete: diagnosis and treatment. Clin Sports Med 2004;23:643–663.
8. Gosheger G, Liem D, Ludwig K, Greshake O, Winkelmann W. Injuries and overuse syndromes in golf. Am J Sports Med 2003;31:438–443.
9. Cooper C, Dennison EM, Leufkens HG, Bishop N, van Staa TP. Epidemiology of childhood fractures in Britain: a study using the general practice research database. J Bone Miner Res 2004;19:1976–81.
10. Cain EL, Jr., Dugas JR, Wolf RS, Andrews JR. Elbow injuries in throwing athletes: a current concepts review. Am J Sports Med 2003;31:621–635.
11. Beighton P, Solomon L, Soskolne CL. Articular mobility in an African population. Ann Rheum Dis 1973;32:413–418.
12. Do T, Herrera-Soto J. Elbow injuries in children. Curr Opin Pediatr 2003; 15:68–73.
13. Difelice GS, Meunier MJ, Paletta Jr. GA. Elbow injury in the adolescent athlete. In: Altchek DW, Andrews JR, eds. The Athlete's Elbow. Philadelphia: Lippincott Williams & Wilkins; 2001:231–248.

14. Morrey BF. Anatomy of the elbow joint. In: Morrey BF, ed. The Elbow and Its Disorders. Philadelphia: Saunders; 2000:13–42.
15. O'Driscoll SW, Bell DF, Morrey BF. Posterolateral rotatory instability of the elbow: clinical and radiographic features. J Bone Joint Surg 1991;73A:440–446.
16. Olsen BS, Sojbjerg JO, Nielsen KK, Vaesel MT, Dalstra M, Sneppen O. Posterolateral elbow joint instability: the basic kinematics. J Shoulder Elbow Surg 1998;7:19–29.
17. Safran MR, Baillargeon D. Soft-tissue stabilizers of the elbow. J Shoulder Elbow Surg 2005;14:179S–185S.
18. Safran MR, McGarry MH, Shin S, Han S, Lee TQ. Effects of elbow flexion and forearm rotation on valgus laxity of the elbow. J Bone Joint Surg Am 2005;87:2065–2074.
19. Cohen MS, Hastings H, 2nd. Rotatory instability of the elbow. The anatomy and role of the lateral stabilizers. J Bone Joint Surg Am 1997:79(2):225–233.
20. Keefe DT, Lintner DM. Nerve injuries in the throwing elbow. Clin Sports Med 2004;23:723–742.
21. Busch M. Sports medicine in children and adolescents. In: Morrissy RT, Weinstein SW, eds. Lovell and Winter's Pediatric Orthopaedics. Philadelphia: Lippincott Williams & Wilkins; 2001:1287–1289.
22. Rudzki JR, Galetta PA, Jr. Juvenile and adolescent elbow injuries in sports. Clin Sports Med 2004;23:581–608.
23. Stoane JM, Poplausku MR, Haller JO, Berdon WE. Panner's disease: X-ray, MR imaging findings and review of the literature. Comput Med Imaging Graphics 1996;19:473–476.
24. Haraldsson S. On osteochondrosis deformas juvenilis capituli humeri including investigation of intra-osseous vasculature in distal humerus. Acta Orthop Scand 1959;Suppl 38:1–232.
25. Safran MR. Elbow injuries in athletes. A review. Clin Orthop Relat Res 1995;310:257–277.
26. Morrey BF. Biomechanics of the elbow and forearm. In: DeLee JC, Drez Jr. D, Miller MD, eds. DeLee & Drez's Orthopaedic Sports Medicine. Philadelphia: Elsevier Science; 2003:1213–1220.
27. Mihata T, Safran MR, McGarry MH, Abe M, Lee TQ. Effect of Humeral Rotation On Elbow Valgus Laxity: Cadaveric Study. Presented at the 5th Annual Meeting of the International Society of Ligament and Tendons, Washington, D.C., February 19, 2005.
28. O'Driscoll SWLR, Smith AM: The "moving valgus stress test" for medial collateral ligament tears of the elbow. Am J Sport Med 2005;33:231–239.
29. Shaw JL, O'Connor FG. Elbow injuries. In: Birrer RB, Griesemer BA, Cataletto MB, eds. Pediatric Sports Medicine for Primary Care. Philadelphia: Lippincott Williams & Wilkins; 2002:350–366.
30. O'Driscoll SW. Classification and evaluation of recurrent instability of the elbow. Clin Orthop 2000;370:34–43.
31. Kobayashi KBK, Rodner C, Smith B, Caputo AE. Lateral compression injuries in the pediatric elbow: Panner's disease and osteochondritis dissecans of the capitellum. J Am Acad Orthop Surg 2004;12:246–254.

32. Kibler WB, Sciascia A. Kinetic chain contributions to elbow function and dysfunction in sports. Clin Sports Med 2004;23:545–552.
33. Kibler WB, Chandler TJ. Range of motion in junior tennis players participating in a risk modification program. J Sci Med Sports 2003;5:51–52.
34. Kissoon N, Galpin R, Gayle M, Chacon D, Brown T. Evaluation of the role of comparison radiographs in the diagnosis of traumatic elbow injuries. J Pediatr Orthop 1995;15:449–453.
35. Chacon D, Kissoon N, Brown T, Galpin R. Use of comparison radiographs in the diagnosis of traumatic injuries of the elbow. Ann Emerg Med 1992;21:895–899.
36. Skaggs DL, Mirzayan R. The posterior fat pad sign in association with occult fracture of the elbow in children. J Bone Joint Surg Am 1999;81:1429–433.
37. Pudas T, Hurme T, Mattila K, Svedstrom E. Magnetic resonance imaging in pediatric elbow fractures. Acta Radiol 2005;46:636–644.
38. Schwartz ML, Al-Zahrani S, Morwessel RM, et al. Ulnar collateral ligament injury in the throwing athlete: Evaluation with saline-enhanced MR arthrography. Radiology 1995;197:297–299.
39. Sofka CM, Potter HG. Imaging of elbow injuries in the child and adult athlete. Radiol Clin North Am 2002;40:251–65.
40. Lazar RD, Waters PM, Jaramillo D. The use of ultrasonography in the diagnosis of occult fracture of the radial neck. A case report. J Bone Joint Surg Am 1998;80:1361–4.
41. O'Driscoll SW, Morrey BF, Korinek S, An KN. Elbow subluxation and dislocation. A spectrum of instability. Clin Orthop 1992;280:186–197.
42. Price CT, Phillips JH, Devito DP. Management of fractures. In: Morrissy RT, Weinstein SL, eds. Lovell and Winter's Pediatric Orthopaedics. Philadelphia: Lippincott Willians & Wilkins; 2001:1338–1356.
43. de las Heras J, Duran D, de la Cerda J, Romanillos O, Martinez-Miranda J, Rodriquez-Merchan EC. Supracondylar fractures of the humerus in children. Clin Orthop 2005;432:57–64.
44. Rasool M. Dislocations of the elbow in children. J Bone Joint Surg Br 2003;86:1050–1058.
45. Josefsson PO, Nilsson BE. Incidence of elbow dislocation. Acta Orthop Scand 1986;57:537–538.
46. Thompson GH. Dislocations of the elbow. In: Beaty JH, Kasser JR, eds. Rockwood and Wilkins' Fractures in Children. Philadelphia: Lippincott Williams & Wilkins; 2001:530–562.
47. Sanchez-Sotelo J, Morrey BF, O'Driscoll SW. Ligamentous repair and reconstruction for posterolateral rotatory instability of the elbow. J Bone Joint Surg Br 2005;87:54–61.
48. Singleton SB, Conway JE. PLRI: posterolateral rotatory instability of the elbow. Clin Sports Med 2004;23:629–642.
49. Ring D, Jupiter JB, Waters PM. Monteggia Fractures in Children and Adults. J Am Acad Orthop Surg 1998;6:215–224.
50. Noonan KJ, Price CT. Forearm and distal radius fractures in children. J Am Acad Orthop Surg 1998;6:146–156.
51. Rodriguez-Merchan EC. Pediatric fractures of the forearm. Clin Orthop Relat Res 2005;432:65–72.

52. Farsetti P, Potenza V, Caterini R, Ippolito E. Long-term results of treatment of fractures of the medial humeral epicondyle in children. J Bone Joint Surg Am 2001;83-A:1299–305.

53. Wilkins KE. Fractures involving the medial epicondylar apophysis. In: Rockwood CA Jr., Wilkins KE, King RE, eds. Fractures in Children. 3rd ed. Philadelphia: JB Lippincott; 1991:509–828.

54. Woods GW, Tullos HS. Elbow instability and medial epicondyle fractures. Am J Sports Med 1977;5:23–30.

55. Hugheds PE, Paletta GA, Jr. Little Leaguer's Elbow, medial epicondyle injury and osteochondritis dissecans. Sports Med Arthroscopy Review 2003;11: 30–39.

56. Case SL, Hennrikus WL. Surgical treatment of displaced medial epicondyle fractures in adolescent athletes. Am J Sports Med 1997;25:682–686.

57. D'Hemecourt PD, Micheli LJ. In: Chan KM, Micheli LJ, eds. Sports and children. Hong Kong: Williams and Wilkins Asia; 1998:4.

58. Adams JE. Injury to the throwing arm. A study of traumatic changes in the elbow joints of boy baseball players. Calif Med 1965;102:127–132.

59. Baumgarten TE, Andrews JR, Satterwhite YE. The arthroscopic classification and treatment of osteochondritis dissecans of the capitellum. Am J Sports Med 1998;26:520–523.

60. Kandemir U, Fu FH, McMahon PJ. Elbow injuries. Current Opin Rheumatol 2002;14:160–167.

61. Bowen RE, Otsuka NY, Yoon ST, Lang P. Osteochondral lesions of the capitellum in pediatric patients: role of magnetic resonance imaging. J Pediatr Orthop 2001;21:298–301.

62. Stubbs MJ, Field LD, Savoie FH 3rd. Osteochondritis dissecans of the elbow. Clin Sports Med 2001;20:1–9.

63. Chen FS, Diaz VA, Loebenberg M, Rosen JE. Shoulder and elbow injuries in the skeletally immature athlete. J Am Acad Orthop Surg 2005;13:172–185.

64. Rudzki JR, Paletta GA, Jr. Juvenile and adolescent elbow injuries in sports. Clin Sports Med 2004;23:581–608.

65. Takahara M, Ogino T, Takagi M, Tsuchida H, Orui H, Nambu T. Natural progression of osteochondritis dissecans of the humeral capitellum: initial observations. Radiology 2000;216:207–212.

66. Takahara M, Ogino T, Tsuchida H, Takagi M, Kashiwa H, Nambu T: Sonographic assessment of osteochondritis dissecans of the humeral capitellum. AJR Am J Roentgenol 2000;174:411–415.

67. Takahara M, Ogino T, Fukushima S, Tsuchida H, Kaneda K. Nonoperative treatment of osteochondritis dissecans of the humeral capitellum. Am J Sports Med 1999;27:728–32.

68. Takahara M, Ogino T, Sasaki I, Kato H, Minami A, Kaneda K. Long term outcome of osteochondritis dissecans of the humeral capitellum. Clin Orthop Relat Res 1999;363:108–115.

69. Ruch DS, Cory JW, Poehling GG. The arthroscopic management of osteochondritis dissecans of the adolescent elbow. Arthroscopy 1998;14:797–803.

70. Micheli LJ, Luke AC, Mintzer CM, Waters PM. Elbow arthroscopy in the pediatric and adolescent population. Arthroscopy 2001;17:694–699.

71. McManama BG, Micheli LJ, Berry MV, Sohn RS. The surgical treatment of osteochondritis of the capitellum. Am J Sports Med 1985;13:11–21.

72. Yamamoto Y, Ishibashi Y, Tsuda E, Sato H, Toh S. Osteochondral Autograft Transplantation for Osteochondritis Dissecans of the Elbow in Juvenile Baseball Players: Minimum 2-Year Follow-up. Am J Sports Med 2005;34: 714–720.
73. Woodward AH, Bianco AJ, Jr. Osteochondritis dissecans of the elbow. Clin Orthop Relat Res 1975;110:35–41.
74. Kaeding CC, Whitehead R. Musculoskeletal injuries in adolescents. Prim Care 1998;25:211–213.
75. Ireland ML, Andrews JR. Shoulder and elbow injuries in the young athlete. Clin Sports Med 1988;7:473–494.
76. Petty DH, Andrews JR, Fleisig GS, Cain EL. Ulnar collateral ligament reconstruction in high school baseball players: Clinical results and injury risk factors. Am J Sports Med 2004;32:1158–1164.
77. Conway JE, Jobe FW, Glousman RE, Pink M. Medial instability of the elbow in throwing athletes: treatment by repair or reconstruction of the ulnar collateral ligament. J Bone Joint Surg Am 1992;74:67–83.
78. Timmerman LA, Schwartz ML, Andrews JR. Preoperative evaluation of the ulnar collateral ligament by magnetic resonance imaging and computed tomography arthrography: evaluation in 25 baseball players with surgical confirmation. Am J Sports Med 1994;22:26–31.
79. Sugimoto H, Ohsawa T. Ulnar collateral ligament in the growing elbow: MR imaging of normal development and throwing injuries. Radiology 1994;192: 417–422.
80. Mirowitz SA, London SL. Ulnar collateral ligament injury in baseball pitchers: MR imaging evaluation. Radiology 1992;185:573–576.
81. Rettig AC, Sherrill C, Snead DS, Mendler JC, Mieling P. Nonoperative treatment of ulnar collateral ligament injuries in throwing athletes. Am J Sports Med 2001;29:15–17.
82. Ahmad CS, ElAttrache NS. Valgus extension overload syndrome and stress injury of the olecranon. Clin Sports Med 2004;23:665–676.
83. Wilson FD, Andrews JR, Blackburn TA. Valgus extension overload in the pitching elbow. Am J Sports Med 1983;11:83–88.
84. Keppler P, Salem K, Schwarting B, Kinzl L. The effectiveness of physiotherapy after operative treatment of supracondylar humeral fractures in children. J Pediatr Orthop 2005;25:314–316.
85. Kottke FJ, Pauley DL, Ptak RA. The rationale for prolonged stretching for correction of shortening of connective tissue. Arch Phys Med Rehabil 1966;47:345–352.
86. Green DP, McCoy H. Turnbuckle orthotic correction of elbow-flexion contractures after acute injuries. J Bone Joint Surg Am 1979;61:1092–1095.
87. Wilk KE, Reinold MM, Andrews JR. Rehabilitation of the thrower's elbow. Clin Sports Med 2004;23:765–801.
88. Kelly EW, Morrey BF, O'Driscoll SW. Complications of elbow arthroscopy. J Bone Joint Surg Am 2001;83-A;1:25–34.
89. Schmittenbecher, PP. What must we respect in articular fractures in childhood? Injury, 2005;36: SA35–SA43.
90. Lyman S, Fleisig GS, Andrews JR, Osinski ED. Effect of pitch type, pitch count, and pitching mechanics on risk of elbow and shoulder pain in youth baseball players. Am J Sports Med 2002;30(4):463–468.

91. Olsen SJ, 2nd, Fleisig GS, Dun S, Loftice J, Andrews JR. Risk factors for shoulder and elbow injuries in adolescent baseball pitchers. Am J Sports Med 2006;34:905–912.
92. Pratt M. Strength, flexibility, and maturity in adolescent athletes. Am J Dis Child 1989;143:560–563.
93. Mulligan IJ, Biddington WB, Barnhart BD, Ellenbecker TS. Isokinetic profile of shoulder internal and external rotators of high school aged baseball pitchers. J Strength Cond Res 2004;18:861–866.
94. Hinton RY. Isokinetic evaluation of shoulder rotational strength in high school baseball pitchers. Am J Sports Med 1988;16:274–279.

9
Injuries to the Wrist, Hand, and Fingers

Donald S. Bae

Wrist and hand injuries in the adolescent athlete present many unique challenges for treating physicians, therapists, trainers, and coaches. The spectrum of injuries, varying degrees of acuity and chronicity, and involvement of multiple anatomic systems (e.g., bone, ligament, tendon, and nerve) add to their complexity. Furthermore, injuries to the adolescent athlete must be managed in the context of continued musculoskeletal growth and development. The use of protective and/or assistive devices (e.g., tape, braces, splints, and casts), timing of return-to-play, and postinjury performance expectations must be carefully weighed in the treatment of these injuries. Finally, the psychosocial and financial consequences of these injuries cannot be ignored.

The purpose of this chapter is to review the epidemiology, prevention, and treatment of common wrist and hand injuries in the young athlete. As a comprehensive review of all injuries is beyond the scope of this chapter, emphasis will be placed on acute traumatic injuries, and particular attention will be made to those injuries requiring specialized nonoperative and/or surgical treatment.

Epidemiology

Hand and wrist injuries are thought to comprise between 3 and 20% of all athletic injuries in this younger patient population (1–10). Indeed, several published studies have suggested that hand and wrist injuries are more common in children and adolescents than adult sports participants. Potential reasons for this include the following: increased sports participation in younger athletes; the increased popularity of "extreme" sports; the inherent inability of the musculoskeletal system in younger athletes to withstand the frequency or intensity of certain sport-specific activities; the use of age- or size-inappropriate equipment; and poor supervision, coaching, and/or athletic technique (11). Sprains are thought to be the most common injury sustained to the hand and wrist, comprising 20–50% of all injuries, followed by contusions (15–30%) and fractures (5–35%) (8,12).

The Athlete's Wrist and Hand

Ryu et al. have established that most adult activities of daily living can be performed with 40 degrees of wrist extension, 40 degrees of wrist flexion, a 40-degree arc of radial-ulnar deviation, and a 100-degree arc of forearm pronation/supination (13). However, greater ranges of wrist motion, force generation, and angular velocities are required for sports participation. Professional baseball pitchers, for example, require over 90 degrees of wrist flexion during the throwing motion (14). In Olympic-level tennis players, maximum angular velocities of 1,950 degrees/s have been recorded for wrist flexion (15). Average mechanical loads across the wrist during pommel horse exercises in high-level gymnasts have been recorded at two times body weight, with peak loading rates of up to 130 times the body weight per second during certain maneuvers (16,17). Similar observations have been made in other sports, highlighting the biomechanical demands placed upon the hand and wrist during athletic activity.

Anatomy

An understanding of anatomy is essential for proper diagnosis, treatment, and ultimate return to sports for athletes with hand and wrist injuries. A brief overview of this anatomy is provided here to serve as a framework for the subsequent discussion of specific injuries.

Twenty-nine bones comprise the hand and wrist. In addition to their osteology and radiographic appearance, awareness of the location of the physes is essential for appropriate care of athletic hand and wrist injuries (Figure 9.1). The physes of the phalanges are located proximally in the digits and the thumb, and the closure of the epiphyseal plates do not typically occur until 14–16yr of age. Conversely, the physes of the metacarpals, with the exception of the thumb, are located distally in the metacarpal neck region. The thumb metacarpal has its physis proximally, near the carpometacarpal joint.

The ossification centers of the carpal bones become radiographically apparent in a predictable pattern, beginning with the capitate at less than 1yr of age, and then proceeding sequentially to the hamate, triquetrum, lunate, scaphoid, trapezius, trapezoid, and pisiform. All ossification centers are visible radiographically by the 10th year of life. The distal radial and distal ulnar epiphyses become visible by 1 and 6–7yr of age, respectively. These physes close between the ages of 16–18yr, at the completion of skeletal growth.

Awareness of the appearance of these physeal zones will avoid confusion between these normal structures and possible fractures and bony injuries.

FIGURE 9.1. Bones of the hand. Anteroposterior radiographic image of the normal hand and wrist in a skeletally immature patient. Note the proximal locations of the phalangeal physes. The physes of the index, long, ring, and small finger metacarpals are distal, whereas the thumb metacarpal has a proximal physis. Courtesy of the Children's Orthopedic Surgery Foundation, Boston, MA.

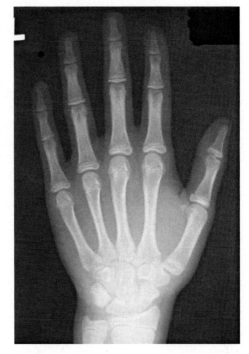

Furthermore, remodeling potential, or the capacity for bony deformity to correct with skeletal growth, is dependent on the amount of remaining growth, degree of deformity, and proximity of deformity to the adjacent physis. Knowledge of the physeal location, therefore, is essential to avoid false assumptions regarding bony healing after an acute injury.

In addition to the bony structures, joint stability in the hand and wrist is conferred by ligaments. At the interphalangeal joints, the collateral ligaments restrict excessive radial and ulnar deviation. These collaterals insert broadly on both the epiphysis and metaphysis, accounting for the infrequency in which avulsion fractures of the epiphysis occur. Conversely, at the metacarpophalangeal (MCP) joints, the collateral ligaments insert on the epiphysis of the more distal phalanx. For this reason, Salter–Harris III avulsion type fractures are much more common at the MCP joint level.

Similarly, wrist stability is imparted by several extrinsic and intrinsic ligaments, which help to stabilize the carpus and allow for the efficient transmission of forces across the wrist. Although a description of these ligamentous structures is beyond the scope of this chapter, special mention will be made regarding the triangular fibrocartilage complex in the ensuing text, owing to its frequent contribution to pain and functional limitations in the adolescent athlete.

Finally, there are a total of 25 extrinsic tendons that traverse the hand and wrist. These include three wrist flexors (flexor carpi radialis, palmaris longus, flexor carpi ulnaris), four wrist extensors (brachioradialis, extensor carpi radialis longus, extensor carpi radialis brevis, extensor carpi ulnaris), the thumb flexor and extensors (flexor pollicis longus, extensor pollicis longus, extensor pollicis brevis), extrinsic digital extensors (extensor digitorum comminus, extensor indicis proprius, extensor digiti quinti), extrinsic digital flexors (flexor digitorum profundus and superficialis), and the long thumb abductor (abductor pollicis longus). In addition to these musculotendinous units, there are 18 intrinsic muscles of the hand, including the thenar, hypothenar, lumbrical, interossei, and adductor pollicis muscles. Because of the number of musculotendinous units and the compensatory abilities of the hand, in cases of suspected injury, precise evaluation of isolated muscle function should be performed to rule out a complete tendon rupture or laceration. For example, when assessing for a possible flexor tendon injury in the finger, assessment of independent distal and proximal interphalangeal joint flexion must be made to check both flexor digitorum profundus and flexor digitorum superficialis integrity, respectively.

Clinical Evaluation

History

Treatment of any injury to the hand or wrist begins with a thorough history and physical examination. Background information, including hand dominance, type of sport(s) played, position and/or events, and level of performance, are critical to provide appropriate sport-specific care. Details of the exact mechanism of injury, including position of the hand or wrist, direction and magnitude of the applied force, and subsequent complaints of pain, weakness, and instability, will provide clues to the diagnosis. In the office setting, athletes should be asked regarding the initial on-field management of the injury in question, such as manipulation, reduction maneuvers, and splinting. Finally, inquiring whether the athlete was able to return immediately to practice or competition will provide insight on the severity of the injury.

Physical Exam

Inspection for the presence of swelling, ecchymosis, lacerations, abrasions, or wounds will help guide the examiner to the anatomic region of interest and rule out the possibility of an open fracture or dislocation. Careful palpation of all the anatomic structures in the zone of injury is essential. Musculoskeletal injuries hurt, and reproducible bony tenderness should be considered a fracture until otherwise proven. In addition to bony tenderness, all adjacent joints should be assessed for motion and stability. Finally, a comprehensive neurovascular examination is performed to assess for possible nerve or vascular injury.

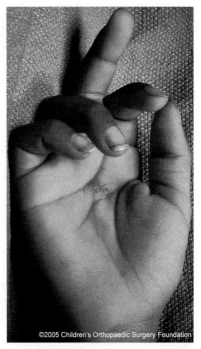

FIGURE 9.2. Clinical photograph depicting a patient with a flexor tendon injury to the long finger due to a traumatic laceration in the palm. Note is made of loss of tenodesis effect, resulting in an extended resting position of the affected digit in relation to the adjacent fingers.

©2005 Children's Orthopaedic Surgery Foundation

The presence of angular or rotational deformity should also raise suspicion for a bony or joint injury. The principle of tenodesis is helpful in these situations. In the normal hand and wrist, passive wrist extension results in obligate passive digital flexion, with all the fingers roughly parallel, pointing toward the scaphoid tubercle. In cases of rotational deformity through a fracture, the affected digit will overlap or underlap the adjacent fingers. After the same principles, in patients with a flexor tendon injury, the affected digit will not passively flex with the adjacent digits in the resting position or with passive wrist extension (Figure 9.2).

Plain radiographs should be obtained in the evaluation of any possible bony or joint injury. In addition to orthogonal views of the region in question, oblique radiographs will often identify bony injuries not readily apparent on anteroposterior (AP) or lateral projections. In cases of suspected carpal, articular, or ligamentous injury, additional magnetic resonance imaging (MRI) or computed tomography (CT) may be warranted; specific situations in which these studies are helpful are discussed below.

Wrist Injuries

Distal Radius Fractures

Distal radius fractures are among the most common injuries in skeletally immature patients, comprising between 20 and 35% of all childhood

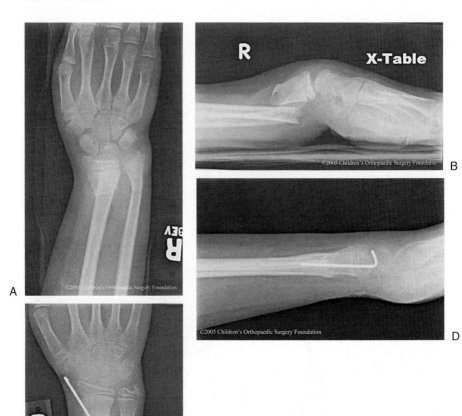

FIGURE 9.3. **(A and B)** Anteroposterior and lateral radiographs of a displaced distal radial metaphyseal fracture. **(C and D)** Anteroposterior and lateral radiographs after closed reduction and percutaneous pin fixation and subsequent bony healing. Courtesy of the Children's Orthopaedic Surgery Foundation, Boston, MA.

fractures (18–20). Approximately one third of these fractures involve the distal radial physis (21,22). With increases in sports participation among younger children, the incidence of forearm, wrist, and hand injuries has risen (11,23). Furthermore, recent analyses suggest that increased body weight may also be contributing to rising rates of pediatric forearm and wrist fractures (24,25).

Anatomy

The distal radial physis contributes approximately 80% of the longitudinal growth of the radius. For this reason, fractures of the distal radius have tremendous remodeling potential, and up to 10 degrees per year of dorsal-volar angulation may remodel with skeletal growth (26–29). In general, younger patients with fractures close to the physis in the plane of adjacent joint motion have the greatest remodeling potential. Rotational deformities, however, have limited remodeling potential. Based on these principles, 20–25 degrees of dorsal-volar angulation, 50% translational displacement, and 10 degrees of radial-ulnar deviation may be expected to remodel with continued skeletal growth in younger patients (less than 12 yr old). Conversely, older adolescents nearing skeletal maturity do not have the same remodeling capacity. In these older patients, treatment recommendations are made as would be for adults.

Clinical and Radiographic Evaluation

Patients will typically present with pain, swelling, and/or deformity of the affected wrist, typically after a fall onto the outstretched upper extremity. Plain radiographs will confirm the diagnosis and guide treatment. An understanding of the normal radiographic appearance of the skeletally immature hand and wrist is paramount (Figure 9.1). In general, the wrist, forearm, and elbow are imaged to rule out ipsilateral injuries of the affected limb.

Distal radius fractures are generally categorized according to their anatomic location, pattern of injury, and degree of displacement, angulation, and/or rotation. These injuries may occur at the distal radial metaphysis, involve the distal radial physis, or extend into the radiocarpal joint.

Management

Distal metaphyseal fractures in skeletally immature patients are generally divided into torus or bicortical fractures. Torus, or "buckle," fractures are characteristic injuries of childhood, owing to the increased porosity of metaphyseal bone during accelerated skeletal growth. Cortical failure occurs in compression, and as a result, these injuries are inherently stable. Immobilization in a short-arm cast or removable wrist splint for 3 wk provides adequate symptomatic relief and prevents further injury. Recent randomized prospective studies have demonstrated that true torus fractures may be effectively and safely treated with splint immobilization, which is removed by parents after 3 wk with no need for subsequent clinical or radiographic evaluation (30–33). Typically, there is little associated fracture displacement, and given the capacity for remodeling, fracture manipulation is not required.

Bicortical fractures of the distal radial metaphysis may occur because of bending, rotational, and/or shear forces sustained by the wrist during injury. Displaced fractures with unacceptable alignment may be treated with closed reduction and cast immobilization. Recent prospective randomized controlled trials have shown that a well-molded below-elbow cast is as effective as above-elbow casts in the treatment of displaced injuries (34,35). Athletes are allowed to return to sports after confirmation of fracture healing and return of motion and strength.

The published recommendations of what constitutes "acceptable" alignment are highly variable, and there continues to be discussion and controversy regarding the indications for fracture manipulation and surgical treatment. In general, most authorities agree that up to 20–25 degrees of angulation in the sagittal plane and translational displacement of up to 50% of the cortical diameter will reliably remodel and may be accepted in patients with greater than 2–3 yr of remaining skeletal growth. In older patients, up to 10 degrees of angulation in the sagittal plane and up to 10 degrees of radioulnar deviation may be accepted.

It is important to recognize, however, that late displacement after initial fracture reduction occurs in roughly one-third of cases (36–38). Inadequate reduction, poor casting techniques, resolution of soft-tissue swelling, muscle atrophy, and initial periosteal disruption have all been implicated as contributing factors. In skeletally mature patients, greater than 20 degrees of apex volar angulation, greater than 5 mm of radial shortening, comminution beyond the midaxial line, and intraarticular fracture extension have all been identified as radiographic predictors of fracture instability (39–42). If the resultant deformity is deemed unacceptable, intervention is warranted.

Current indications for surgical treatment include irreducible or unstable fractures, open fractures, "floating elbow injuries," neurovascular compromise, or soft-tissue swelling precluding circumferential cast immobilization. Percutaneous smooth pin fixation may be performed after closed reduction to maintain appropriate fracture alignment (Figure 9.3).

Some advocate percutaneous pin fixation for all displaced metaphyseal fractures in older children to avoid loss of reduction and need for remanipulation. However, pin fixation carries the concomitant risks of infection, neurovascular injury, and general anesthesia. Randomized, prospective studies comparing the two treatment methods cite similar complication rates and no significant outcomes differences (36,43).

The majority of distal radial physeal fractures are Salter–Harris type II fractures, and are amenable to closed reduction and cast immobilization. Closed reduction should be performed atraumatically with adequate analgesia and/or anesthesia. Because of concerns regarding iatrogenic physeal injury, repeated reduction attempts or attempts at late reduction (greater than 5–7 d from injury) are discouraged. Indications for surgical treatment include significant soft-tissue swelling or concomitant neurovascular compromise (e.g., compartment syndrome or acute carpal tunnel syndrome) precluding circumferential cast immobilization or intraarticular fractures with joint incongruity (e.g., Salter–Harris III fractures).

Scaphoid Fractures

The scaphoid is the most commonly injured carpal bone, comprising approximately 70–80% of all carpal fractures, and it is most commonly seen in young males in the second and third decades of life. Despite our increased awareness of the prevalence of these injuries, the diagnosis and treatment of scaphoid fractures remain challenging, due, in part, to its complex anatomy, tenuous vascular supply, and role in wrist biomechanics. Indeed, few injuries in the adolescent athlete provide as many diagnostic challenges, treatment options, and potential complications for the treating care provider.

Anatomy

The scaphoid has a complex three-dimensional shape, resembling a peanut that is twisted and bent (44). The majority of the scaphoid surface is covered by cartilage. For this reason, the vascularity of the scaphoid is imparted by a limited number of vessels. Seventy to eighty percent of the scaphoid's intraosseous vascularity, including the entire proximal pole, is provided by branches of the radial artery that enter the dorsal ridge of the scaphoid and travel in a retrograde fashion (45); 20–30%, in the region of the scaphoid tubercle, is supplied by volar radial artery branches. This vascular pattern accounts for the high predisposition for scaphoid nonunions and osteonecrosis of the proximal pole after fractures of the scaphoid waist.

With radial deviation of the wrist, the scaphoid moves with the proximal carpal row into flexion. Conversely, with ulnar deviation of the wrist, the scaphoid will extend. Displaced scaphoid fractures will result in abnormal wrist kinematics, allowing the distal pole to flex while the proximal pole extends. This results in apex dorsal and radial angulation of the scaphoid fracture, the so-called "humpback deformity (46)." Even with fracture healing, this flexion deformity will alter normal wrist kinematics, often leading to pain, stiffness, weakness, and progressive radiocarpal arthrosis (46–48). As a result, bony healing in anatomic alignment is critical for restoration of function.

Clinical Evaluation

Patients will typically present with radial-sided wrist pain after a fall onto an outstretched hand. Often, the clinical manifestations are subtle, demanding careful evaluation. In addition to a thorough physical examination, specific testing of the scaphoid should be performed. Tenderness may be elicited from palpation of the "anatomic snuffbox" or scaphoid tubercle. Axial loading the thumb across the carpometacarpal joint, the so-called "grind test," may also produce pain. The scaphoid compression test, in

TABLE 9.1. Radiographic evaluation of suspected scaphoid fractures.

Radiographic evaluation of suspected scaphoid fractures	Anteroposterior (AP) x-ray of wrist
	AP x-ray of wrist in ulnar deviation
	Lateral x-ray of wrist
	45 degrees pronated and supinated views
	CT or MRI
Radiographic findings in acute displaced scaphoid fractures	Fracture displacement >1–2 mm
	Scapholunate angle greater than 60 degrees on lateral view
	Radiolunate angle >10–15 degrees on lateral view
	Intrascaphoid angle >45 degrees
	Presence of "cortical ring sign" on AP view

which the examiner compresses the scaphoid between the proximal and distal poles with his/her thumb and index finger, may be the most accurate provocative sign on examination (49).

Radiographs

Appropriate radiographic imaging should be performed in all suspected cases of scaphoid fracture (Table 9.1). Routine anteroposterior (AP) and lateral plain radiographs of the wrist alone do not suffice. Because the scaphoid normally extends and lies more parallel to the plane of the hand with ulnar deviation of the wrist, an AP view in ulnar deviation should be obtained. Furthermore, the middle third of the scaphoid may be better visualized with a 45-degree semipronated view, whereas the dorsal ridge may be best seen on a semisupinated view (50). In addition to confirming the diagnosis, radiographs will identify fracture displacement, defined as a gap greater than 1–2 mm, a scapholunate angle greater than 60 degrees, a radiolunate angle greater than 10–15 degrees, or an intrascaphoid angle of greater than 45 degrees (46,51) (Table 9.1).

Plain radiographs may not always identify fractures, however. Treating physicians, trainers, and coaches are often confronted with a patient with radial wrist pain, but negative radiographs. Appropriate evaluation and treatment of these patients remains a subject of debate. Traditionally, patients with scaphoid tenderness but normal x-rays were treated for 1–2 wk in a thumb spica cast, followed by repeat plain radiographs to evaluate for possible bony injury. This approach has several limitations, particularly in the young, active working or athletic population. Unnecessary casting results in loss of work or sports participation, and repeat radiographs may not adequately visualize subtle injuries, particularly nondisplaced fractures.

Bone scintigraphy has been advocated in these situations; however, isotope scans may be positive in settings of synovitis or early arthrosis. In addition, bone scintigraphy will not provide information regarding bony anatomy, which is needed to make the appropriate treatment recommendations. For these reasons, early CT (Figure 9.4) or MRI is advocated to make the diagnosis and define the fracture pattern. Indeed, early studies suggest that MRI may be more cost effective than serial plain radiographs and cast immobilization, particularly in the younger athletic or working population (52,53). A diagnostic algorithm is proposed (Figure 9.5) for the evaluation of suspected scaphoid injuries.

Nonoperative Treatment

Cast immobilization will result in successful healing in over 90% of acute, nondisplaced scaphoid fractures. However, scaphoid fractures require longer periods of immobilization until bony union is achieved, and it is not uncommon for these injuries to take 8–12 wk to heal.

Methods of cast immobilization continue to be debated. Incorporation of the thumb into a spica cast has been advocated to eliminate forces across the scaphoid that may inhibit healing or cause displacement. Clay et al. performed a randomized prospective study of 392 patients comparing short-arm casting with or without a thumb spica component for the treatment of acute nondisplaced injuries (54). At the 6-mo follow-up, rates of bony healing did not differ between the two treatment groups. Immobilization of the elbow eliminates forearm rotation, which has previously been shown to cause scaphoid fracture motion (55). Gellman et al. performed a prospective randomized study comparing long- versus short-arm thumb spica casting for the treatment of acute nondisplaced scaphoid waist fractures (56). Patients treated with long-arm casts for the first 6 wk have a faster healing time (9.5 vs. 12.7 wk) and lower nonunion and delayed union rate than those treated with short-arm casts alone. Finally, several biomechanical and clinical studies have evaluated the effect of wrist position on scaphoid healing during casting. Arguments have been made for wrist extension, wrist flexion, and radial and ulnar deviation. Hambidge et al. performed a prospective, randomized study comparing cast immobilization in 20 degrees wrist flexion and 20 degrees wrist extension (57). No difference was found in fracture healing, although patients immobilized in flexion had restrictions in motion at early follow-up. The author's current preferred method of casting for nondisplaced scaphoid waist fractures is long-arm thumb-spica cast for 4–6 wk, followed by short-arm thumb-spica casting until clinical and radiographic healing.

It is important to remember that fractures of the scaphoid tubercle and distal pole are extraarticular and have a more robust vascular supply. Bony healing is reliable and more rapid. For this reason, short-arm thumb-spica casting for 3–6 wk in nondisplaced or minimally displaced injuries will usually suffice.

234   D.S. Bae

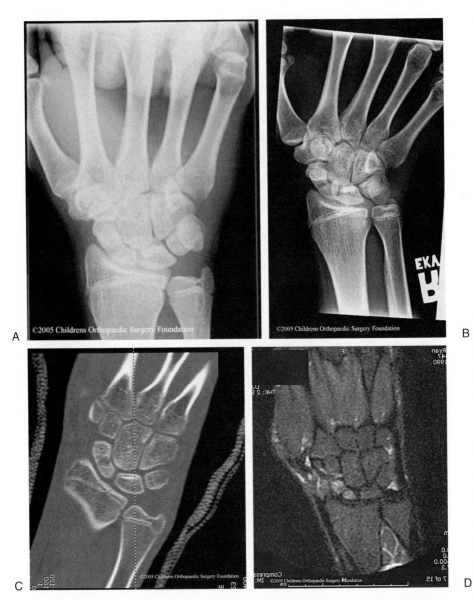

FIGURE 9.4. **(A)** Anteroposterior view of the wrist in a patient with radial wrist pain. **(B)** Anteroposterior view of the wrist in ulnar deviation, in which the fracture of the scaphoid waist is more apparent. **(C)** Computed tomography scan and **(D)** MRI of the wrist, confirming the diagnosis. **(E)** Postoperative AP view of the wrist after open reduction and internal fixation with a compression screw. Courtesy of the Children's Orthopedic Surgery Foundation, Boston, MA.

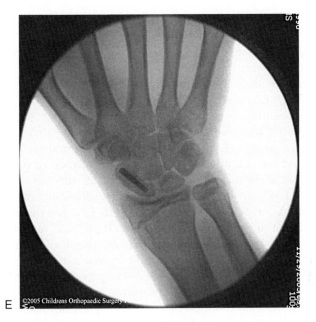

FIGURE 9.4. *Continued*

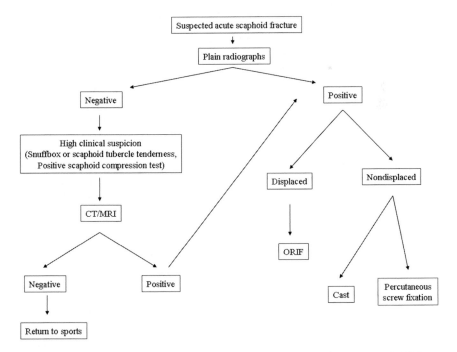

FIGURE 9.5. Clinical algorithm in the evaluation of suspected acute scaphoid fracture. ORIF, open reduction and internal fixation. Courtesy of the Children's Orthopedic Surgery Foundation, Boston, MA.

Surgical Treatment

Established indications for surgical treatment include displaced fractures of the scaphoid waist, proximal pole fractures, fractures with associated injuries (e.g., distal radius fractures and carpal instability), and fractures that have failed nonoperative treatment (Figure 9.4).

There is a continuing debate regarding the most appropriate treatment for nondisplaced scaphoid waist fractures in the young athletes. Because of the prolonged period of immobilization often required for successful cast treatment and the risk of nonunion, some have advocated surgical fixation of nondisplaced injuries. The enthusiasm for surgical treatment has increased recently, given advances in techniques for minimally invasive and percutaneous approaches to screw fixation (58–61). The theoretical advantages of surgical stabilization for nondisplaced fractures include more rapid healing, shorter cast immobilization, decreased risk of nonunion or late displacement, and more expedient return to sports or work.

Several studies have shown more rapid bony healing and faster return to activity with surgery. Bond et al. performed a prospective, randomized study comparing cast immobilization to percutaneous screw fixation for nondisplaced scaphoid waist fractures in young naval personnel, average age 24 yr (62). Average fracture healing time was 7 wk in the screw fixation group, compared to 12 wk in the casting group; return to military duty was 8 wk compared with 15 wk, respectively. In a similar study, Adolfsson et al. performed a randomized study of 53 patients comparing percutaneous screw fixation to cast immobilization for nondisplaced scaphoid waist fractures (63). Although there were no differences in rate of bony union or time to healing, patients who underwent surgical fixation had significantly better range of motion at the 16-wk follow-up. More recently, Dias et al. performed a randomized controlled trial of 88 patients comparing short-arm casting (with the thumb left free) to screw fixation without supplemental casting or splinting (64). Range of motion and grip strength were higher in the surgically treated group at 8 wk; however, at longer follow-up, patients had equivalent motion and function. Both groups returned to work at 5–6 wk after injury. Notably, 10 out of 44 patients in the casting group had no evidence of healing after 12 wk of casting and ultimately required additional treatment. This high percentage of casting failures may be caused by the casting technique (i.e., failure to incorporate the thumb and/or elbow in the cast).

Given the improvements in imaging and surgical techniques, as well as the data suggesting that early screw fixation may lead to more rapid bony healing and return to sports participation, patients with non-displaced scaphoid waist fractures should be counseled regarding the advantages and disadvantages of cast immobilization versus screw fixation.

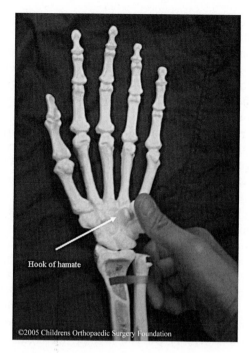

Hook of hamate

©2005 Childrens Orthopaedic Surgery Foundation

FIGURE 9.6. Illustration demonstrating palpation of the hook of the hamate. The examiner places the interphalangeal joint of his/her thumb over the pisiform, allowing the tip of the thumb to fall upon the hook of the hamate. Courtesy of the Children's Orthopedic Surgery Foundation, Boston, MA.

Other Carpal Fractures

Hook of Hamate Fractures

Hook of hamate fractures represent approximately 2–4% of all carpal fractures (65). The hook of hamate is a bony projection of the hamate, lying just distal and radial to the pisiform (Figure 9.6). Despite its location beneath palmar fibrofatty tissue, it may reliably be located if the examiner places the interphalangeal joint of his/her thumb on the pisiform; by flexing the interphalangeal joint, the thumb tip will fall over the hamate hook (Figure 9.6). Anatomically, it serves as the attachment for the pisohamate and transverse carpal ligaments, origin of the flexor digiti quinti and opponens digiti quinti muscles, and forms the radial border of Guyon's canal (the ulnar tunnel). In addition, it lies in close proximity to the flexor tendons of the small and ring fingers and the sensory and deep motor branches of the ulnar nerve.

Classically, these injuries occur because of direct force applied to the hamate hook, either from a fall onto an extended wrist or from the impact of the butt of a baseball bat or racquet, which rests adjacent to the hamate's bony process (66). Acutely, hook of hamate fractures present with localized tenderness, swelling, and ecchymosis. There may be pain with resisted small and ring finger flexion, as well as paresthesias or dysesthesias in the ulnar nerve distribution.

Specific radiographic studies must be performed to confirm the diagnosis. The carpal tunnel and supinated oblique views of the wrist may be obtained to better visualize the hook of hamate in suspected cases (67,68). Computed tomography, however, will best provide visualization of the hook of hamate to make the diagnosis of fracture and guide treatment.

Acute nondisplaced or minimally displaced fractures may be successfully treated with splint or cast immobilization when diagnosed early (69). Acute displaced fractures may be treated with cast immobilization or surgery. Although a stable fibrous union may form after casting, there is a risk for development of a painful nonunion. For this reason, many have recommended either open reduction and internal fixation (ORIF) or hamate hook excision in displaced injuries (70,71). Several published reports have documented rapid return to sports with little, if any, disability after hook of hamate excision (66,70,71). Chronic hamate hook fractures may present with tenosynovitis or rupture of the flexor tendons and ulnar nerve symptoms. Although some have advocated open reduction and internal fixation with the use of bone graft, hook of hamate excision may provide the most reliable means of symptomatic improvement and expedient return to activities (72).

Dorsal Triquetrum Avulsion Fractures

Triquetral fractures are commonly seen in young athletes. Dorsal avulsion fractures may be seen after a fall onto an outstretched hand or hyperflexion injuries of the wrist. These represent avulsion of the dorsal intercarpal and radiotriquetral ligaments from their insertion on the triquetrum. Patients will typically present with dorsal wrist pain, swelling, and tenderness after a fall. Radiographs will confirm the diagnosis. A comprehensive examination is critical to rule out associated bony or ligamentous injury. In the absence of associated pathology, these may be successfully treated with a short-arm cast or splint immobilization for 3–6 wk.

Triangular Fibrocartilage Injuries

Though descriptions of triangular fibrocartilage complex (TFCC) injuries in adults have been widespread since the 1980s, only recently has there been increased understanding of similar injuries in the pediatric and adolescent patient population (73,74). Although this may be attributed to increased awareness, increased sports participation in younger athletes may also be contributing to the increased prevalence. Furthermore, as the use of diagnostic tools such as high-resolution MRI become more widespread, so too may our appreciation of the frequency of these injuries (75,76). When present, TFCC injuries may be the source of ulnar-sided wrist pain and functional limitations in the adolescent athlete.

Anatomy

The TFCC refers to a convergence of structures on the ulnar side of the wrist that serve to support the ulnocarpal articulation and stabilize the distal radioulnar joint (DRUJ). First described by Palmer and Werner, these structures include the triangular fibrocartilage, the dorsal and volar radioulnar ligaments, the meniscal homologue, the ulnolunate and ulnotriquetral ligaments, and the subsheath of the extensor carpi ulnaris (ECU) tendon (73). Functionally, the TFCC provides a smooth articular surface between the radius and ulna, transmits and absorbs axial loads across the ulnocarpal articulation, and contributes stability to the ulnar wrist and DRUJ. Previous studies have demonstrated that approximately 20% of the axial load is transmitted across the ulnocarpal joint in wrists with neutral ulnar variance (77). Small changes in ulnar variance may result in significant alterations in axial loads borne by the TFCC.

Clinical Presentation

Most patients with TFCC tears present with ulnar-sided wrist pain, which is exacerbated with forceful grip and twisting-type activities, often in the setting of prior wrist trauma. It is thought that most TFCC injuries arise from axially loading of/fall onto the extended and pronated wrist (78). The symptoms of TFCC injury may be subtle, particularly in the child or adolescent. Indeed, patients may complain of wrist pain only during specific sports-related activity and be free of pain or functional limitations during activities of daily living (74).

Physical examination findings may also be subtle. Usually there is tenderness over the ulnar aspect of the wrist. The TFCC compression test, in which the wrist is axially loaded, ulnarly deviated, and rotated, is a helpful provocative test. Stability of the DRUJ must be assessed, as TFCC disruption may be associated with DRUJ instability.

All patients with suspected TFCC injury should be evaluated with plain radiographs to identify potential coexisting wrist pathology, including distal radial fracture malunion, ulnar styloid nonunion, positive ulnar variance

TABLE 9.2. Classification of triangular fibrocartilage tears.

Class 1: traumatic	
A	Central perforation
B	Ulnar avulsion
C	Distal avulsion
D	Radial avulsion

Class 2: degenerative	
A	TFCC wear
B	TFCC wear, lunate/ulnar chondromalacia
C	TFCC perforation, lunate/ulnar chondromalacia
D	TFCC perforation, lunate/ulnar chondromalacia, LT ligament perforation
E	TFCC perforation, lunate/ulnar chondromalacia, LT ligament perforation, ulnocarpal arthritis

with ulnocarpal impaction, and DRUJ instability. As the apparent length of the distal ulna can vary with forearm rotation, standardized views should be obtained and variance measured according to the technique of perpendiculars (79). Comparison radiographs of the contralateral wrist may be useful in these situations. Magnetic resonance imaging may be used to assess the integrity of the TFCC. Though early reports of this imaging modality noted significant limitations in the evaluation of the TFCC, the sensitivity and specificity of MRI has improved (75,76).

The Palmer classification is the most commonly used system to describe TFCC injuries (80). In the pediatric population, traumatic (class 1) injuries represent the vast majority of TFCC tears; as expected, degenerative (class 2) tears of the TFCC are far less common. Injuries to the TFCC are further classified based on the location of the cartilage complex tear (Table 9.2).

Based on previously published reports, there is an apparent increased prevalence of Palmer 1B tears in pediatric patients compared with adults (74,81). Indeed, tears from the ulnar attachment, with or without associated ulnar styloid fractures, represent the most common variety of TFCC injuries in children and adolescents.

Tears of the radial attachment (Palmer 1D tears) represent the second most common type. Care should be made during preoperative evaluation, MRI analysis, and intraoperative arthroscopic survey to ensure accurate diagnosis of these radial-sided tears. If mistaken for a central traumatic tear (Palmer 1A), simple debridement alone may result in persistent pain, instability, and functional limitations.

Patients with persistent pain and functional limitations associated with TFCC injury despite rest, activity modification, and physical/occupational therapy are candidates for surgical treatment.

Surgical Management

In appropriate patients with peripheral TFCC tears, repair of the TFCC to its ulnar or radial attachments is recommended. Surgical repair typically consists of wrist arthroscopy, debridement of the tear, and subsequent suture fixation of the TFCC edge to either its ulnar or radial attachments (82). Coexisting wrist pathology, such as ulnar styloid fractures, ulnocarpal impaction in the setting of positive ulnar variance, and DRUJ instability, are addressed at the time of TFCC repair.

Postoperatively, patients are immobilized in long-arm casts with the elbow flexed 90 degrees and the forearm in supination for 4 wk, followed by short-arm casts or splints for an additional 2 wk. Range-of-motion and strengthening exercises are then initiated. Sports participation is allowed after 3 mo.

Compared to the extensive published data regarding the surgical management of TFCC injuries in adults, relatively little has been written about the results of treatment in the pediatric patient population. Terry and Waters reviewed a series of 29 children and adolescents treated for posttraumatic, surgically documented TFCC injuries at an average age of 13 yr (74). All patients presented for evaluation of ulnar wrist pain. Over three-fourths had Palmer 1B lesions. Eighty-six percent of patients had coexisting wrist pathology, most commonly being ulnar styloid nonunion, DRUJ instability, distal radial fracture malunion, and/or ulnocarpal impaction. All Palmer 1B, 1C, and 1D tears were repaired using the principles and techniques outlined above. At average follow-up of 21 mo, over 85% of patients had good to excellent results as assessed by the modified Mayo Wrist score, which assesses pain, motion, and wrist function (74,81–83).

The Gymnast's Wrist and Ulnocarpal Impaction

Repetitive axial loading of the wrist during sports participation may cause growth disturbance of the distal radial physis in skeletally immature athletes, leading to relative ulnar overgrowth and altered wrist biomechanics. As noted previously, a change in ulnar variance by 2 mm can increase the axial loads borne across the ulnocarpal joint from 20 to 41% (77). This may lead to ulnar wrist pain, TFCC tears, and DRUJ instability.

This constellation of findings is commonly seen in gymnasts because of the repetitive weight bearing performed with the wrist in dorsiflexion. Indeed, studies of high-level gymnasts have demonstrated a higher incidence of ulnar positive variance and distal radial physeal stress changes compared to nongymnasts (84,85).

In patients with pain and functional limitations despite splinting, therapy, and activity modification, surgical treatment may be warranted. Depending

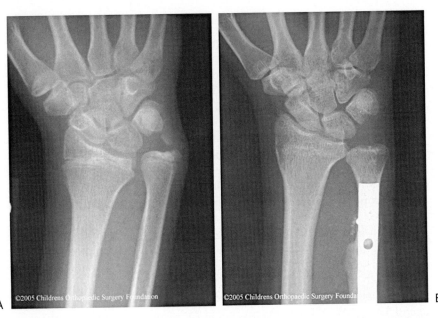

A
B

©2005 Childrens Orthopaedic Surgery Foundation
©2005 Childrens Orthopaedic Surgery Founda

FIGURE 9.7. **(A)** Anteroposterior radiograph of the wrist in a patient with ulnocarpal impaction. Note the ulnar styloid fracture nonunion and positive ulnar variance. **(B)** AP radiograph after ulnar styloid nonunion excision and ulnar shortening osteotomy. Courtesy of the Children's Orthopaedic Surgery Foundation, Boston, MA.

on the degree of deformity and amount of skeletal growth remaining, surgery may consist of arthroscopic-assisted TFCC repair, distal ulnar epiphyseodesis, ulnar-shortening osteotomy, corrective radial osteotomy, or combinations thereof (86) (Figure 9.7).

Hand Injuries

Metacarpal Fractures

Although the majority of metacarpal fractures may be successfully treated with nonoperative means, care providers should have an understanding of fundamental treatment principles and indications for surgical intervention. Not all metacarpal fractures are the same, and treatment is predicated on the location of injury, digit involved, degree of associated displacement, and presence of associated injury.

Patients will present with pain, swelling, and deformity after hand trauma. Fractures may occur because of direct blow or indirect trauma, such as when the limb or body pivots around a planted hand. A comprehensive physical examination is performed to assess for associated neurovascular or tendinous injury, as well as to assess the adjacent soft tissues and skin integrity.

Perhaps the most important component of the physical examination is to assess for rotational deformity of the affected digit. This may be best assessed using the principle of tenodesis, as described earlier in the chapter. In cases of a malrotated metacarpal fracture, the tenodesis maneuver may result in over- or underlapping of the affected digit with respect to the adjacent fingers. Malrotation is important to identify, as such deformity compromises hand function and does not remodel, even in skeletally immature patients. Radiographs will confirm the diagnosis; AP, lateral, and oblique views of the hand are recommended.

Metacarpal Shaft Fractures

Isolated fractures of the metacarpal shaft often demonstrate little displacement or angulation. This is, in part, caused by the presence of the intermetacarpal ligaments, which connect the distal metacarpals to one another, and the keystone configuration of the carpometacarpal (CMC) joint. Mild deformity may be accepted with no adverse effect on hand function. In addition, because of the compensatory motion present in the CMC joints of the ring and small fingers, more angular deformity may be accepted in the ring and small fingers than the index and long fingers. Most authorities agree that up to 20–30 degrees of angulation may be accepted in the ring and small metacarpals, whereas only 10 degrees of angulation or less should be accepted in the index and long metacarpals (87).

In cases of unacceptable deformity, closed reduction and cast immobilization is recommended. Casts are typically maintained for 3–4 wk, with interval radiographs performed to confirm maintenance of acceptable alignment. Several modified cast gloves and splints have been proposed in athletes with these injuries to provide expedited return to play (88). Although the exact form of immobilization may be modified for each individual, the principles of treatment remain the same.

Indications for surgical treatment of metacarpal shaft fractures include the following: open fractures, multiple metacarpal fractures (in which the stabilizing effects of the adjacent metacarpals are lost), rotational malalignment, and unstable fractures in which acceptable alignment cannot be maintained with cast or splint immobilization. In these situations, surgical stabilization may be accomplished by several different techniques, including percutaneous smooth wires, intramedullary wires, interfragmentary compression screws, or plate-and-screw constructs, depending on fracture pattern and associated injuries (Figure 9.8).

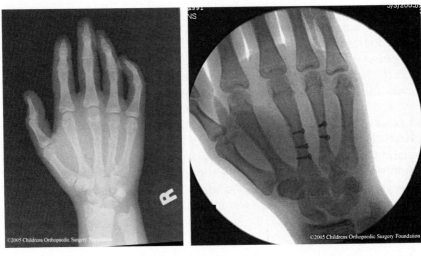

FIGURE 9.8. **(A)** Anteroposterior radiograph of the hand demonstrating fractures of the long and ring finger metacarpal shafts in a 13-yr-old gymnast. **(B)** Because of malrotation of the digits seen on clinical examination, as well as the fact that multiple adjacent metacarpals were involved, the injury was treated with open reduction and internal fixation using interfragmentary compression screws. The patient returned to gymnastics at 3 mo. Courtesy of the Children's Orthopedic Surgery Foundation, Boston, MA.

Metacarpal Neck Fractures

Fractures of the metacarpal neck are also common injuries, typically affecting the ring and small rays. Though often referred to as "boxer's fractures," these injuries are rarely seen in high-level boxing athletes. The mechanism of injury involves a direct axial load across a flexed MCP joint.

Patients will present with pain, swelling, and deformity. Radiographs will confirm the diagnosis, typically demonstrating apex dorsal angulation caused by the position of the hand during injury and the deforming forces imparted by the intrinsic muscles of the hand. Because of the compensatory motion present in the ring and small MCP and CMC joints, considerable amounts of angulation may be accepted with no adverse effects on hand function. Although there is no consensus, most authorities would agree that up to 30–40 degrees of apex dorsal angulation may be accepted in the ring and small metacarpals (87). As with metacarpal shaft fractures, less deformity may be accepted in the index and long fingers, and most authors agree that only 10–15 degrees of angulation may be accepted in these digits (87).

In cases of unacceptable angulation, closed reduction may be performed, followed by application of a well-molded cast or splint to maintain alignment during bony healing. The reduction maneuver consists of longitudinal traction, followed by MCP joint flexion and dorsally directed pressure on the metacarpal head to correct the angular deformity. Several different cast configurations have been recommended. A recent study of 263 patients with extraarticular metacarpal fractures treated with three different cast configurations (with the MCP joint flexed or extended, with the interphalangeal [IP] joints included, or with the IP joints free) demonstrated no difference in bony healing, grip strength, or final range of motion (89).

Indications for surgical treatment include presence of angular or rotational malalignment refractory to closed reduction and immobilization. Options for surgical stabilization include percutaneous smooth wire fixation or formal open reduction and internal fixation. In these instances, early range of motion exercises are recommended to avoid long-term stiffness. Return to athletic participation is restricted until there is clinical and radiographic evidence of healing.

Metacarpal Head Fractures

Metacarpal head fractures are intraarticular injuries. In cases when there is more than 25% of articular surface involvement or any evidence of articular surface incongruity, surgical treatment is recommended to reconstitute the MCP joint.

Phalangeal Fractures

Patients with phalangeal fractures will typically present with pain, swelling, and deformity after direct or indirect hand trauma. In young athletes, these injuries are commonly seen in contact or ball sports. Again, evaluation for possible rotational malalignment must be performed. In cases in which the patient is unable to make a fist or flex the affected digit, the tenodesis maneuver may be utilized. AP, lateral, and oblique radiographs of the affected digit are recommended to confirm the diagnosis. Fractures are classified according to location, displacement, angulation, and malrotation. The presence of intraarticular extension or comminution should be noted.

Extraarticular fractures of the distal phalanx commonly occur after crushing injuries. In the absence of associated wounds or nail bed injuries, tuft fractures may be treated symptomatically, with the expectation of clinical healing in 2–4 wk. Splinting or taping may allow for better symptomatic control and earlier return to sports. Fractures involving the distal phalangeal shaft are typically stable and may be treated according to similar principles. In rare instances, unstable shaft fractures with excessive angulation may be treated with closed reduction and percutaneous pin fixation.

Displaced physeal fractures of the distal phalanx are typically treated with closed reduction and splint immobilization. Careful examination of the affected digit is paramount, as the presence of an associated nail bed laceration may signify an open fracture (the so-called Seymour's fracture) (90,91). In these injuries, surgical treatment with nail plate removal, irrigation and debridement of the fracture site, open reduction, and nail bed repair are recommended to ensure bony healing and prevent complications of infection and growth disturbance.

Fractures of the middle and proximal phalangeal shaft are treated according to their fracture stability. Stable fractures that are minimally displaced may be treated with buddy-taping or splinting and early digital mobilization. Serial radiographs are recommended, however, to detect late displacement. In fractures with excessive angulation (greater than 10 degrees) or any malrotation, closed reduction with or without surgical stabilization is recommended (87) (Figure 9.9). Types of surgical fixation will depend on the fracture location, pattern, and degree of deformity. Early referral to a hand surgeon is recommended in these instances.

Articular fractures of the phalanges merit special attention. Nondisplaced unicondylar fractures may heal with immobilization alone; however, these injuries are prone to late displacement and must be evaluated with serial radiographs to ensure healing in proper alignment. Any displaced or comminuted articular fractures of the middle or proximal phalanx warrant hand surgery consultation and consideration for operative treatment.

Proximal Interphalangeal Joint Dislocations

The proximal interphalangeal joint (PIP) is the most commonly dislocated joint, particularly among participants in contact and ball sports. Patients will present with acute pain, deformity, and limitations in digital motion after a "jamming" or "catching" injury. An axial load combined with hyperextension of the fingertip typically results in a dorsal dislocation of the middle phalanx.

Knowledge of the functional anatomy of the PIP joint is needed to understand treatment principles (Figure 9.10). The PIP joint is a diarthroidal joint that relies on adjacent soft-tissue for stability. The collateral ligaments arise from the concave collateral recess along the radial and ulnar aspects of the proximal phalanx and pass distally and palmarly to insert on the volar and lateral aspects of the middle phalanx. The palmar-most fibers of the collateral ligaments blend in with fibers of the volar plate. The volar plate is a stout ligamentous structure that forms the floor of the PIP joint and serves to resist PIP hyperextension.

Initial management consists of reduction of the obvious deformity via traction and flexion of the dorsally dislocated digit. Often, this is performed on

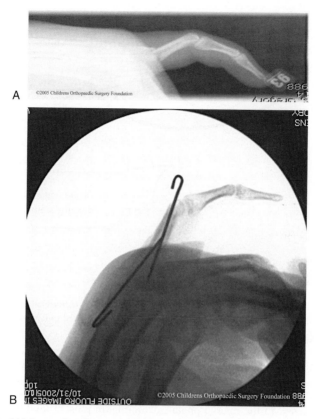

FIGURE 9.9. **(A)** Lateral radiograph of the small finger depicting a proximal phalanx fracture with apex volar angulation in a 16-yr-old football player. **(B)** This injury was treated with closed reduction and percutaneous pin fixation. Pins were removed after 3 wk, and the patient returned to sports 6 wk after surgery. Courtesy of the Children's Orthopedic Surgery Foundation, Boston, MA.

the field by the athlete, teammate, coach, or trainer. Subsequent pain, swelling, and diminished range of motion of the affected joint are the norm.

A careful evaluation of the dislocated PIP joint is required to rule out associated injury, guide postinjury activity, and assess criteria for return to sports participation. Radiographs of the affected digit, including a true lateral view, are essential to assess postreduction joint congruency and to evaluate for associated fractures.

Treatment is predicated on joint congruency and stability. In cases of pure dislocations without associated bony injury, if a congruently reduced joint is confirmed on radiographs and the joint is stable on examination, management may consist of edema control and buddy taping to an adjacent finger for 3–6 wk. Early motion is initiated to decrease the risk of

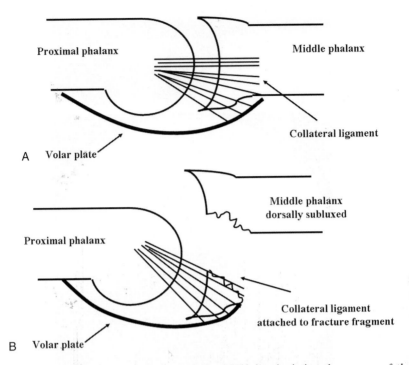

FIGURE 9.10. **(A)** Schematic diagram of the PIP joint depicting the course of the collateral ligament and volar plate. **(B)** Schematic diagram of an unstable PIP joint fracture dislocation; with a large fracture fragment, little or no collateral ligament remains attached to the middle phalanx, resulting in joint instability. Courtesy of the Children's Orthopedic Surgery Foundation, Boston, MA.

long-standing joint stiffness. Athletes may return to practice or competition with appropriate protective taping or splinting.

In the setting of PIP fracture-dislocations, treatment is again dependent on joint congruency and stability. In cases of a small avulsion fracture from the palmar base of the middle phalanx in an otherwise reduced and stable joint, buddy taping and early motion may be initiated. If the associated fracture comprises a greater portion of the articular surface of the middle phalanx, a considerable portion of the collateral ligament insertion will insert on the displaced fracture fragment (Figure 9.10). As a result, the PIP joint may be reducible, but will subluxate or dislocate as the joint moves from a flexed to extended position. In these situations, a dorsal extension-block splint may be used to maintain joint reduction but allow for some protected motion. This splint is typically used for 4–6 wk, with incremental increases in extension over time until full extension is achieved. In those patients with fracture-dislocations in which the joint is not reducible or able to be maintained, even in extreme flexion, surgical treatment is recommended. Surgical treatment may comprise open reduction and internal fixation of the bony fragment. If the fracture is comminuted or irreparable, the bony fragment may be excised and the volar plate advanced to reconstitute joint congruity and stability. In these cases, athletes may expect to remain out of sports participation for a minimum of 4–6 wk, until adequate bony and soft tissue healing has occurred and digital motion has been restored.

Gamekeeper's Thumb

Sprains and tears of the ulnar collateral ligament (UCL) of the MCP joint of the thumb are known as "gamekeeper's" or "skier's" thumb. These injuries result from extreme radially directed force imparted onto the thumb MCP joint, typically during a fall onto an abducted thumb.

The UCL is comprised of two distinct ligamentous expansions, the proper and accessory collateral ligaments. The proper collateral ligament arises from the metacarpal head and inserts on the palmar aspect of the proximal phalanx. The accessory collateral ligament, which is contiguous with the proper, runs more palmarly and attaches to the volar plate (92,93). In flexion, the proper collateral ligament—and to a lesser degree, the dorsal joint capsule—serves as the primary restraint to radial deviation and palmar subluxation of the MCP joint. Conversely, in full extension, the accessory collateral ligament and volar plate are the primary restraints to valgus deviation. When both the accessory and proper collateral ligaments are disrupted, a complete tear results.

In complete tears, the UCL is commonly avulsed from the base of the proximal phalanx and retracts proximal and superficial to the adjacent aponeurosis of the adductor pollicis. In this position, the retracted end of the UCL may be palpated as a tender mass along the ulnar aspect of the UCL, the so-called "Stener lesion (93)." Because of interposition of the adductor aponeurosis, the UCL is not longer in proximity to its bony insertion and will not heal with immobilization alone.

Patients typically present with pain, tenderness, swelling, and ecchymosis around the ulnar aspect of the MCP joint after a fall or valgus injury to the thumb. Anteroposterior, lateral, and oblique radiographs of the thumb should be obtained to rule out fracture or dislocation. In the absence of bony injury, stress testing is performed to distinguish between a partial or complete UCL tear. Excessive laxity to valgus stress with the MCP joint both flexed and extended signifies a complete UCL tear. Although there is great variation in what constitutes "normal" MCP laxity, average valgus laxity is 6 degrees with MCP extension and 15 degrees with MCP flexion (94). Although there is some debate as to what constitutes excessive or pathological laxity, most authorities would agree that 30 degrees or more of valgus laxity, or greater than 15 degrees compared to the contralateral thumb, suggests complete ligamentous disruption (92).

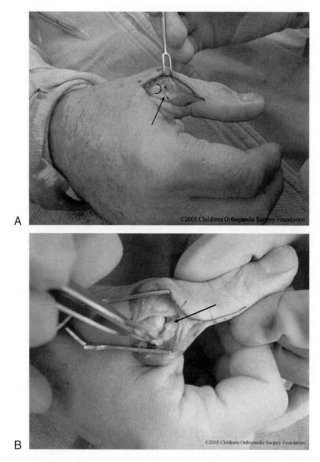

FIGURE 9.11. **(A)** Intraoperative photographs depicting a Stener's lesion. The retracted distal end of the collateral ligament (outlined) lies superficial and proximal to the adductor aponeurosis (arrow). **(B)** After the adductor pollicis is incised and retracted, the collateral ligament (held in forceps) may be repaired to its bony insertion along the base of the proximal phalanx (arrow). Courtesy of the Children's Orthopedic Surgery Foundation, Boston, MA.

Immobilization of the thumb in a thumb spica splint or cast with the inter-phalangeal joint free for 4–6 wk is recommended for partial tears. This is followed by range-of-motion and strengthening exercises and return to activities. However, in cases of complete UCL tears when a Stener lesion is present, surgical treatment is recommended (Figure 9.11). Postoperatively, the thumb is immobilized in a thumb spica cast for 4 wk, followed by a thumb spica splint for an additional 2 wk to allow for ligament healing.

In skeletally immature patients, avulsion fractures of the ulnar base of the proximal phalanx may occur, rather than purely ligamentous injuries.

Although these injuries are most accurately described as Salter–Harris III fractures of the proximal phalanx, they are the pediatric equivalent of the "gamekeeper's thumb" (Figure 9.12). Surgical treatment using smooth pin fixation is recommended in these instances to restore articular surface congruity and provide for MCP joint stability. A thumb spica cast is applied for 4 wk, at which point the Kirschner wires are removed if there is adequate radiographic bony healing. Splint immobilization is utilized for an additional 2 wk, followed by range-of-motion and strengthening exercises.

Mallet Finger

Also known as "baseball" or "drop" finger, mallet fingers are so named because of the characteristic appearance of the digital tip, with the flexed distal IP (DIP) joint resembling the end of a hammer (95) (Figure 9.13). This deformity is caused by a disruption of the extensor tendon mechanism in the region of the DIP joint, typically resulting from an axial load and/or sudden DIP joint flexion moment imparted on the extended fingertip.

When identified in a timely fashion, the acute mallet finger without associated laceration, fracture, or joint instability may be successfully treated by splinting the affected DIP joint in full extension for 6–8 wk, followed by splinting at nighttime and during athletic activity for an additional 2–4 wk (95–97). The PIP joint need not be immobilized. Although several different custom and commercially available splints are available, adherence to these treatment principles results in successful healing of the extensor tendon mechanism and correction of the mallet finger deformity in the vast majority of patients (98,99).

Young athletes may also present with "mallet fractures," in which the extensor tendon insertion is avulsed from the dorsal base of the distal phalanx with a bony fragment. A lateral radiograph of the affected digit will confirm the diagnosis. In instances when the avulsed bony fragment comprises less than 30% of the articular surface and there is no associated DIP joint subluxation, extension splinting is recommended, as previously described (100). In cases where there is significant articular surface involvement or palmar subluxation of the distal phalanx in relationship to the middle phalanx, surgical treatment is advised. Percutaneous pinning, "extension block" pinning, and formal open reduction with internal fixation of the bony fragment have all been proposed in these situations (95).

Several challenges exist, however, in the treatment of young athletes with mallet finger injuries. Compliance with full-time digital splinting is often difficult to achieve in the young, active patient, resulting in a higher incidence of failed nonoperative treatment. Furthermore, as these injuries often arise from relatively minor trauma and do not always cause immediate functional impairment, adolescents with mallet finger injuries may not present acutely for evaluation or treatment. As a consequence, the diagnosis of mallet finger injury is often delayed beyond the acute injury period.

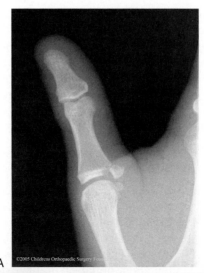

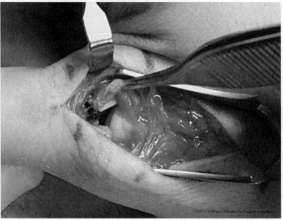

FIGURE 9.12. **(A)** Radiograph depicting a Salter–Harris III fracture of the base of the thumb proximal phalanx, the "pediatric gamekeeper's" injury. **(B)** Intraoperative photograph demonstrating the fracture fragment (held by forceps) with its attached ulnar collateral ligament. **(C)** Reduction and internal fixation is performed with smooth wires. **(D)** Postoperative radiograph depicting anatomic reduction and a congruent thumb metacarpal phalangeal joint. Courtesy of the Children's Orthopedic Surgery Foundation, Boston, MA.

Several studies have supported the use of extension splinting in subacute and chronic mallet fingers (101,102). Splinting in these situations may be successful in compliant patients and should be considered. Several surgical techniques have also been advocated for the treatment of chronic mallet finger deformities, including tenodermodesis, oblique retinacular ligament

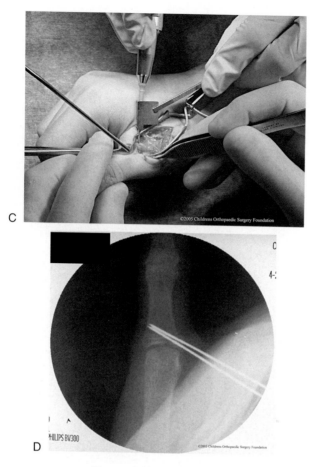

FIGURE 9.12. *Continued*

reconstruction, central slip tenotomy, and even DIP joint arthrodesis (103–109). Although the technical aspects of these procedures, their indications, and results of treatment are beyond the scope of this chapter, it is recommended that patients with chronic mallet fingers failing splinting therapy be referred to a hand surgeon for consultation regarding potential treatment options.

Jersey Finger

Avulsion injuries of the flexor digitorum profundus (FDP) tendon from its bony insertion onto the base of the distal phalanx commonly occur in young athletes. These injuries typically occur during forced extension of a maximally flexed finger, such as when an athlete grabs another player's jersey

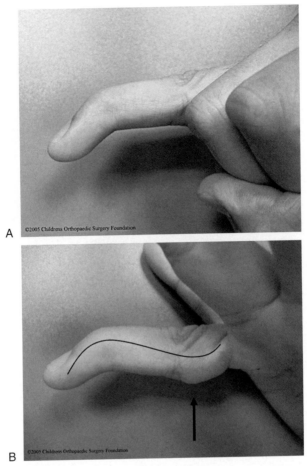

FIGURE 9.13. **(A)** Clinical photograph of the mallet finger deformity. **(B)** Secondary swan-neck deformity (outlined) characterized by hyperextension at the proximal interphalangeal joint (arrow). Courtesy of the Children's Orthopedic Surgery Foundation, Boston, MA.

while attempting to make a tackle in football or rugby; it is from this common mechanism that this clinical entity derives its colloquial name, "jersey finger" (110). Patients will typically present with pain, swelling, and inability to fully flex the affected digit, often after a relatively innocuous injury. The ring finger is affected approximately 70% of the time (111,112). A careful physical examination is imperative, as active PIP joint flexion may be apparent from the intact flexor digitorum superficialis (FDS). Anteroposterior, lateral, and oblique radiographs of the affected digits should be obtained to rule out a concomitant bony avulsion, particularly in the skeletally immature.

Leddy and Packer have classified these injuries into 3 types, depending on the level of tendon retraction and presence or absence of a bony fragment (110). Type I injuries are soft tissue avulsions with retraction of the tendon stump into the palm. In these instances, the vinculae have been disrupted, depriving the FDP tendon of its vascular supply and allowing for tendon retraction. Given the degree of retraction and loss of vascular supply, primary repair of the tendon avulsion is recommended within 7–10 d of injury. Delay in diagnosis and treatment leads to inability to perform a primary repair because of scar formation and contraction of the proximal muscle belly. In type II injuries, the tendon stump retracts to the level of the PIP joint. It is thought that intact vinculae help to prevent complete retraction. If the tendon is avulsed with a small bony fragment, radiographs may depict a bony "fleck" at the level of the PIP joint. Repair after 1–2 wk may be possible because of the intact blood supply and preservation of tendon and muscle belly length. In type III avulsions, the FDP tendon is avulsed with a large bony fragment, which is entrapped by the A4 tendon pulley. As a result, the tendon stump retracts minimally, just proximal to the DIP joint. Radiographs confirm the diagnosis. Treatment consists of open reduction and internal fixation of the bony fragment to the base of the distal phalanx, which restores the FDP tendon insertion to its anatomic location.

Avulsion injuries of the FDP tendon are not amenable to nonoperative treatment and require surgical repair. Accurate diagnosis and timely referral to a hand surgeon is critical. With prompt surgical repair and appropriate rehabilitation, near-normal restoration of digital motion and strength may be expected. However, athletes may expect to be out of sports for a minimum of 8–12 wk.

Unfortunately, jersey finger injuries are often diagnosed late, as young athletes often will not seek immediate medical attention and continue to participate in sports, despite pain and limitations in digital motion and strength. If enough time has elapsed such that primary repair is not feasible, treatment options include flexor tendon reconstruction with free tendon graft, arthrodesis of the DIP joint, or abandoning attempts at any reconstructive procedure, particularly if the affected digit provides little functional impairment.

Prevention

There is no better treatment than prevention, and many hand and wrist injuries may be averted with appropriate preventative measures. The high incidence of wrist fractures in snowboarders and in-line skaters, for example, has prompted many to advocate the use of protective wrist guards to prevent injury. In a review of 7,430 snowboarding injuries sustained over a 10-yr period, Idzikowski et al. reported that approximately half involved the upper extremity and 21% involved the wrist (113). Snowboarders who wore protective wrist guards were found to be half as likely to sustain wrist injuries compared to those without wrist protection. Ronning et al. came to similar conclusions in their prospective randomized study of over 5,000 snowboarders (114). Over three times as many wrist injuries (sprains and fractures) occurred in snowboarders without wrist braces as in those who wore protectors. No additional injuries were related to the use of the wrist braces.

Schieber et al. conducted a case-control study of over 200 in-line skaters in efforts to identify risk factors for injury (115). Almost half of the study participants reported that they did not wear any kind of protective equipment (e.g. wrist guards, elbow pads, helmets). The odds ratio for wrist injury, adjusted for age and sex, was 10.4 for those athletes who did not wear wrist guards as compared with those who did. Similarly, the odds ratio for elbow injury was 9.5 for those who did not wear elbow pads. Similar conclusions and recommendations for protective equipment have been recommended by others, particularly for athletes involved in snowboarding, in-line skating, and skateboarding (10,116–118).

With increased sports participation among younger children, there has been a rising awareness of the need for age- and size-appropriate equipment to aid injury prevention. Boyd et al. recently studied the relationship between ball size and environmental conditions and the rate of distal radius fractures among young soccer goalkeepers, highlighting this concern (11). In this study of athletes between the ages of 6–15 yr, there was a statistically significant higher rate of distal radius fracture in younger children using an adult-sized ball compared to a junior ball, during both organized and informal game settings. This study raised the question of whether some sports injuries in younger athletes may be prevented by using age- and size-appropriate equipment. Similar considerations are being applied to other sports.

Return to Play Guidelines

Recommendations regarding return-to-play guidelines vary according to the type of hand/wrist injury, treatment modality, acuity or chronicity, and sport-specific demands of the individual athlete. Although no universal guidelines exist, the following principles should be considered. Bony or ligamentous injuries typically require 3–6 wk to heal; participation in practice or competition, particularly contact sports, should only be allowed if there is appropriate cast or splint immobilization of the zone of injury, including the joints proximal and distal. In cases where the injury is inherently stable, or has been stabilized with internal fixation, athletes may work on edema control, scar management, and gentle range-of-motion exercises when not participating in athletic activities. In general, full unprotected return to sports is not allowed until the athlete demonstrates full active and passive motion and near full strength of the affected hand or wrist. Athletes should be counseled regarding the potential for delayed or failed healing requiring subsequent surgical intervention inherent to all hand and wrist injuries, regardless of the measures of immobilization and protection utilized. For this reason, early referral and serial evaluations by a hand surgeon are recommended. Finally, the safety of the particular athlete and other sports participants must be considered; permission for return to play with protective devices must be obtained by the appropriate coaches, trainers, and officials.

Clinical Pearls

- Physical examination: Use the tenodesis effect to evaluate for rotational deformity and/or musculotendinous injuries to the hand. In the normal hand and wrist, passive wrist extension results in obligate passive digital flexion, with all the fingers roughly parallel, pointing toward the scaphoid tubercle.
- Radiographic evaluation: AP, lateral, and oblique views of the *specific part* of the wrist or hand should be obtained during injury evaluation. Failure to obtain appropriate imaging may result in missed diagnoses.
- Scaphoid fractures: Evaluation of all wrist injuries should include palpation of the anatomic snuffbox, palpation of the scaphoid tubercle, and the "scaphoid compression test" to assess for a possible scaphoid fracture.
- Scaphoid fractures: Consider obtaining MRI or CT imaging of patients with radial wrist pain and negative plain radiographs to rule out possible scaphoid fractures.
- TFCC injuries: The symptoms of TFCC injury may be subtle; patients complaining of persistent ulnar wrist pain during specific sports-related activity despite rest and strengthening should be evaluated for possible TFCC injury.
- Metacarpal fractures: Indications for manipulative reduction or surgical treatment of metacarpal fractures include open injuries, any rotational malalignment, or excessive angulation. Providers should remember that more angulation can be accepted in neck than shaft fractures, and more deformity is acceptable in the small and ring metacarpals compared with the long and index metacarpals.
- Intraarticular fractures of the metacarpals and phalanges: All intraarticular fractures of the hand and wrist warrant early referral to a hand surgeon.
- PIP fracture-dislocations: Treatment of fracture-dislocations of the PIP joint depends on congruity of the joint reduction, joint stability, and size of the intraarticular fracture fragment. Small avulsion fractures from the palmar base of the middle phalanx in otherwise reduced and stable joints should be treated with buddy taping and early motion to avoid long-term stiffness.

258   D.S. Bae

- Salter–Harris III fractures of the thumb proximal phalanx: These injuries represent the pediatric equivalent of the adult "gamekeeper's thumb." Open reduction and internal fixation is recommended for displaced injuries to restore joint congruity and stability.
- Jersey finger: Careful evaluation of isolated DIP joint flexion should be performed in the evaluation of a "jammed" or "pulled" finger to rule out an FDP tendon avulsion. Early hand surgery referral should be made for all flexor tendon injuries.

References

1. Adickes MS, Stuart MJ. Youth football injuries. Sports Med 2004;34: 201–207.
2. Bergfeld JA, Weiker GC, Andrish JT, et al. Soft playing splint for protection of significant hand and wrist injuries in sports. Am J Sports Med 1982; 10:293–296.
3. Boyce SH, Quigley MA. An audit of sports injuries in children attending an accident and emergency department. Scott Med J 2003;48:88–90.
4. DeHaven KE, Lintner DM. Athletic injuries: comparison by age, sport, and gender. Am J Sports Med 1986;14:218–224.
5. Jacobson BH, Hubbard M, Redus B, et al. An assessment of high school cheerleading: injury distribution, frequency, and associated factors. J Orthop Sports Phys Ther 2004;34:261–265.
6. McKay GD, Goldie PA, Payne WR, et al. A prospective study of injuries in basketball: a total profile and comparison by gender and standard of competition. J Sci Med Sport 2001;4:196–211.
7. Rettig AC. Athletic injuries of the wrist and hand. Am J Sports Med 2003;31:1038–1048.
8. Rettig AC, Ryan RO, Stone JA. Epidemiology of hand injuries in sports. In: Strickland JW, Rettig AC, eds. Hand Injuries in Athletes. Philadelphia: WB Saunders; 1992:37–44.
9. Torjussen J, Bahr R. Injuries among competitive snowboarders at the national elite level. Am J Sports Med 2005;33:370–377.
10. Zalavras C, Nikolopoulou G, Essin D, et al. Pediatric fractures during skateboarding, roller skating, and scooter riding. Am J Sports Med 2005;33:568–573.
11. Boyd KT, Brownson P, Hunter JB. Distal radial fractures in young goalkeepers: a case for an appropriately sized soccer ball. Br J Sports Med 2001;35:409–411.
12. Damore DT, Metzl JD, Ramundo M, et al. Patterns in childhood sports injury. Pediatr Emerg Care 2003;19:65–67.
13. Ryu JY, Cooney WP, Askew JL, et al. Functional ranges of motion of the wrist joint. J Hand Surg Am 1991;16:409–419.
14. Pappas AM, Morgan WJ, Schulz LA, et al. Wrist kinematics during pitching. A preliminary report. Am J Sports Med 1995;23:312–315.
15. Fleisig G, Nicholls R, Elliott B, et al. Kinematics used by world class tennis players to produce high-velocity serves. Sports Biomech 2003;2:51–64.

16. Davidson PL, Mahar B, Chalmers DJ, et al. Impact modeling of gymnastic back-handsprings and dive-rolls in children. J Appl Biomech 2005;21:115–128.
17. Markolf KL, Shapiro MS, Mandelbaum BR, et al. Wrist loading patterns during pommel horse exercises. J Biomech. 1990;23(10):1001–1011
18. Cheng JCY, Shen WY. Limb fracture pattern in different age groups: a study of 3,350 children. J Orthop Trauma 1993;7:15–22.
19. Landin LA. Fracture patterns in children. Acta Orthop Scand 1983; 202:1–109.
20. Worlock P, Stower M. Fracture patterns in Nottingham children. J Pediatr Orthop Am 1986;6:656–660.
21. Mann DC, Rajmaira S. Distribution of physeal and nonphyseal fractures of long bones in children aged 0 to 16 years. J Pediatr Orthop Am 1990;10:713–716.
22. Peterson HA, Madhok R, Benson JT, et al. Physeal fractures: part 1. Epidemiology in Olmsted County, Minnesota, 1979–1988. J Pediatr Orthop Am 1994;14:423–430.
23. Taylor BL, Attia MW. Sports-related injuries in children. Acad Emerg Med 2000;7:1376–1382.
24. Khosla S, Melton LJ, Dekutoski MB, et al. Incidence of childhood distal forearm fractures over 30 years: a population-based study. JAMA 2003;290:1479–1485.
25. Skaggs DL, Loro ML, Pitukcheewanont P, et al. Increased body weight and decreased radial cross-sectional dimensions in girls with forearm fractures. J Bone Miner Res 2001;16:1337–1342.
26. Friberg KS. Remodelling after distal forearm fractures in children. III. Correction of residual angulation in fractures of the radius. Acta Orthop Scand 1979;50:741–749.
27. Houshian S, Holst AK, Larsen MS, et al. Remodeling of Salter-Harris type II epiphyseal plate injury of the distal radius. J Pediatr Orthop Am 2004;24:472–476.
28. Younger ASE, Tredwell SJ, Mackenzie WG. Factors affecting fracture position at cast removal after pediatric forearm fracture. J Pediatr Orthop Am 1997;17:332–336.
29. Zimmermann R, Gschwentner M, Pechlaner S, et al. Remodeling capacity and functional outcome of palmarly versus dorsally displaced pediatric radius fractures in the distal one-third. Arch Orthop Trauma Surg 2004;124:42–48.
30. Davidson JS, Brown DJ, Barnes SN, et al. Simple treatment for torus fractures of the distal radius. J Bone Joint Surg Br 2001;83:1173–1175.
31. Solan MC, Rees R, Daly K. Current management of torus fractures7 of the distal radius. Injury 2002;33:503–505.
32. Symons S, Rowsell M, Bhowal B, et al. Hospital versus home management of children with buckle fractures of the distal radius. A prospective, randomized trial. J Bone Joint Surg Br 2001;83:556–560.
33. West S, Andrews J, Bebbington A, et al. Buckle fractures of the distal radius are safely treated in a soft bandage: a randomized prospective trial of bandage versus plaster cast. J Pediatr Orthop Am 2005;25:322–325.
34. Bohm ER, Bubbar V, Yong Hing K, Dzus A. Above and below-the-elbow plaster casts for distal forearm fractures in children. A randomized controlled trial. J Bone Joint Surg Am 2006;88:1–8.

35. Webb GR, Galpin RD, Armstrong DG. Comparison of short and long arm plaster casts for displaced fractures in the distal third of the forearm in children. J Bone Joint Surg Am 2006;88:9–17.

36. Gibbons CL, Woods DA, Pailthorpe C, et al. The management of isolated distal radius fractures in children. J Pediatr Orthop Am 1994;14:207–210.

37. Miller BS, Taylor B, Widmann RF, et al. Cast immobilization versus percutaneous pin fixation of displaced distal radius fractures in children: a prospective, randomized study. J Pediatr Orthop Am 2005;25:490–494.

38. Proctor MT, Moore DJ, Paterson JM. Redisplacement after manipulation of distal radial fractures in children. J Bone Joint Surg Br 1993;75:453–454.

39. Abbaszadegan H, Jonsson U, von Sivers K. Prediction of instability of Colles' fractures. Acta Orthop Scand. 1989;60:646–650.

40. Altissimi M, Mancini GB, Azzara A, et al. Early and late displacement of fractures of the distal radius. The prediction of instability. Int Orthop. 1994;18: 61–65.

41. Hove LM, Solheim E, Skjeie R, et al. Prediction of secondary displacement in Colles' fracture. J Hand Surg Br 1994;19:731–736.

42. Lafontaine M, Hardy D, Delince P. Stability assessment of distal radius fractures. Injury. 1989;20:208–210.

43. McLauchlan GJ, Cowan B, Annan IH, et al. Management of completely displaced metaphyseal fractures of the distal radius in children. A prospective, randomized controlled trial. J Bone Joint Surg Br 2002;84:413–417.

44. Gleberman RH, Worlock BS, Siegel DB. Fractures and nonunions of the carpal scaphoid. J Bone Joint Surg Am 1989;71:1560–1565.

45. Gelberman RH, Menon J. The vascularity of the scaphoid. J Hand Surg Am 1980;5:508–13.

46. Amadio PC, Berquist TH, Smith DK, et al. Scaphoid malunion. J Hand Surg Am 1989;14:679–687.

47. Burgess RC. The effect of a simulated scaphoid malunion on wrist motion. J Hand Surg Am 1987;12(2 pt 1):774–776.

48. Vender MI, Watson HK, Wiener BD, et al. Degenerative change in symptomatic scaphoid nonunion. J Hand Surg Am 1987;12:514–519.

49. Grover R. Clinical assessment of scaphoid injuries and the detection of fractures. J Hand Surg Br 1996;21:341–343.

50. Cheung GC, Lever CJ, Morris AD. X-ray diagnosis of acute scaphoid fractures. J Hand Surg Br 2005;in press.

51. Cooney WP, Dobyns JH, Linscheid RL. Fractures of the scaphoid: a rational approach to management. Clin Orthop 1980;149:90–97.

52. Dorsay TA, Major NM, Helms CA. Cost-effectiveness of immediate MR imaging versus traditional follow-up for revealing radiographically occult scaphoid fractures. Am J Roentgenol 2001;177:1257–1263.

53. Gooding A, Coates M, Rothwell A. Accident Compensation Corporation. Cost analysis of traditional follow-up protocol versus MRI for radiographically occult scaphoid fractures: a pilot study for the Accident Compensation Corporation. N Z Med J. 2004;117:U1049.

54. Clay NR, Dias JJ, Costigan PS, et al. Need the thumb be immobilised in scaphoid fractures? A randomised prospective trial. J Bone Joint Surg Br 1991;73:828–832.

55. Falkenberg P. An experimental study of instability during supination and pronation of the fractured scaphoid. J Hand Surg Br 1985;10:211–213.

56. Gellman H, Caputo RJ, Carter V, et al. Comparison of short and long thumb-spica casts for non-displaced fractures of the carpal scaphoid. J Bone Joint Surg Am 1989;71:354–357.
57. Hambidge JE, Desai VV, Schranz PJ, et al. Acute fractures of the scaphoid. Treatment by cast immobilisation with the wrist in flexion or extension? J Bone Joint Surg Br 1999;81:91–92.
58. Haddad FS, Goddard NJ. Acute percutaneous scaphoid fixation: a pilot study. J Bone Joint Surg Br 1998;80:95–99.
59. Kamineni S, Lavy CBD. Percutaneous fixation of scaphoid fractures: an anatomical study. J Hand Surg Br 1999;24:85–88.
60. Slade JF, Gutow AP, Geissler WB. Percutaneous internal fixation of scaphoid fractures via an arthroscopically assisted dorsal approach. J Bone Joint Surg Am 2002;84 (suppl 2):21–36.
61. Yip HSF, Wu WC, Chang RYP, et al. Percutaneous cannulated screw fixation of acute scaphoid waist fracture. J Hand Surg Br 2002;27:42–46.
62. Bond CD, Shin AY, McBride MT, et al. Percutaneous screw fixation or cast immobilization for nondisplaced scaphoid fractures. J Bone Joint Surg Am 2001;83:483–488.
63. Adolfsson L, Lindau T, Arner M. Acutrak screw fixation versus cast immobilization for undisplaced scaphoid waist fractures. J Hand Surg Br 2001;26:192–195.
64. Dias JJ, Wildin CJ, Bhowal B, et al. Should acute scaphoid fractures be fixed? J Bone Joint Surg Am 2005;87;2160–2168.
65. Walsh JJ, Bishop AT. Diagnosis and management of hamate hook fractures. Hand Clin 2000;16:397–403.
66. Stark HH, Jobe FW, Boyes JH, et al. Fracture of the hook of the hamate in athletes. J Bone Joint Surg Am 1977;59:575–582.
67. Hart V, Graynor V. Roentogenographic study of the carpal canal. J Bone Joint Surg 1941;23:382–383.
68. Papilion JD, DuPuy TE, Aulicine PL, et al. Radiographic evaluation of the hook of the hamate. J Hand Surg Am 1988;13:437–439.
69. Whalen JL, Bishop AT, Linscheid RL. Nonoperative treatment of acute hamate hook fractures. J Hand Surg Am 1992;17:507–511.
70. Bishop AT, Beckenbaugh RD. Fracture of the hamate hook. J Hand Surg Am 1988;13:135–139.
71. Foucher G, Schuind F, Merle M, et al. Fractures of the hook of the hamate. J Hand Surg Br 1985;10:205–210.
72. Watson HK, Rogers WD. Nonunion of the hook of the hamate: an argument for bone grafting the non-union. J Hand Surg Am 1989;14:486–490.
73. Palmer AK, Werner FW. The triangular fibrocartilage complex of the wrist: anatomy and function. J Hand Surg Am 1981;6:153–162.
74. Terry CL, Waters PM. Triangular fibrocartilage injuries in pediatric and adolescent patients. J Hand Surg Am 1998;23:626–634.
75. Kato H, Nakamura R, Shionoya K, et al. Does high-resolution MR imaging have better accuracy than standard MR imaging for evaluation of the triangular fibrocartilage complex? J Hand Surg Br 2000;25:487–491.
76. Saupe N, Prussmann KP, Luechinger R, et al. MR imaging of the wrist: comparison between 1.5- and 3-T MR imaging—preliminary experience. Radiology 2005;234:256–264.
77. Palmer AK, Werner FW. Biomechanics of the distal radioulnar joint. Clin Orthop 1984;187:26–35.

78. Palmer AK. The distal radioulnar joint: anatomy, biomechanics, and triangular fibrocartilage complex abnormalities. Hand Clin 1987;3:31–40.
79. Steyers CM, Blair WF. Measuring ulnar variance: a comparison of techniques. J Hand Surg Am 1989;14:607–612.
80. Palmer AK. Triangular fibrocartilage complex lesions: a classification. J Hand Surg Am 1989;14:594–606.
81. Cooney WP, Linscheid RL, Dobyns JH. Triangular fibrocartilage tears. J Hand Surg Am 1994;19:143–154.
82. Bae DS, Waters PM. Pediatric distal radius fractures and triangular fibrocartilage complex injuries. Hand Clin 22:43–53.
83. Cooney WP, Bussey R, Dobyns JH, Linscheid RL. Difficult wrist fractures: perilunate fracture-dislocations of the wrist. Clin Orthop 1987;214:136–147.
84. De Smet L, Claessens A, Lefevre J, et al. Gymnast wrist: an epidemiologic survey of ulnar variance and stress changes of the radial physis in elite female gymnasts. Am J Sports Med. 1994;22:846–850.
85. DiFiori JP, Puffer JC, Mandelbaum BR, et al. Distal radial growth plate injury and positive ulnar variance in nonelite gymnasts. Am J Sports Med. 1997;25:763–768.
86. Waters PM, Bae DS, Montgomery KD. Surgical management of posttraumatic distal radial growth arrest in adolescents. J Pediatr Orthop. 2002;22:717–724.
87. Stern PJ. Fractures of the metacarpals and phalanges. In: Green DP, Hotchkiss RN, Pederson WC, Wolfe SW, eds. Green's Operative Hand Surgery. 5th ed. Philadelphia: Elsevier; 2005: 277–342.
88. Toronto R, Donovan PJ, Macintyre J. An alternative method of treatment for metacarpal fractures in athletes. Clin J Sport Med 1996;6:4–8.
89. Tavassoli J, Ruland RT, Hogan CJ, et al. Three cast techniques for the treatment of extra-articular metacarpal fractures. Comparison of short-term outcomes and final fracture alignments. J Bone Joint Surg Am 2005;87:2196–2201.
90. Al-Qattan MM. Juxta-epiphyseal fractures of the base of the proximal phalanx of the fingers in children and adolescents. J Hand Surg Br 2002;27:24–30.
91. Seymour N. Juxta-epiphyseal fracture of the terminal phalanx of the finger. J Bone Joint Surg Br 1966;48:347–349.
92. Heyman P, Gelbermann RH, Duncan K, et al. Injuries of the ulnar collateral ligament of the thumb metacarpophalangeal joint: biomechanical and prospective clinical studies on the usefulness of valgus stress testing. Clin Orthop 1993;292:165–171.
93. Stener B. Displacement of the ruptured ulnar collateral ligament of the metacarpo-phalangeal joint of the thumb: a clinical and anatomical study. J Bone Joint Surg Br 1962;44:869–879.
94. Coonrad RW, Goldner JL. A study of the pathological findings and treatment in soft-tissue injury of the thumb metacarpophalangeal joint. With a clinical study of the normal range of motion in one thousand thumbs and a study of post mortem findings of ligamentous structures in relation to function. J Bone Joint Surg Am 1968;50:439–451.
95. Bendre AA, Hartigan BJ, Kalainov DM. Mallet finger. J Am Acad Orthop Surg 2005;13:336–344.
96. Brzezienski MA, Schneider LH. Extensor tendon injuries at the distal interphalangeal joint. Hand Clin 1995;11:373–386.

97. Katzman BM, Klein DM, Mesa J, et al. Immobilization of the mallet finger: effects on the extensor tendon. J Hand Surg Br 1999;24:80–84.
98. Okafor B, Mbubaegbu C, Munshi I, et al. Mallet deformity of the finger: five-year follow-up of conservative treatment. J Bone Joint Surg Br 1997;79: 544–547.
99. Foucher G, Binhamer P, Cange S, et al. Long term results of splintage for mallet finger. Int Orthop 1996;20:129–131.
100. Wehbe MA, Schnieder LH. Mallet fractures. J Bone Joint Surg Am 1984;66: 658–669.
101. Garberman SF, Diao E, Peimer CA. Mallet finger: results of early versus delayed closed treatment. J Hand Surg Am 1994;19:850–852.
102. Patel MR, Desai SS, Bassini-Lipson L. Conservative treatment of chronic mallet finger. J Hand Surg Am 1986;11:570–573.
103. De Boeck H, Jaeken R. Treatment of chronic mallet finger deformity in children by tenodermodesis. J Pediatr Orthop 1992;12:351–354.
104. Ferrari GP, Fama G, Maran R. Dermatotenodesis in the treatment of "mallet finger." Arch Putti Chir Organi Mov. 1991;39:315–319.
105. Thompson JS, Littler JW, Upton J. The spiral oblique retinacular ligament (SORL). J Hand Surg Am 1978;3:482–487.
106. Kleinman WB, Petersen DP. Oblique retinacular ligament reconstruction for chronic mallet finger deformity. J Hand Surg Am 1984;9:399–404.
107. Houpt P, Dijkstra R, Storm Van Leeuwen JB. Fowler's tenotomy for mallet deformity. J Hand Surg Br 1993;18:499–500.
108. Grundberg AB, Reagan DS. Central slip tenotomy for chronic mallet finger deformity. J Hand Surg Am 1987;12:545–547.
109. Katzman SS, Gibeault JD, Dickson K, Thompson JD. Use of a Herbert screw for interphalangeal joint arthrodesis. Clin Orthop 1993;296:127–132.
110. Leddy JP, Packer JW. Avulsion of the profundus insertion in athletes. J Hand Surg Am 1977;2:66–69.
111. Gunter GS. Traumatic avulsion of the insertion of flexor digitorum profundus. Aust N Z J Surg 1960;30:1.
112. Manske PR, Lesker PA. Avulsion of the ring finger digitorum profundus tendon: an experimental study. Hand 1978;10:52–55.
113. Idzikowski JR, Janes PC, Abbott PJ. Upper extremity snowboarding injuries. Ten-year results from the Colorado snowboard injury survey. Am J Sports Med 2000;28(6):825–832.
114. Ronning R, Ronning I, Gerner T, et al. The efficacy of wrist protectors in preventing snowboarding injuries. Am J Sports Med 2001;29:581–585.
115. Schieber RA, Branche-Dorsey CM, Ryan GW, et al. Risk factors for injuries from in-line skating and the effectiveness of safety gear. N Engl J Med 1996;28: 1630–1635.
116. Beirness DJ, Foss RD, Desmond KJ. Use of protective equipment by in-line skaters: an observational study. Inj Prev 2001;7:51–55.
117. Matsumoto K, Sumi H, Sumi Y, et al. Wrist fractures from snowboarding: a prospective study for 3 seasons from 1998 to 2001. Clin J Sport Med 2004;14: 64–71.
118. Schuster M, Israeli A. Survey of injuries and protective gear worn by in-line skaters in public parks. Am J Phys Med Rehabil 1999;78:7–10.

10
Pelvic, Hip, and Thigh Injuries

Jason H. Nielson

Pelvic, hip, and thigh injuries are relatively rare in the young athlete (1). The young athlete with pelvic or hip pain may present with an acute injury necessitating immediate treatment. An acute injury may cause pain in the pelvic, hip, thigh, or even knee region. More commonly, the young athlete will have a chronic injury that will limit activities during or after sporting activities. The spectrum of injury can range from osseous tumors, masked by injury (2), to simple strains. Apophyseal avulsions and stress fractures are the most commonly encountered skeletal injuries of the hip and pelvis. These injuries can result in substantial amount of injury time for the young athlete. Diagnosis and treatment of the pelvis, hip, and thigh injuries is one of the most difficult clinical tasks for the sports physician, and one of possibly great frustration for the young athlete. Therefore, careful clinical diagnosis with considerations of broad differentials and appropriate treatment in this age group is crucial.

Anatomy

The hip joint has two separate and unique development patterns, the femoral head and the acetabulum, which have been well described by Ogden (3). The acetabulum is created by the normal development of the triradiate cartilage. With normal development, a congruent and stable joint is formed. Injuries to the developing triradiate cartilage could have long-lasting effects for the young athlete such as acetabular dysplasia and degenerative hip disease later in life (3). The femoral side of the hip joint has three separate ossification centers: the capital femoral epiphysis, the greater trochanter, and the lesser trochanter. The growth and progression of these ossification centers contribute to the biomechanics of the proximal femur and its injury patterns. The hip and pelvis have several apophyses, all of which have large muscle attachments (Figure 10.1). These apophyses contain secondary ossification centers, which allow circumferential growth, but do not add to longitudinal growth of the skeleton. The secondary

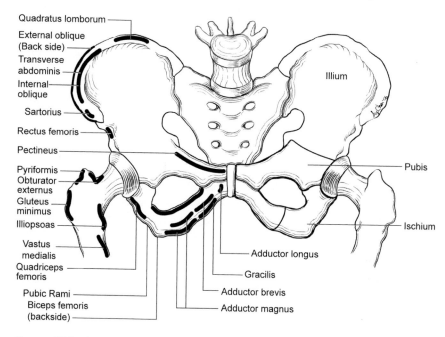

Quadratus lomborum
External oblique (Back side)
Transverse abdominis
Internal oblique
Sartorius
Rectus femoris
Pectineus
Pyriformis
Obturator externus
Gluteus minimus
Illiopsoas
Vastus medialis
Quadriceps femoris
Pubic Rami
Biceps femoris (backside)

Illium
Pubis
Ischium
Adductor longus
Gracilis
Adductor brevis
Adductor magnus

FIGURE 10.1. Anatomy of the hip. (Adapted from Safran M, Stone D, Zachazewski J. Instructions for Sports Medicine Patients. Philadelphia: W.B. Saunders; 2003. With permission from Elsevier.)

ossifications centers appear between the ages of 11 and 15 yr of age (3). These apophyses are weaker then the surrounding soft tissues and, hence, allow for the avulsion fractures seen in adolescent athletes, in contrast to muscle or tendon strains and tears in the older athlete.

There are several muscle groups in the thigh, including flexors, extensors, abductors, and adductors. The quadriceps muscles (sartorius, rectus femoris, vastus lateralis, and vastus medialis) are the strongest muscles in the anterior thigh and are responsible for knee extension. On the posterior aspect, the hamstring complex is composed of three muscles: the biceps femoris (a short and long head), the semitendinosus, and the semimembranosus. The hamstrings span two joints, causing hip extension and knee flexion. The long head of the biceps, semitendinosus, and semimembranosis originate on the ischial tuberosity.

Clinical Evaluation

History

The type and extent of injury to the young athlete is dependent on several factors. Eliciting details of these factors can be very helpful in making an accurate diagnosis. These factors include the patient's age, the mechanism of injury, the physiologic condition of the young athlete, and the type of sport or activity engaged in at the time of injury. The history should also evaluate potential risk factors that contribute to overuse injuries. These include inappropriate rate, intensity, and duration of training; the patient's age, to assess developmental muscle tendon imbalances; footwear; and surface conditions (4).

Physical Examination

The sports physician on the field must be able to identify the urgency of an acute injury. Injuries with deformity, obvious dislocations, and inability to bear weight should be managed by splinting the injured limb and arranging transport to the appropriate emergency facility. Reductions should not routinely be done on the field, unless there is an obvious and serious neurovascular compromise noted in the distal extremity. The examination should include a thorough, but brief, evaluation of the alignment, stability, neurologic state, and vascular state of the pelvis and extremity. In a stable injury in the office setting, a more detailed examination can be done. Special attention should be given to the hip exam in a young patient, as well as to the determination of muscle tendon imbalances, specific sites of bony tenderness, and extent of range of motion. When treating young athletes, who are more prone to bony avulsions and possible pathologic lesions, radiographic evaluation of the pelvis, hip, and femur should be included in the standard work-up of the injury. Magnetic resonance imaging (MRI) is very helpful to evaluate soft tissue injury and give more detail concerning bony injuries.

Acute Injuries of the Pelvis, Hip, and Thigh

Iliac Crest Contusion

Iliac crest contusion or a hip pointer is a common injury and, potentially, a debilitating condition. A hip pointer is a contusion of the iliac crest and the surrounding subcutaneous soft tissues. This injury is common in contact sports, such as football, rugby, and soccer, and is caused by a direct blow. Adjacent soft tissues may also be injured, causing localized pain, swelling, and difficulty with gait.

The athlete typically presents with localized pain, ecchymosis, and antalgic gait. Focal tenderness is common along the iliac crest. Because of the multiple muscle attachments of the abdominal and gluteal muscles at the iliac crest, leg elevations and muscle contractions may be painful. The diagnosis is usually made clinically, but AP and oblique pelvic radiographs can be very helpful in the young athlete to rule out apophyseal avulsions or wing fractures.

Initially, rest from aggravating activities, ice, and nonsteriodal antiinflammatory drug (NSAIDs) are used to treat hip pointers. In the clinical scenario of a large hematoma, aspiration can relieve pain and possibly speed up recovery time. After the acute pain has resolved, a progressive rehabilitation program is begun that includes hip range of motion, stretching, and, ultimately, strengthening. Typical recovery time is 2–4 wk, with return to sport when the pain has resolved and the athlete is able to perform sport-specific activities. Additional padding may be required for further protection. Myositis ossificans traumatica, muscle fibrosis, and muscle soreness are possible complications of hip pointers.

Avulsion Injuries of the Pelvis

Apophyseal avulsion fractures are common in the young athlete (5). These avulsion fractures are secondary to either a sudden pull of the large muscle attachments on the apophysis or an excessive stretch injury of the tendon and osseous junction on an open apophysis. The apophyses of the pelvis in an immature skeleton appear and fuse later than the growth plates in the long bones. This delay in ossific maturation places the young athlete at increased risk for bony avulsion injures. The physis is the weakest structure of the immature skeleton, and is more vulnerable to avulsions and direct trauma. This usually happens in adolescent male athletes between 14–17 yr of age and in female athletes between 12–15 yr of age, with a male preponderance (5). Avulsions of the apophyses routinely occur during a growth spurt with corresponding tight soft tissues, and "musculoskeletally tight" athletes are more prone to this injury (6).

The more common sites of avulsions are at the iliac crest (insertion of the abdominal muscles), anterior superior iliac spine (origin of the sartorius), anterior inferior iliac spine (origin of the rectus), ischial tuberosity (origin of the hamstrings), and lesser trochanter (insertion of the iliopsoas) (7,8) (Figure 10.1) This can occur in many different sports, but often occurs with extreme exertion, particularly in sprinters and jumpers. Localized pain, swelling, and limitation of motion are common with presentation. Pain may be extreme, with point tenderness at the site of avulsion. Plain radiographs are diagnostic, but specific views, such as pelvic Judet and inlet and outlet views, may be required to identify the avulsion (Figure 10.2).

Treatment is usually nonoperative for avulsion fractures, and includes rest, ice, and avoidance of aggravating activities. Rehabilitation begins with gentle stretching and range of motion exercises with progressive strengthening (9). Return to sport is allowed after full range of motion and 90% of strength is achieved, which is usually within 4–8 wk. For displaced ischial

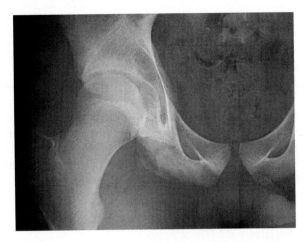

FIGURE 10.2. A proximal hamstring avulsion injury in a 15-yr-old soccer player. He was injured as he flexed the lower extremity going in for a ball. This injury was missed with initial evaluation, as films were not taken. He never fully recovered from his initial injury. Upon subsequent proximal hamstring injury, radiographs were obtained and noted to have had a previous avulsion injury of the proximal hamstrings.

tuberosity avulsion fractures (more than 3 cm), open reduction and internal fixation may be required to avoid late sequelae, such as proximal hamstring syndrome and sciatic nerve irritation, and to improve hamstring strength (10). Displaced anterior inferior iliac spine avulsions may block hip range of motion if the fragment is large.

Chondral Injury of the Hip

Chondral injuries of the hip may occur in the young athletic patient and can be a source of disabling hip pain. Such injuries can be seen with trauma or underlying pathologic conditions. Traumatic history may include a frank dislocation, but more commonly involves a direct blow to the greater trochanter or a fall onto the lateral hip. In thin young athletes, the force of a direct blow to the hip is not cushioned by soft tissue and is transferred directly to the chondral surface. The resultant force can cause an array of injuries, from a superficial articular surface lesion, to a full-thickness articular defect with production of a traumatic loose fragment. The cartilage damage is often at the labral junction of the acetabulum and can be associated with labral tears.

Athletes will often present with a popping sensation, pain, and failure to fully recover after injury. Symptoms are often mildly limiting, but become increasingly painful with movement of the hip. Mechanical symptoms, such as clicking and catching, can be common and are favorable prognostic indicators for arthroscopic treatment (11). Imaging of the hip is often helpful. Images from MRI can reveal specific injury, such as articular defects or loose fragments or simply increased bony edema, which are suggestive of trauma to the femoral head or the acetabulum. In acute lesions with intact articular cartilage, initial management should include protected weight bearing and early range of motion. If symptoms continue, or if there are loose bodies or unstable articular fragments, hip arthroscopy can be very helpful in managing the mechanical symptoms (11–13).

Adductor Injuries

Adductor strains are common, and result from repetitive contractions or a sudden forceful contraction with the lower extremity in an externally rotated and abducted position. This is often seen in the soccer player who uses the medial foot for ball advancement and control. Muscular imbalance can be a predisposing factor to groin injuries (14). The athlete might complain of a sharp tearing pain with a known incident and subsequent pain with contraction of the inner thigh musculature. The adductor muscle may be tender along its course, and pain is present with resisted adduction of the leg. In acute injuries, there may be some swelling and ecchymosis at the muscular origin at the pubic symphysis.

Radiographs should be taken to exclude other causes of pubic pain, such as avulsion injuries or an intrapelvic lesion, which can be common in this age group. Images from MRI can help to identify the degree of injury to the adductor musculature, and the images correlate well with symptoms (15). Severity of injury can be classified with a scale of I–III. Grade I strains are painful without loss of function or mobility. Grade II strains have some loss of strength and mobility. Grade III strains have complete loss of function. Treatment is conservative with rest, ice, NSAIDs, and avoidance of aggravating activities. Protective weight bearing for a few days for low-grade injuries, and a few weeks for high-grade injuries, is helpful. Physical therapy is very important, and can lessen pain, as well as maintain range of motion and strength. Therapy has been shown to decrease the amount of adductor strength loss in young athletes (14), and should include stretching and strengthening. Return to sport is allowed after symptoms resolve, full range of motion is regained, and adductor strength has recovered.

Hamstring Injuries

Hamstring injuries are common in athletes, and are seen in the young athlete especially during the adolescent growth spurt. Skeletal growth can outpace the muscle–tendon unit growth during the adolescent growth spurt, resulting in loss of muscular flexibility. With the immature skeleton, avulsion injuries must always be in the differential because the apophysis is the weakest portion of the hamstring complex, with the majority of the hamstrings muscles originating from the ischial tuberosity.

Injuries commonly occur with eccentric elongation during the swing and heel-strike phases. The biceps femoris is the most commonly injured hamstring muscle (16). Failure most often occurs at the proximal musculotendinous junction of the biceps femoris. Multiple risk factors have been described for hamstring injuries, such as previous hamstring injury, flawed technique, lack of flexibility (17), improper warm-up exercises, and strength imbalance, with the hamstring being significantly weaker than the quadriceps muscle (18). Some studies have reported that athletes with proper strengthening, stretching, and warm-up activities have a decreased incidence of hamstring injuries (19). Hamstring injuries are typically classified into three groups, based on severity. Grade I injuries are minor and have only a small degree of disruption of the integrity of the musculotendinous unit. Grade II injuries are more severe, with partial tearing of the musculotendinous unit, with some fibers left intact. Grade III hamstring injuries are complete tears of the hamstring musculature, with a subset of Grade III B injuries with a bony avulsion injury at the origin.

The young athlete may present with an acute injury or chronic pain in the proximal posterior thigh. Athletes may report a sudden tearing or popping sensation with strenuous activity, often with sprinting. With a more prolonged course, athletes may complain of a posterior thigh tightness and dull pain at the proximal hamstring origin. Physical examination may reveal posterior thigh swelling, ecchymosis, and tenderness at the proximal muscle origin, musculotendinous junction, and the muscle belly. Often, the athlete will be reluctant to fully extend the knee in an acute injury. With complete rupture, the biceps may retract distally and a mass may be noted, with a defect seen proximally (20). Pain with passive hip flexion and resisted knee flexion are very common in the acute setting, and less striking with chronic injuries. In the young athlete, plain films of the pelvis should be obtained to rule out a bony avulsion or in chronic and recurrent cases. This is important because young patients are at higher risk of pelvic tumors, which can be masked by ongoing athletic injuries. An MRI is helpful when the diagnosis is unclear or in the setting of a severe injury to determine the extent of the hamstring tear and to evaluate for potential repair.

Treatment of hamstring injuries is conservative and based on injury severity. The mainstay of treatment consists of rest, ice, and compression, followed by a well-supervised physical therapy program. Hamstring stretching and strengthening should be initiated after the acute pain has subsided. The goal of therapy is to provide strength for the hamstring during its most vulnerable time of activities, i.e., eccentric elongation. Mild eccentric strengthening is most helpful in treatment and prevention (21,22). Return to activities is allowed when the athlete has regained full, painless range of hip motion and almost full strength. In addition, correction of muscle imbalances is of great importance in avoiding reinjury and chronic conditions. With complete hamstring rupture, surgical repair of the musculotendinous junction or the bony avulsion may be required to return the athlete to his/her previous level of sport participation (23).

Quadriceps Strain

The quadriceps can have a wide range of injury, from tendonitis to rupture of the tendon, and blunt trauma. These injuries are similar to the adult counterpart, but are less common in the young athlete. Although not common, quadriceps ruptures have been reported in adolescents (24). These injuries can be secondary to repetitive microtrauma or overuse. More commonly, the young athlete will have an acute episode of anterior thigh pain. This is accompanied by various degrees of swelling of the thigh. MR imaging is helpful in predicting the prognosis for acute quadriceps strains (25). Treatment is conservative, with rest and avoidance of aggravating activities. Early rehabilitation is very helpful to regain knee motion and maintain muscle tone. Return to sports is allowed after resolution of symptoms, return of knee range of motion, and adequate muscle strength.

Quadriceps Contusions and Myositis Ossificans Traumatica

Athletes engaged in contact sports often have injuries secondary to blunt trauma of the thigh. After a traumatic blunt injury, the normal healing response of hemorrhage and inflammation can lead to granulation tissue and, eventually, scar tissue formation. Athletes usually can recall a specific incident of injury and present with localized thigh pain, tenderness, swelling of the thigh, loss of knee flexion and, occasionally, a knee effusion. Plain films are useful to rule out any bony injury initially, but might show signs of calcifications 2–4 wk after injury. Contusions can be treated similarly to muscle strains. An effort to limit the hematoma formation should be attempted through initial use of the RICE protocol (rest, ice, compression, elevation). In addition, therapy with gentle and gradual range of motion exercises, followed by stretching and strengthening, is helpful (26,27).

A potential sequela of blunt trauma to the thigh is myositis ossificans, which results from significant compressive trauma to the soft tissues of the thigh. The heterotopic ossification in usually noted at the anterior aspect of the femur and suggests a more substantial injury, but rarely will it change the subsequent treatment (27). In young cadets, the incidence of myositis ossificans was 9–20% (26), but the incidence is thought to be much lower in young athletes (28). The differential diagnosis must include infection and malignancies, such as osteosarcoma, synovial sarcomas, and chondrosarcomas. The initial radiographs might appear similar to a malignant process, but a history of recent blunt trauma, anterior location, and intact cortex suggest a posttraumatic injury. These lesions tend to stabilize radiographically in 3–4 mo (29). MR and computed tomography (CT) have been used to further analyze calcifications. The appearance of these lesions can vary depending on the maturity of the lesion (30). Long-term limitations are rare in the young athlete. Rarely, symptoms continue and become limiting. In these rare cases after failure of conservative treatment, excision of the bony mass can be done, but preferably not until 6 mo after initial injury (29).

Overuse Injuries

Stress Fractures

Stress fractures are a result of repetitive improper or overtraining, with resultant microtrauma to the supporting skeleton (31–33). The female athlete is at higher risk, especially in the context of disordered eating, amenorrhea, and osteoporosis (31,32,34,35). The prevalence and pattern of stress fractures in children differs from their adult counterparts, as does the response of the growing skeleton to the repetitive stresses applied to it (36). Multiple risks factors will increase the likelihood of overuse injuries in young athletes, such as training errors, muscle tendon imbalances, anatomic alignment, footwear, playing surface, nutritional factors, medical conditions, and deconditioning (36). Usually, two or more risk factors can be identified. Training errors tend to be the most common, and include rapid increase in volume or intensity of training (36). Restrictions of the young athlete's training progression should be limited to no more than a 10% increase per week (36).

Pelvic Stress Fractures

Stress fractures in the pelvis in young athletes are quite uncommon. Stress fractures in the pelvis and hip are more commonly reported in young female distance runners or athletes involved in jumping sports (35). Iliac crest stress injuries have been reported in young athletes as a result of repetitive training (5). Much more commonly in this age group, stresses around the pelvis will result in frank apophyseal avulsions (37). Stress fractures of the pubic rami (Figure 10.3) and sacrum are the most commonly encountered, and are most commonly seen in distance runners (31).

Athletes will complain of pain with weight bearing or activity-related pain in the hip or pelvis, which decreases with rest. Localized pain to the

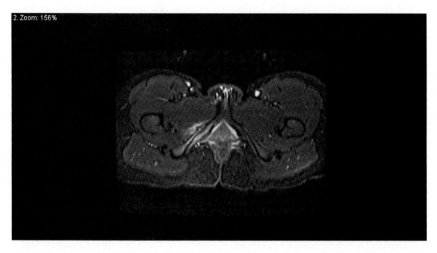

FIGURE 10.3. Axial MRI of the pelvis in a young patient with an inferior pubic rami stress fracture.

inguinal or adductor region is common. Range of motion is often painful and limited. Axial loading and internal rotation of the extremity is likewise painful. Plain radiographs may initially be negative (38). If suspicion of a stress fracture is high, particularly if there is persistent pain in the light of negative x-rays, bone scan or MRI should be obtained (38).

Pelvic stress fractures are usually stable and are treated conservatively with rest and protected weight bearing while symptomatic. Progressive rehabilitation with hydrotherapy can be helpful (38). Complete recovery may take 3–5 mo (31).

Femoral Neck (Hip) Stress Fractures

Femoral neck stress fractures and proximal femur stress fractures occur most commonly in endurance athletes, such as distance runners and tri-athletes. Femoral neck stress fractures in the young athlete with open physes are rare (39). Occasionally, however, hip pain in the young athlete will ultimately be found secondary to a fracture of the base of the neck of the femur (40,41). The athlete may describe pain at the hip, anterior thigh, or groin region, as well as nonspecific muscle pain. Examination often reveals pain with axial loading. In addition, pain in the proximal thigh, pelvis, or groin can occur with internal rotation. Plain radiographs may be normal, but with a high index of suspicion a bone scan should be obtained.

Treatment of femoral neck stress fractures depends on the location of the fracture (42). Compression-type stress fractures involving the inferior aspect of the medial portion of the femoral neck are the most common, and are inherently more stable (43). Treatment consists of non weight bearing until pain resolves, with a slow, gradual return to full weight bearing. Rehabilitation with hydrotherapy for maintaining muscle mass during the partial weight bearing period can be helpful. Tension-type femoral neck stress fractures occur superiorly at the lateral aspect of the femoral neck and are inherently unstable (44). These are routinely treated with early surgical intervention with multiple screw fixations through the femoral neck (45).

Femoral Stress Fractures

Stress injuries of the femur in young athletes are not common, representing 3–12% of the stress fractures found in this age group (41,44). Femoral stress fractures often occur in such sports that require cyclical loading of the lower extremities, such as endurance activities, distance running, and dancing (Figure 10.4) (46). Stress fractures can occur anywhere in the femur, even at the distal femoral physis (47). In the young athlete, these are often compression-type stress fractures at the base of the femur.

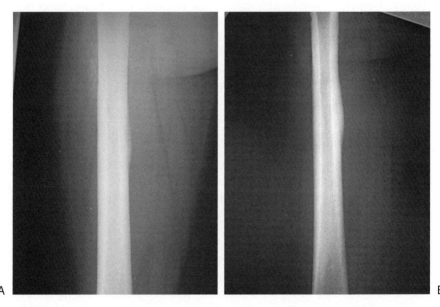

A   B

FIGURE 10.4. A femoral stress fracture in a 16-yr-old female cross-country runner. Her symptoms began after increasing her mileage and changing running surfaces. (A) Initial presentation for activity-related thigh pain. (B) After 6wk of rest with limited activities.

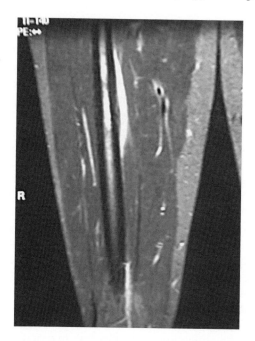

FIGURE 10.5. A femoral stress reaction in a 15-yr-old female distance runner. She had a history of amenorrhea, eating disorders, and right thigh pain with weight-bearing activities. A coronal MR reveals marrow edema, as well as edema in the surrounding periosteum.

Symptoms of a femoral stress fracture are usually activity related, and are relieved with rest. Vague, dull exertional pain is often the presenting complaint. Proximal femoral neck fractures may present with referred pain to the knee and inner thigh. If the athlete presents late in the course of injury, an antalgic gait may be present. Pain with three-point stress of the femur is common, as well as pain with axial loading. Radiographic presentation of a stress fracture may differ from adults secondary to the presence of a thick periosteum (36,48). Because of the healing response, radiographic findings may be mistaken for a tumor (49). Further imaging studies, such as MRI or bone scan, can be used if radiographs are negative (Figure 10.5). Often, simple changes in training technique and intensity can allow healing in most stress fractures, but a course of modified weight bearing is required for femoral stress fractures. Cases of complete fracture displacement have been reported. Progressive protected weight bearing is advanced as the clinical symptoms abate. Usually, 6–10 wk is required for complete healing. Return to sport can occur with complete resolution of pain and adjustment of the precipitating risk factors. Physical therapy during the recovery phase can be helpful to avoid disuse atrophy, bone demineralization, and stiffness.

Labral Tears

In the young athlete, new onset of hip pain should warrant a high suspicion for the more common causes of pediatric hip pain, even with reported athletic trauma. These include infection, Legg–Calve–Perthes disease, developmental dysplasia, and slipped capital femoral epiphysis (SCFE) (50). After these entities have been ruled out, further diagnoses, including loose bodies, labral tears, and chondral injury, should be considered (51). Labral tears are common lesions in the hip joint of young athletes. Athletes with labral tears usually present after rotational trauma to the hip joint, which can range from mild to severe. The labrum is more susceptible to tearing with underlying hip dysplasia or degeneration (52). Tears commonly occur at the junction between the acetabulum and the labrum, and they can be associated with chondral injury (53). Labral tears commonly occur in dancers, golfers, and activities requiring significant hip rotation.

The young athlete with a labral tear will complain of hip or groin pain, and often, report a painful clicking and catching sensation with pivoting, twisting activities, or flexed and internally rotated positions (54). Examination of the athlete often reveals pain with provocative hip flexion, as well as with hyperflexion, adduction, and internal rotation for anterior labral tears. Extension and abduction of the hip with external rotation can cause symptoms with posterior labral tears. Imaging begins with plain radiographs to assess for acetabular dysplasia. MR imaging is helpful for diagnosing labral tears, and MR arthrograms (Figure 10.6) have been reported to have a sensitivity of greater than 90% (55).

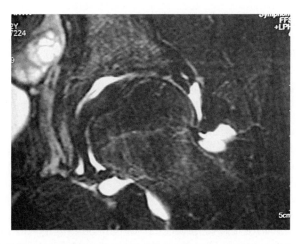

FIGURE 10.6. MR arthrogram of a torn labrum in a young 14-yr-old synchronized swimmer. This injury occurred after performing the splits. She had subsequent mechanical symptoms of the hip and a catching sensation with "egg-beater" swimming activities.

Treatment of the young athlete with a labral tear should begin with a period of protected weight bearing for 4 wk. Only a small portion of these patients (13%) will become asymptomatic (56). In the presence of reproducible mechanical symptoms after a twisting or axial loading event during athletics, arthroscopic evaluation should be considered with persistent symptoms if therapy fails (51,57). Most commonly, the anterior labrum is torn. The torn labrum can either be repaired or debrided arthroscopically (58). Good outcomes have been reported after hip arthroscopy, especially in patients with preoperative mechanical symptoms (11,56). In addition, hip arthroscopy has been found to be a safe and efficacious treatment option for children and adolescents with hip pathology (59). Postoperative protocols differ significantly in the literature, but should include a brief period of protected weight bearing and early onset of controlled hip range of motion exercises and strengthening activities.

Osteitis Pubis

Osteitis pubis is a chronic painful inflammatory condition that affects the pubic symphysis (60). This condition is caused by repetitive microtrauma in the young athlete with overuse of the adductors and gracilis muscles, but can be a result of nontraumatic etiology as well. It has been reported in athletes such as distance runners, weightlifters, fencers, soccer players, and football players (61,62). There is usually a gradual onset of pubic pain, which may radiate to the groin at the medial thigh region. Athletes may also complain of vague muscular symptoms and spasms of the hip adductors.

It can be difficult to distinguish osteitis pubis from an adductor strain, but focal tenderness over the anterior pubis symphysis is noted in osteitis pubis. Plain radiographs may reveal symmetrical bone resorption at the medial symphysis, widening of the symphysis, and sclerosis along the pubic rami or degenerative changes at the medial symphysis in chronic cases (61,62). Bone scans may show diffuse increased uptake in the region.

Osteitis pubis normally responds well to conservative treatment, and it is usually self-limited. Rest, avoidance of aggravating activities, and NSAIDs are the first-line treatment options (61). Rehabilitation utilizing hydrotherapy is usually successful, but can be prolonged, often lasting 3–9 mo for complete resolution. Careful use of steroid injections under fluoroscopy can be helpful in patients who do not respond favorably to conservative treatments. More recently, prolotherapy has been used for treatment (63). Surgical treatments have been described (64), but are rarely indicated in the young athlete. Return to sport is allowed as symptoms permit.

Sacroiliitis

Sacroiliitis or sacral iliac sprains are relatively rare, and hence, often over-looked (65). The sacroiliac ligaments are strong and motion at this joint is limited. This joint is important in the dissipation of forces between the spine and the lower extremities (66). Forces at this joint can be increased with forceful hamstring muscle contractions, sudden torsional motions, direct blows, and forceful straightening from a squatting position (66). The young athlete will complain of low back pain in the region of the sacroiliac joint, as well as possible radiation to the buttock or thigh (31).

The athlete with sacroiliitis typically has focal tenderness over the sacroiliac joint. The Faber test (the ipsilateral hip is flexed, abducted, and externally rotated), Sacroiliac Compression test, and the Gaenslen's test (hyperflexion of the contralateral hip to lock the pelvis and hyperextension of the affected hip) are commonly used for diagnosis (13,65). Painful response from these maneuvers indicates a positive result. Radiologic evaluation is more helpful to rule out other types of pathology, such as stress fractures, tumors, infection, and inflammatory conditions, but MRI images can detect injury and abnormality at the sacroiliac joint (Figure 10.7). Treatment includes rest, heat, and NSAIDs. A restrictive elastic bandage is often helpful after the acute phase. Steroid injections under fluoroscopy can be both diagnostic and useful in refractory cases. Healing normally takes 4–6 wk, and might require protective range of motion for healing to occur (13,65,67). Rehabilitation is useful for peripelvic stability and pelvic girdle strengthening. The athlete may return to sport after reso-

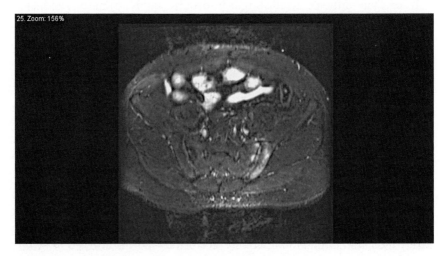

FIGURE 10.7. Axial MRI of the sacroiliac joints revealing inflammation of the left sacroiliac joint.

lution of symptoms, return of range of motion, and normalization of strength.

Snapping Hip

Snapping hip syndrome is a condition with a painful audible snap in the hip with flexion and extension. This is often seen in dancers and gymnasts, as well as football and soccer players. Causes of a snapping hip can include abnormal contact of the iliotibial band over the greater trochanter (68). Localized lateral tenderness at the greater trochanter and posterior to it can be noted secondary to the inflamed trochanteric bursa. The athlete can often reproduce these symptoms voluntarily. The Ober test is often positive secondary to tightening of the iliotibial band over the symptomatic greater trochanter. The most common cause of snapping hip is usually caused by the iliopsoas tendon snapping over the pectineal prominence of the femoral neck (68,69). With extension of the hip, the iliopsoas tendon slides from a lateral position to a more medial position in relation to the femoral head (68). In addition, loose bodies in the hip joint, labral tears, or synovial chondromatosis of the hip joint may cause intraarticular snapping.

With a prolonged history of snapping hip, a scenario of significant contractures of the hip flexors and hamstrings are often noted. Diagnosis is made on the basis of the history and can be confirmed with the physical examination. Provocative testing can be helpful for diagnosis. Progressive passive hyper flexion of the hip will cause pain, as well as resisted flexion and adduction with the leg in the figure of four position. In addition, hyperextension and abduction of the hip with internal rotation can be painful. MR imaging can be helpful to exclude intraarticular causes of hip pain and can identify inflammation of the corresponding tendons or bursa.

The treatment for snapping hip is conservative. Rest and avoidance of aggravating activities can be very helpful. Physical therapy should include stretching of the iliotibial band and any contractures or tightness in the hip region. In addition, core strengthening can be helpful. Ultrasound and iontophoresis can be very effective in decreasing pain. Greater trochanteric bursitis can likewise be treated with ultrasound and stretching. In recalcitrant cases, an injection of a corticosteroid is helpful in relieving symptoms enough to effectively benefit from physical therapy. For refractory cases of external snapping, bursal excision and Z-plasty of the iliotibial band has been described in adolescents (70). Internal snapping of the hip can be treated with surgical tendon lengthening for recalcitrant cases (71). Intraarticular sources of snapping hip usually require surgical treatment with arthroscopy or an open approach if there is a large loose body of synovial chondromatosis (68). Return to sport is allowed as symptoms permit and when strength and range of motion allow safe participation.

Proximal Hamstring Syndrome

Proximal hamstring syndrome was first described by Puranene (10). After a hamstring injury, the inflammatory and reparative process can inflame and constrict the sciatic nerve, causing local buttock pain with radiation down the thigh. Patients often complain of gluteal or proximal posterior thigh pain, which increases with stretching of the hamstring muscle or fast running. The pain can be relentless with sitting and improves in the supine position. The ischial tuberosity is often tender, and passive stretching of the hamstring causes pain. The diagnosis is mostly made by history, but imaging studies are very helpful in ruling out other causes of buttock pain. MR images can show inflammation at the proximal hamstrings, but are often negative. Treatment is conservative, with activity modifications and NSAIDs. Physical therapy can be initiated for hamstring stretching. Injections under fluoroscopy can be used to settle the inflammatory process and allow physical therapy to be attempted. Chronic proximal hamstring syndrome often cannot be alleviated through conservative means. Surgical release of the lateral portion of the proximal hamstring tendon has been reported to have a favorable outcome (10).

Piriformis Syndrome

The piriformis muscle can cause compression of the sciatic nerve and is a common cause of buttock and proximal posterior thigh or hamstring pain. Piriformis syndrome is thought to be a more recognized cause of low back pain and sciatica (72). History often reveals blunt trauma to the gluteal or sacroiliac region. Patients complain of pain in the SI joint region, at the greater sciatic notch, with occasional radiation to the lower leg. This pain is often "crampy" or described to be similar to a tight posterior hamstring. Stooping over, as well as lifting heavy objects, tends to aggravate symptoms. A palpable mass may be detected. Physical exam commonly reveals buttock pain with hip flexion, adduction, and internal rotation. It is important to rule out other more common causes of low back and radicular pain.

Imaging studies of the spine and pelvis are important to rule out other pathology. Atrophy and fibrosis of the piriformis muscle can be suggestive of piriformis syndrome (73). Treatment of piriformis syndrome includes NSAIDs and local steroid and anesthetic injections, along with physical therapy for stretching of the piriformis muscle and local modalities to reduce pain. In recalcitrant cases, a new arthroscopic procedure releasing the piriformis has been described with immediate relief of pain and quick return to normal activities (74).

Trochanteric Bursitis

Trochanteric bursitis is secondary to irritation of the iliotibial band (ITB) over the greater trochanter (GT). Continual repetitive motions, such as running, leg length discrepancy, a broad pelvis in females, and increased foot pronation, can irritate the bursa deep to the ITB. Tenderness is found at the greater trochanter, and pain can be elicited by external rotation and adduction of the hip.

Treatment focuses on physical therapy. Antiinflammatory medications are often helpful to allow the athlete to undergo more effective therapy. Exercises to stretch the ITB and strengthen the gluteal musculature can resolve symptoms. Often, local injection of a corticosteroid helps to allow symptomatic relief. In recalcitrant cases, a proximal release of the ITB with debridement of the fibrotic bursa can relieve symptoms (75). This condition is one of irritation, and the athlete may continue to play as desired, with the aid of NSAIDs, ice, and stretching exercises.

Acquired Conditions

Slipped Capital Femoral Epiphysis

An acute Slipped capital femoral epiphysis (SCFE) is an uncommon sports-related injury, but is the most common hip disorder in adolescence (76). The sports physician treating young athletes must always keep in mind that hip pathology can manifest itself with knee symptoms. In the scenario with vague knee complaints and negative findings on physical examination of the knee, hip pathology must be excluded. A SFCE rarely occurs as an acute fracture with an identified injury. More commonly, this is a chronic injury of the preadolescent and adolescent during growth spurts, secondary to mechanical failure of the proximal femoral physis during normal physiologic loading of the hip (77).

The physical examination will reveal a normal knee with limitation of internal rotation of the hip. With hip flexion, the leg tends to externally rotate. Both anteroposterior and lateral plain films of both hips are indicated. Radiographs commonly reveal a widened and blurred physis, and increased sclerosis of the femoral neck secondary to the posterior overlap of the epiphysis. Treatment for SCFE is surgical and involves stabilization of the physis using transphyseal screws.

Nerve Entrapments

Nerve entrapments are not common, but are often overlooked and can cause symptoms in young athletes. These nerve entrapments should be ruled out in the differential of chronic pelvic girdle pain and can be treated definitively.

Obturator Nerve Entrapment

The obturator nerve can be compressed in multiple sites. It arises from the lumbar plexus and travels through the true pelvis. It can be compressed by pregnancy, pelvic trauma, and intrapelvic masses, such as a hematoma or infectious collection. In addition, retroperitoneal masses or collections can compress the nerve (78). In athletes, the nerve is more at risk of compression after it exits the pelvis, by a fascial band at the distal end of the obturator canal (78,79). Sporting activities, including repetitive kicking, as well as lateral and twisting motions, appear to be additional factors in the development of symptoms. The athlete describes exercise-induced medial groin and thigh pain, which decreases with rest (78). Sensation remains intact. Abductor weakness and mild muscle spasm may be present. Reproducible pain is often present with external rotation and adduction of the affected hip while standing. Diagnosis is based on the history and examination. Routine radiographs are usually normal, and MRI findings are usually within normal limits. Needle electromyographic studies in the adductor muscles often show chronic denervation patterns (80).

Conservative management, consisting of rest, avoidance of aggravating activities, NSAIDs, and adductor muscle strengthening in physical therapy should be initiated. This appears to be more helpful in acute mild cases; however it has not been found to be helpful in chronic injuries that have resulted in denervation (78). Surgical release is necessary to treat chronic cases of obturator entrapment, and can provide permanent relief of symptoms with timely return to full activities (78).

Lateral Femoral Cutaneous Nerve Entrapment

Lateral femoral cutaneous nerve entrapment (meralgia paresthetica) is a common problem. Symptoms can present in any age group with various activities. Sports that require tight belts, pads, or bracing over the iliac crest, causing mechanical compression, are at higher risk for nerve entrapment. The lateral femoral cutaneous nerve is purely sensory, and it supplies the skin from the anterior lateral aspect of the thigh to the knee. The course of the nerve is superficial as it exits the pelvis over the lateral iliac crest. Patients complain of unilateral pain or sensory changes at the lateral thigh region. Diagnosis is mainly by history and examination. Sensory changes should be confirmatory, and a Tinel's sign is often noted just inferior and medial to the ASIS (81). Local nerve blocks provide temporary relief, and can be helpful in diagnosis and prediction of which patients with chronic symptoms might benefit from surgical release. Relief of symptoms with nerve blocks is a good predictor of successful operative management (82).

Conservative treatment includes NSAIDs and minimizing aggravating activities, such as wearing tight clothing or equipment around the hip region and long periods of standing (81). The athlete who does not have a resolution of symptoms with conservative management may benefit from surgical decompression of the nerve, with over 90% of patients receiving complete or partial resolution of symptoms (83).

Prevention

Acute injuries of the pelvis, hip, and femur can be difficult to prevent. However, some measures can be employed. The appropriate equipment and padding should always be used during sporting activities. Many acute injuries can be prevented with proper stretching, adequate strengthening, and proper warm up. In addition, playing with similarly skilled athletes can avoid many acute traumatic injuries. Chronic injuries can be prevented by addressing proper training regimens and avoiding training errors. These include inappropriate progression of rate, intensity, and duration of training (4,6,7,84). Addressing anatomic factors such as lower extremity alignment, muscle–tendon imbalances of strength, endurance, or flexibility can decrease injuries (4,6,84). Additional risk factors including footwear, playing surfaces, associated disease states, nutritional factors, and deconditioning can be addressed with education of athletes, coaches, and parents (4,84).

Return to Play

Returning to play is dependent on several factors, including whether the athlete is able to return safely and effectively to sport. Before returning to sport, flexibility and strength should return to within 80–90% of normal to prevent further injury and allow effective movement with activities. Therapy can be very useful to monitor and gage the athlete's readiness to return to play.

For most minor injuries of the pelvis, hip, and thigh, such as strains, bursitis, nerve entrapments, and mild avulsion injuries, a period of rest followed by appropriate therapy entailing stretching and strengthening will allow athletes to regain strength and flexibility. Sport can be resumed once the pain has subsided. Return to play after acute fractures and stress fractures must be delayed until pain has resolved, there is radiologic evidence of a healed fracture, and there has been modification of the contributing risk factor.

Clinical Pearls

- Contusions and musculotendinous injuries are the most common injuries around the pelvis and hip.
- Apophyseal avulsion fractures are common in the young athlete, particularly during growth spurts.
- The majority of these injures can be treated successfully with physical therapy after conservative management including rest, ice, elevation, and antiinflammatories until the athlete is functionally pain free.

- Physical therapy should focus on return of range of motion, stretching, and strengthening before return to sports.
- Young athletes with hip pain during activities must be evaluated for more concerning causes of hip pathology, including SCFE, Perthes disease, hip dysplasia, infection, and tumor.

References

1. Waters PM, Millis MB. Hip and pelvic injuries in the young athlete. Clin Sports Med 1988;7:513–526.
2. Joyce MJ, Mankin HJ. Caveat arthroscopos: Extra-articular lesions of bone simulating intra-articular pathology of the knee. J Bone Joint Surg Am 1983;65:289–292.
3. Ogden JA. Trauma, hip development, and vascularity. In: Tronzo RG, ed. Surgery of the hip joint. New York: Springer-Verlag; 1984.
4. Outerbridge AR, Micheli LJ. Overuse injuries in the young athlete. Clin Sports Med 1995;14:503–516.
5. Soyuncu Y, Gur S. Avulsion injuries of the pelvis in adolescents. Acta Orthop Traumatol Tur 2004;Suppl 1:88–92.
6. Micheli LJ, Fehlandt AF. Overuse tendon injuries in pediatric sports medicine. Sports Med Arthrosc 1996;4:190–195.
7. Micheli LJ. Lower extremity overuse injuries. Acta Med Scand 1986;Suppl 711:171–177.
8. White KK, Williams SK, Murarack SJ. Definition of two types of anterior superior iliac spine avulsions fractures. J Ped Orthop 2002;22:578–582.
9. Metzmaker JN, Pappas AM. Avulsion fractures of the pelvis. Am J Sports Med 1985;13:349–358.
10. Puranene J, Orava S. The hamstring syndrome: A new diagnosis of gluteal sciatic pain. Am J Sports Med 1988;16:517–521.
11. O'Leary JA, Bernard K, Vail TP. The relationship between diagnosis and outcomes in arthroscopy of the hip. Arthroscopy 2001;17:181–188.
12. Byrd JW. Hip arthroscopy in athletes. Instr Course Lect 2003;52:701–709.
13. Byrd JW. Hip arthroscopy: Patient assessment and indications. Instr Course Lect 2003;52:711–719.
14. Merrifield HH, Cowan RJF. Groin strain injuries in ice hockey. J Sports Med 1973;1:41–42.
15. Cross TM, Gibbs N, Houang MT, et al. Acute quadriceps muscle strains: Magnetic resonance imaging features and prognosis. Am J Sports Med 2004;32:710–719.
16. Hoskins W, Pollard H. Hamstring injury management—Part 2: Treatment. Man Ther 2005;10:189–190.
17. Witvrouw E, Asselman DL, D'Have P, Cambier T. Muscle flexibility as a risk factor for developing muscle injuries in male professional soccer players: A prospective study. Am J Sports Med 2003;31:41–46.
18. Yamamoto T. Relationship between hamstring strains and leg muscle strength: A follow-up study of collegiate track and field athletes. J Sports Med Phys Fitness 1993;33:194–199.

19. Taylor DC, Dalton JD Jr, Seaber AV, et al. Experimental muscle strain injury: Early functional and structural deficits and the increased risk for re-injury. Am J Sport Med 1993;21:190–194.
20. Ishakawa K, Koichi K, Mizuta H. Avulsion of the hamstring muscles from the ischial tuberosity. Clin Orthop 1988;232:153–155.
21. Proske U, Morgan DL, Brockett CL, et al. Identifying athletes of hamstring strains and how to protect them. Clin Exp Pharmacol Physiol 2004;31:546–550.
22. Croisier JL, Forthomme B, Namurois MH, et al. Hamstring muscle strain recurrence and strength performance disorders. Am J Sports Med 2002;30:199–203.
23. Klingele KE, Sallay PI. Surgical repair of complete proximal hamstring tendon rupture. Am J Sports Med 2003;30:742–747.
24. Omololu B, Ogunlade SO, Alonge TO. Quadriceps tendon rupture in an adolescent. West Afr J Med 2001;20:272–273.
25. Cross TM, Gibbs N, Houang MT, et al. Acute quadriceps muscle strains: magnetic resonance imagining features and prognosis. Am J Sports Med 2004;32:710–719.
26. Ryan JB, Wheller JH, Hopkinson WJ, et al. Quadriceps contusions. West Point update. Am J Sports Med 1990;19:299–304.
27. Jackson DW, Feagin JA. Quadriceps contusions in young athletes: Relation of severity of injury to treatment and prognosis. J Bone Joint Surg Am 1973;55:95–105.
28. Nalley J, Jay MS, Durant RH. Myositis ossificans in an adolescent following sports injury. J Adolesc Health Care 1985;6:460–462.
29. Brown, TD, Brunet ME. Pediatric Thigh. In: DeLee, Drez, Miller, eds. Orthopaedic Sports Medicine: Principles and Practice. 2003:1517–1519.
30. Kransforf MJ, Meis JM, Jeliniek JS. Myositis Ossificans: MR appearance with radiographic-pathologic correlation. Am J Roentgenol 1991;157:1243–1248.
31. Nuccion SL, Junter DM, Finnerman GA. Hip and pelvis: adult. In: DeLee, Drez and Miller, eds. Orthopedic Sports Medicine: Principles and Practice. 2003:1443–1462.
32. Nelson C. Which athletes are most at risk for stress fractures? Sports Med Dig 2001;23:1–5.
33. Coady CM, Micheli LJ. Stress fractures in the pediatric athlete. Clin Sports Med 1997;16:225–238.
34. Yeager KK, Agostini R, Nattiv A, et al. The female athlete triad: Disordered eating, amenorrhea, osteoporosis. Med Sci Sports Exerc 1993;25:775–777.
35. Loud KJ, Micheli LJ. Correlates of stress fractures among preadolescent and adolescent girls. Pediatrics 2005;115:399–406.
36. Micheli LJ. Overuse injuries in the young athlete. In: Bar-Or O, ed. The Child and Adolescent. Champaign IL: Blackwell Science Ltd; 1996:189–201.
37. Micheli LJ. Injuries to the hip and pelvis. In: Sullivan JA, Grana WA, eds. The Pediatric Athlete. American Academy of Orthopedic Surgeons. Park Ridge, IL: 1990:167–172.
38. Miller C, Major N, Toth A. Pelvic stress injuries in the athlete: Management and prevention. Sports Med 2003;33:1003–1012.
39. Roman M, Recio R, Moreno JC, et al. Stress fractures of femoral neck in a child. Acta Orthop Belg 2001;67:286–289.

40. Bettin D, Pankalla T, Bohm H, et al. Hip pain related to femoral neck stress fracture in a 12-year-old boy performing intensive soccer playing activities: A case report. Int J Sports Med 2003;24:593–596.
41. St Pierre P, Shaheli LT, Smith JB, Green NE. Femoral neck stress fractures in children and adolescents. J Ped Orthop 1995;15:470–473.
42. Clough TM. Femoral neck stress fracture: The importance of clinical suspicion and early review. Br J Sports Med 2002;36:308–309.
43. Maezawa K, Nozawa M, Sugimoto M, et al. Stress fractures of the femoral neck in a child with open capital femoral epiphysis. J Pediatr Orthop B 2004;13: 407–411.
44. Meaney JEM, Carty H. Femoral stress fractures in children. Skeletal Radiology 1992;21:173–176.
45. Johansson C, Ekenman I, Tornkvist H, et al. Stress fractures of the femoral neck in athletes. The consequence of a delayed diagnosis. Am J Sports Med 1990;18:524–528.
46. Micheli LJ, Santopietro F, Gerbino P, et al. Etiologic assessment of overuse stress fractures in athletes. Nova Scotia Med Bull 1980;59:43–47.
47. Weber PC. Salter Harris type II stress fracture in a young athlete. A case report. Orthopedics 1988;11:309–311.
48. Engh CA, Robinson R, Milgram J. Stress fractures in children. J Trauma 1970; 10:532–541.
49. Davies AM, Carter SR, Grimmer RJ, et al. Fatigue fractures of the femoral diaphysis in the skeletally immature simulating malignancy. Br J Radiol 1989;62:893–896.
50. Waters PM, Millis MB. Hip and pelvic injuries in the young athlete. Clin Sports Med 1988;7:513–526.
51. Berend KR, Vail TP. Hip arthroscopy in the adolescent and pediatric athlete. Clin Sports Med 2001;20:763–778.
52. Dorell J, Catterall A. The torn acetabular labrum. J Bone Joint Surg Am 1986;68:400–404.
53. McCarthy JC, Noble PC, Schuck MR, et al. The watershed labral lesion: Its relationship to early arthritis of the hip. J Arthorplasty 2001;16:81–87.
54. Fitzgerald RH. Acetabular labral tears. Diagnosis and treatment. Clin Orthop 1995;311:60–68.
55. Erb RE. Current concepts in the adult hip. Clin Sports Med 2001;20: 661–696.
56. Byrd JW. Labral lesions: An elusive source of hip pain. Arthroscopy 1996;12:603–612.
57. Kelly BT, Williams RJ, Phillipon MJ. Hip arthroscopy: Current indications, treatment options, and management issues. Am J Sports Med 2003;31:1020–1037.
58. Kelly BT, Weiland DE, Schenker ML, et al. Arthroscopic labral repair in the hip: surgical technique options, and management issues. Arthroscopy 2005;21: 1496–1502.
59. Kocher MS, Kim YJ, Millis MB, et al. Hip arthroscopy in children and adolescents. J Ped Orthop 2005;25:680–686.
60. Anderson K, Strickland SM, Warren R. Hip and groin injuries in athletes. Am J Sports Med 2001;27:521–533.

61. Johnson R. Osteitis pubis. Curr Sports Med Rep 2003;2:98–102.
62. Koch R, Jackson D. Pubic symphysis in runners. Am J Sports Med 1981;9: 62–63.
63. Topol GA, Reeves KD, Hassanein KM. Efficacy of dextrose prolotherapy in elite male kicking-sport athletes with chronic groin pain. Arch Phys Med Rehabil 2005;86:697–702.
64. Paajanen H, Heikkinen J, Hermunen H, et al. Successful treatment of osteitis pubis by using totally extra peritoneal endoscopic technique. Int J Sports Med 2005;26:303–306.
65. LeBlanc KE. Sacroiliac sprain: an overlooked cause of back pain. Am Fam Physician 1992;46:1459–1463.
66. Harrison DE, Harrison DD, Troyanovich SJ. The sacroiliac joint: A review of anatomy and biomechanics with clinical implications. J Manipulative Physiol Ther 1997;20:607–617.
67. Brolinson PG, Kozar AJ, Cibor G. Sacroiliac joint dysfunction in athletes. Curr Sports Med Rep 2003;2:47–56.
68. Allen WC, Cope R. Coxa Saltans: the snapping hip syndrome. J Am Acad Othop Surg 1995;3:303–308.
69. Jacobson T, Allen WC. Surgical correction of the snapping iliopsoas tendon. Am J Sports Med 1990;18:470–474.
70. Dobbs MB, Gordon JE, Luhmann SJ, et al. Surgical correction of the snapping iliopsoas tendon in adolescent. J Bone Joint Surg AM 2002;84:420–424.
71. Gruen GS, Scioscia TN, Lowenstein JE. The surgical treatment of internal snapping hip. Am J Sports Med 2002;30:606–613.
72. Broadhurst NA, Simmons DN, Bond MJ. Piriformis syndrome: Correlation of muscle morphology with symptoms and signs. Arch Phys Med Rehab 2004;85: 2036–2039.
73. Lee EY, Margherita AJ, Gierada DS, et al. MRI of piriformis syndrome. Am J Roentgenol 2004;183:63–68.
74. Dezawa A, Kusano S, Miki H. Arthroscopic release for the piriformis muscle under local anesthesia for piriformis syndrome. Arthroscopy 2003; 19:554–557.
75. Zoltan DJ, Clancy WG, Keene JS. A new operative approach to snapping hip and refractory trochanteric bursitis in athletes. Am J Sports Med 1986;14: 201–204.
76. Arsonson J. Osteorarthritis of the young adult hip: Etiology and treatment. Instr Course Lect 1986;35:119–128.
77. Carney BT, Weinstein SL, Noble J. Long-term follow up of slipped capital femoral epiphysis. J Bone Joint Surg AM 1991;73:667–674
78. Bradshaw C, McCrory P, Bell S, et al. Obturator nerve entrapment. A case of groin pain in athletes. Am J Sports Med 1997;25:402–408.
79. Harvey G, Bell S. Obturator neuropathy. An anatomic perspective. Clin Orthop 1999;363:203–211.
80. Delagi EF, Perotto A. Anatomical Guide for the Electromyographer: The Limb. 2nd ed. Springfield, Ill.: Charles C. Thomas; 1980:207.
81. Grossman MG, Ducey SA, Nadler SS, et al. Meralgia pareasthetica: Diagnosis and treatment. J Am Acad Orthop Surg 2001;9:336–334.

82. Nahabedian MY, Delton AL. Meralgia Pareasthetica: Etiology, diagnosis and outcome of surgical decompression. Ann Plast Surg 1995;35:590–595.
83. Sui TL, Chandran KN. Neurolysis for meralgia pareasthetica: an operative series of 45 cases. Surg Neurol 2005;63:19–23.
84. O'Neill DB, Micheli LJ. Overuse injuries in the young athlete. Clin Sports Med 1988;7:591–610.

11
Knee Injuries

Michelle McTimoney

Injuries to the knee are common among young athletes. Three percent of all injuries in children between 5–9 yr of age occur at the knee. This rate is doubled in children between the ages of 10–14 (5.9%) and 15–19 (6.2%) (1). The number of knee injuries can be partially attributed to the increase in organized youth sport.

Both acute and chronic injuries are seen in youth. Acute knee injuries occur frequently in sports such as basketball, hockey, soccer, skiing, and football. Chronic or overuse knee injuries, such as patellofemoral pain syndrome and Osgood–Schlatter disease (OSD), are seen in running and jumping sports (2). Some knee injuries can potentially be quite debilitating if not properly managed. Therefore, it is essential that practitioners taking care of young athletes have an understanding of knee injuries that are unique to children and the anatomy that results in different injury patterns in children as compared to adults.

Anatomy

The knee joint is composed of the femur superiorly, the tibia inferiorly, and the patella anteriorly (Figure 11.1 A). The proximal fibula articulates with the proximal tibia, but does not articulate with the femur. The fibula ends just distal to the joint, underneath the lateral tibial plateau. The medial and lateral prominences of the distal femur are referred to as the medial and lateral femoral condyles, and the depression between these two condyles is the intercondylar notch or trochlear groove, in which the patella articulates. The flared articular surface of the tibia is referred to as the tibial plateau. The tibial spine is a bony eminence in the center of the tibial plateau. The articular surfaces of these bones are covered with articular cartilage.

In the young athlete, each of these bones has a growth plate. The distal femoral growth plate and the proximal tibial growth plate each contribute over half of longitudinal growth for each of these bones (3). Injury to either

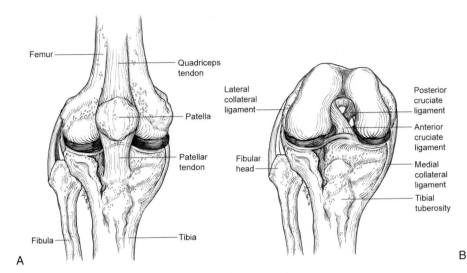

FIGURE 11.1. Anatomy of the knee. **(A)** The bones of the knee. **(B)** The ligaments of the knee.

of these growth plates has the potential to significantly impact the growth of the young athlete. The proximal tibia also has an apophysis anteriorly called the tibial tubercle. This is the site of attachment of the patellar tendon and another location of growing bone in the tibia.

The patella is a triangular-shaped bone, with its wider base superiorly oriented. There are two apophyses at each of the superior-lateral aspects of the patella and one apophysis at the inferior pole of the patella. The quadriceps tendon attaches at these apophyses as it crosses the patella. Distally, the quadriceps tendon becomes the patellar tendon as it leaves the patella at the inferior apophysis. These bony areas of tendinous insertion are areas of bone growth and susceptible to injury in the growing athlete. The patella functions to increase the mechanical advantage of the knee by increasing the distance of the extensor mechanism (quads and patella) from the axis of rotation through the knee joint. As a result, the quadriceps can generate a more powerful knee extension.

The quadriceps muscle group extends the knee. It is composed of the vastus lateralis, vastus medialis obliquus, vastus intermedius, and the rectus femoris. The rectus femoris and the vastus intermedius run between these two muscles with the rectus femoris superficial to the vastus intermedius. The rectus femoris originates on the anterior inferior iliac spine and crosses both the hip and knee joint to insert on the tibial tubercle via the patellar tendon. The vastus lateralis, medialis, and intermedius all originate on the proximal femur and, together with the rectus femoris, insert on the patella via the quadriceps tendon.

The hamstrings are composed of the long and short heads of the biceps femoris, the semimembranosus, and the semitendinosus muscles. This muscle group originates on the ischial tuberosity. The semimembranosus and semitendinosus insert medially on the proximal tibia. The biceps femoris inserts on the head of the fibula. The hamstrings flex the knee. The sartorius and gracilis muscles originate in the pelvis, and they cross the knee medially to insert on the medial aspect of the proximal tibia. These muscles also contribute to knee flexion. The popliteus muscle originates on the distal femur, as does the plantaris and gastrocnemius muscles. These muscles cross the knee joint posteriorly and contribute to knee flexion. Laterally a tight band of fascial tissue crosses the knee as the iliotibial band (ITB). This band emanates from the tensor fasciae latae, gluteus medius, and gluteus maximus muscles. This fascial band inserts at Gerdy's tubercle, just lateral to the tibial tubercle. In knee extension, this band lies anteriorly to the lateral femoral condyle; while in flexion, it lies posteriorly.

Within the joint capsule, there are several structures important to knee function. The medial meniscus (MM) and lateral meniscus (LM) are C-shaped masses of hyaline cartilage on the medial and lateral surfaces of the tibial plateau. They function as shock absorbers, protecting the knee from high mechanical loads. The peripheral vascular zone of the meniscus extends further medially in children than it does in adults. With age, the zone of vascularization recesses. After age 10, only the peripheral one third is vascularized. The anterior cruciate ligament (ACL) originates at the medial aspect of the lateral femoral condyle and inserts in the anteromedial portion of the tibial plateau (Figure 11.1 B). It prevents the excessive anterior translation of the tibia on the femur. The posterior cruciate ligament (PCL) originates on the lateral aspect of the medial femoral condyle and crosses behind the ACL to insert on the posterolateral portion of the central tibial plateau. It prevents excessive posterior translation of the tibia on the femur. The medial collateral ligament (MCL) originates on the distal medial femoral epiphysis and inserts on the proximal tibial epiphysis. It protects against excessive valgus force. The lateral collateral ligament (LCL) originates on the lateral femoral epiphysis and inserts on the proximal fibular epiphysis. It protects the knee against excessive varus forces.

Although seldom injured in the growing athlete, it is also important to be aware of the significant neurovascular structures which course posteriorly to the knee, in the popliteal fossa. The femoral artery courses posteromedially as it becomes the popliteal artery in the popliteal fossa. The sciatic nerve becomes the posterior tibial nerve and the common peroneal nerve while still above the knee. These two nerves cross the knee posteriorly and eventually provide sensation to the plantar and dorsal aspect of the foot, respectively.

Clinical Evaluation

History

An accurate description of the presenting complaint is often the key to correct diagnosis. It is important to know whether the complaint is that of pain, instability, or swelling. The resulting effect on the function of the knee as it relates to daily activities also needs to be explored. In cases of acute injury, a description of the event is helpful. Many practitioners will find, however, that the child or youth is often unable to accurately describe the exact events of the injury. A history of inability to weight bear, swelling, locking, clicking, or giving way after the event suggests significant, often intraarticular, pathology that warrants further investigation.

Chronic complaints of knee pain are common in the pediatric athlete, and may suggest overuse injuries. The location of the pain can point to potential diagnoses, such as OSD. Knee pain can occur at the time of a growth spurt in the young athlete; therefore, enquiry into recent growth patterns may also be helpful.

It is important to assess knee complaints in the context of the athlete. Knowledge of type of sport, hours of training, recent changes in training, and training/performance goals can help guide management. Management of the injured athlete not only includes management of the injury but also of the athlete within the context of their sport. The athlete must be given guidelines on what activities are permitted, as well as what is restricted.

A review of systems must be completed to make sure that the knee complaints are not part of a bigger picture of medical illness in a pediatric athlete. A history of multiple swollen joints, night pain or sweats, unexplained fevers, or changes in weight or growth pattern suggest a possible infectious, rheumatologic, or malignant etiology, rather than a mechanical cause of knee pain.

Physical Exam

The physical examination of the knee in the young athlete begins with observation of stance and gait, looking for abnormalities of biomechanical alignment and asymmetries of gait. Abnormalities commonly observed include genu varum, valgum, or recurvatum; femoral anteversion; kissing patella; and pes planus. The range of motion of the knee must be documented and should be compared with the unaffected side. Because of the prevalence of ligamentous laxity in the pediatric athlete, full knee extension may actually include a few degrees of hyperextension, which might be overlooked if only the affected side is examined. A child should be able to flex the knee so that the heel touches the buttocks when lying prone. The knee is inspected for any bony abnormalities, such as a prominent tibial tubercle or the presence of any visible swelling. Muscle bulk should be inspected for evidence of atrophy and asymmetry. Disuse secondary to injury quickly produces significant atrophy in the quadriceps musculature.

An effusion can be assessed by milking the joint fluid superiorly on the medial aspect of the patella. Next, the suprapatellar communication is occluded with one hand while the other is used to compress the space just lateral to the patella (Figure 11.2). An effusion is present if a bulge of fluid can be appreciated on the medial side of the patella as the effusion is forced from the lateral joint space to the medial joint space. Any effusion in a child is significant and must be evaluated further.

Palpation is performed looking for tenderness of any bony structure. Areas of bone growth may be tender to palpation, as in OSD or Sindig–Larsen–Johansson disease (SLJD). The articular surface of the medial and lateral femoral condyle is easily palpated with the knee in flexion. Tenderness may suggest an osteochondral injury. The joint line is palpated for tenderness that may occur with meniscal injuries.

The patellar tendon can be palpated along its length for tenderness. The MCL is easily palpated on the medial aspect of the joint. The LCL is easier to palpate by putting the knee in a figure of four position. This brings out the LCL so it can be easily palpated between the fibular head and the lateral femoral epiphysis.

Special tests of the knee begin with the anterior drawer and Lachman. Both test the integrity of the ACL. The anterior drawer test (Figure 11.3)

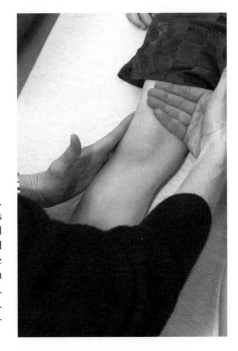

FIGURE 11.2. Assessment for effusion. The examiner's right hand occludes the suprapatellar bursa as the left hand is used to milk any excess joint fluid across the joint from the lateral to the medial side. The presence of fluid seen medially is known as the "bulge" sign. No effusion is present in this patient. (Courtesy of Bruce Carruthers, Carruthers Photography)

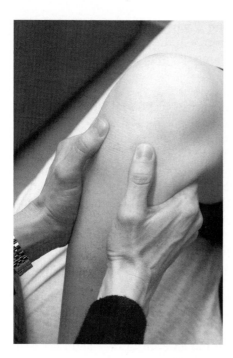

FIGURE 11.3. Anterior drawer test. Note the examiner's hands attempting to glide the tibia anteriorly, while the patient's lower tibia is stabilized by gently sitting on the foot. (Courtesy of Bruce Carruthers, Carruthers Photography)

is performed by having the patient lie supine with the affected knee flexed to 90 degrees. The examiner stabilizes the patient's lower extremity by sitting on the foot. The proximal tibia is held with both hands encircling it. It is essential to remind the patient to relax the hamstrings. This can be verified as the test is performed because the examiners fingers are on the hamstring tendons. Once the hamstrings are relaxed, the examiner attempts to glide the tibia forward. A positive test is indicated by more glide on the affected than unaffected side. With experience, a "soft" endpoint is appreciated rather than the firm endpoint of an intact ACL.

The Lachman test (Figure 11.4) is performed with the patient lying supine with the affected leg extended. This time one hand encircles the distal femur and the other encircles the proximal tibia, again trying to glide the tibia forward on the femur. Excessive glide confirms incompetence of the ACL. Comparison with the uninjured knee is important because of the ligamentous laxity in children.

The integrity of the PCL is tested by the posterior drawer test. This is performed with the patient positioned as for the anterior drawer test. With the same hand positioning, the tibia is forced posteriorly. An injured PCL will allow for posterior translation of the tibia on the femur. Comparison with the unaffected leg is also helpful in this test.

Both McMurray's and Apley's tests are helpful for identifying meniscal injuries. For McMurray's test (Figure 11.5), the patient is positioned supine

FIGURE 11.4. Lachman test. The examiner's lower hand attempts to glide the tibia forward on a stabilized femur. (Courtesy of Bruce Carruthers, Carruthers Photography)

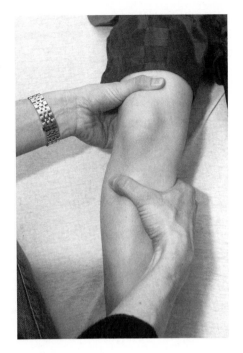

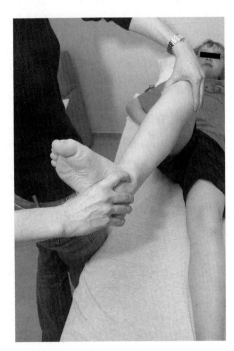

FIGURE 11.5. McMurray's test. Note the positioning of the examiner's fingers along the joint line to feel any pop associated with meniscal pathology. (Courtesy of Bruce Carruthers, Carruthers Photography)

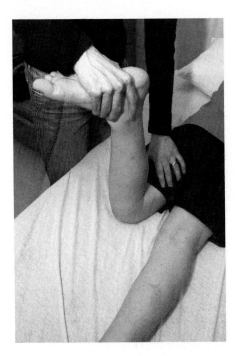

FIGURE 11.6. Apley's compression test. A torn meniscus will produce pain when an axial load and rotation is applied. (Courtesy of Bruce Carruthers, Carruthers Photography)

with legs extended. The examiner holds the heel of the affected side with one hand and flexes the knee. The other hand is placed with fingers along the medial joint line and thumb along the lateral joint line. A valgus force is applied to the knee while externally rotating and extending the knee. The sensation of a click or pop in the joint beneath the examiners hand is a positive result and may indicate meniscal pathology. Apley's compression test (Figure 11.6) is performed by having the patient lie prone with the affected leg flexed to 90 degrees. The heel is held and an axial load is applied while rotating the tibia internally and externally on the femur. A torn meniscus will make this procedure painful.

The collateral ligaments are examined by having the patient lie supine on the examining table (Figure 11.7). The affected knee is flexed slightly to 30 degrees. The ankle can either be held with one hand (Figure 11.7A), or in larger patients, secured between the examiners trunk and upper arm (Figure 11.7B). The other palm is placed first on the lateral side of the knee and a valgus force is applied at the knee with a counter force at the ankle. This stresses the MCL. Laxity and or pain suggest injury to the MCL. The same procedure can be repeated with the palm on the medial surface applying a varus stress to the knee. Again, laxity and/or pain suggests injury to the LCL.

Ober's test (Figure 11.8) is used to evaluate the tightness of the ITB. With the patient lying on the unaffected side, the affected leg is abducted at the hip. A tight ITB will prevent the hip from passively adducting past

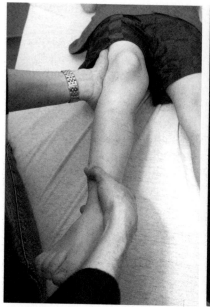
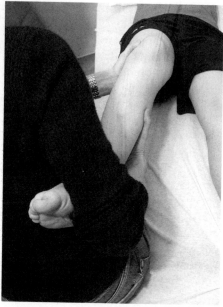

A   B

FIGURES 11.7. **(A)** Medial collateral ligament stability test. Note the different techniques for stabilizing the distal tibia while valgus force is applied more proximally. The underarm technique **(B)** is helpful in larger patients when more stability is required distally. (Courtesy of Bruce Carruthers, Carruthers Photography)

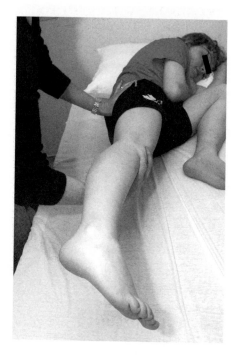

FIGURE 11.8. Ober's Test. In patients with a tight ITB, the extended leg will not fall past horizontal. (Courtesy of Bruce Carruthers, Carruthers Photography)

an imaginary horizontal line. This test is often positive in patients with ITB friction syndrome.

Patellar apprehension (Figure 11.9) can be appreciated by having the patient supine on the examining table with knees extended. The examiner places both thumbs along the medial aspect of the patella with both index fingers along the lateral aspect of the patella. The quadriceps need to be relaxed for this test. While watching the patient's face, force is applied in a lateral direction with the thumbs in an effort to sublux the patella laterally. Patients who have a history of patellar subluxation or dislocation will be apprehensive as the patella is moved laterally.

Once the special tests have been completed, a neurologic examination of the lower extremity, including strength and sensation, must be performed.

No examination of the knee is complete without an examination of the hip. Many pathologies of the hip will present with pain referred to the knee because of the pattern of innervation of the hip and knee. Knee pain without physical findings at the knee is a red flag for possible hip pathology, and a thorough examination of the hip is essential!

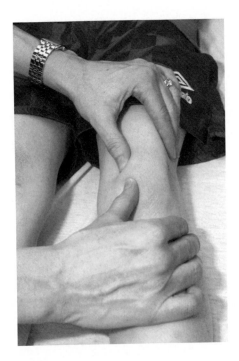

FIGURE 11.9. Patellar apprehension. The thumbs are used to apply a lateral pressure to the medial side of the patellar. (Courtesy of Bruce Carruthers, Carruthers Photography)

Acute Injuries

Patellar Dislocation

Acute patellar dislocation lies at the most severe end of the spectrum of patellar instability. The forces that predispose the athlete to patellar dislocation include a forceful quadriceps contraction, together with a partially flexed knee and a twisting motion that displace the patella laterally, resulting in significant pain, swelling and an obvious deformity of the knee . The risk of patellar dislocation is highest in adolescent girls (4).

Clinical Examination

There may be an obvious deformity of the knee, consistent with a laterally displaced patella. Once the patella has been reduced, there will be a hemarthrosis, decreased range of motion and tenderness (or even palpable defect) of the medial patellar retinaculum. If there is a significant defect of the patellar retinaculum, the hemarthrosis may displace from the knee joint into the quadriceps musculature resulting in an underestimation of the severity of articular injury (5). It is difficult to assess for patellar apprehension acutely because of pain in the patellar retinaculum; however, in the subacute setting, this sign may be positive. Patellar tracking, both actively and passively, can also be assessed. It is essential to have the patient actively extend the knee to ensure the extensor mechanism is intact. Ligamentous testing may be difficult to assess acutely, but will be normal.

Imaging includes an AP, lateral and skyline view of the knee looking for osteochondral fractures and loose bodies. Because both plain films and magnetic resonance imaging (MRI) have a high false-negative rate for loose bodies, if clinical suspicion is high, further investigation with arthroscopy is warranted (5,6). The skyline view can be used to assess the congruity at the patellofemoral articulation.

Management

If the patella has not spontaneously reduced (10% of cases), closed reduction is necessary (7). This can be accomplished by gently extending the patient's knee under mild-to-moderate sedation. Postreduction films are obtained to look for osteochondral injury and document successful reduction. A long leg immobilizer is then applied for 1–2 wk (RJ splint or double-hinged brace immobilized in extension). Maenpaa and Lehto found that patients not immobilized had a three-fold higher risk of redislocation than patients treated with immediate immobilization (8). Weight bearing as tolerated with the immobilizer is allowed. Cryotherapy is initiated immediately. Physiotherapy is essential to restore strength to the quadriceps and knee range of motion. Limited evidence exists to support the ongoing use of a knee brace; however, many patients and physicians find subjective support can be obtained with a J-brace worn at all times during the reha-bilitation phase of recovery, and during sport once return to play has begun.

Recurrence is not unusual. One study found the recurrence rate after primary dislocation to be 17%; for those with multiple episodes of sublux-ation/dislocation, the recurrence rate was 50% (4). Young age was posi-tively associated with reinjury. Immediate surgery has not reduced this risk (9,10).

Anterior Cruciate Ligament Tear

Tears of the ACL are becoming increasingly more common in young athletes. This increase is secondary to increasing athletic participation, awareness of the medical community of these injuries in children, and the capacity to diagnose these injuries with the evolution of imaging techniques (11,12).

Prince et al. found that athletes with completely open physes were more likely to have partial tears of the ACL or an avulsion of the tibial spine than complete ACL tears (13). Tibial spine avulsions were rarely seen in physically mature patients (4%). They also found that children suffer the same concurrent injuries as adults in ACL trauma, including torn meniscus (medial 24%, lateral 13%), sprained MCL (22%), and torn PCL (10%) (13).

In children with open physes, more ACL injuries were seen in boys (6.75:1), but with physical maturity ACL injuries in the female were seen twice as often as in the male athlete. Although various factors, including Q angle, shape, and size of the femoral notch, thickness of the ACL, joint laxity, hormonal influences, and training techniques (14) have been suggested to account for this difference, no definitive cause has been established.

The usual mechanism of injury is cutting or pivoting with a planted foot in order to stop suddenly and change direction. Alternatively, the patient may describe landing a jump on a hyperextended knee. A "pop" is often reported to have been heard at the time of injury. Severe pain and inability to bear weight ensue. Significant swelling follows within hours of the injury.

Clinical Examination

The exam may be most revealing either at the field of play before significant swelling develops or in the subacute phase of injury, once pain and appre-hension have subsided. Findings include a significant effusion, decreased range of motion, a positive anterior drawer, and a positive Lachman. Because of the frequency of concurrent injuries, it is essential to examine the patient carefully to assess the integrity of other structures. Comparison

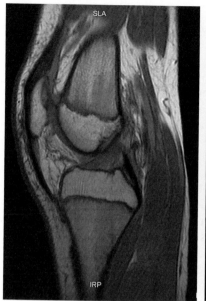
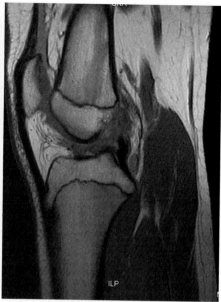

A

B

FIGURE 11.10. **(A)** MRI of intact ACL. Note intact fibers extending between the anterior tibial plateau and the femoral condyle. **(B)** MRI of Torn ACL. Note the mass of shredded fibers in the location of the usually linear ACL. Some buckling of the PCL can also be seen.

with the uninjured leg, which is used as a baseline, is necessary because of the significant ligamentous laxity present in most children. Quadriceps atrophy becomes evident within days of the injury.

Plain films of the knee (AP, lateral, notch and skyline) are obtained to rule out concomitant osseous injury. Particularly in the youngest patients, these films must be meticulously inspected for a fracture of the tibial eminence, which accounts for 26% of all 'ACL' injuries in athletes with open physes (13).

The ACL is best imaged with MRI (Figure 11.10); however, arthroscopy remains the gold standard for assessing its integrity. It is important that the MRI be interpreted by clinicians with significant experience in this area to minimize inaccurate interpretations of the integrity of the ACL and its surrounding structures.

Management

Management of the immature patient with the ACL-deficient knee is difficult and necessitates early involvement of an orthopedist experienced in this area. Initially, weight bearing must be protected with a combination of a hinged knee brace and crutches until the quadriceps and hamstrings have regained their strength. Physiotherapy is initiated early to increase range of motion and diminish the effusion. After the initial phases of healing, more aggressive therapy can be instituted with a goal of regaining the pre-injury ratio of quadriceps to hamstrings muscle strength. Sports requiring running or cutting are discouraged during these first phases of recovery.

There continues to be controversy regarding the definitive management of ACL injuries in the skeletally immature athlete. Current options include conservative management with significant activity restriction until growth has been completed followed by ACL reconstruction; traditional recon-struction in patients with minimal remaining growth, and therefore minimal risk of iatrogenic growth disturbance; or early surgery with a physeal sparing technique. Nonoperative management leaves the patient with an unstable knee with increased risk of further meniscal and chondral injury; however, traditional operative techniques violate the immature physis to varying degrees and may result in increased risk of iatrogenic growth disturbance in the affected tibial and femoral physes. Kocher et al (15) have reported positive functional and growth outcomes of a physeal sparing ACL recon-struction technique. In the absence of universal guidelines, each case must be considered individually in consultation with an experienced orthopedic surgeon.

Meniscal Tears

The incidence of meniscal tears in the pediatric athlete is low, but the exact rate is unknown. Tears in this population are usually traumatic after a twist-ing motion of the knee. Tears in children under the age of 10 are likely to be associated with a discoid meniscus (16).

The pattern of injury to the meniscus differs in the child compared to the adult, with 50–90% of tears being longitudinal in children. Displaced bucket handle tears are also common. Given normal meniscal anatomy, the MM is more likely to be torn. The relative increase in lateral meniscal tears in adolescents can be attributed to the presence of discoid LM (17).

Clinical Examination

The physical exam reveals an effusion and possibly joint line tenderness. The utility of provocative testing (McMurray's and Apley's) for meniscal pathology in children lies in the hands of the examiner. These tests can be up to 86–94% accurate when performed by experienced clinicians (18,19), but have been noted to have accuracies as low as 29–59% in a series using multiple examiners (17,18).

MRI has been shown to be both a sensitive and specific tool to diagnose meniscal tears. Kocher found better sensitivity and specificity (79% and 92%) when looking at medial meniscal tears as opposed to lateral tears (67% sensitive, 83% specific) (19).

Management

Nonoperative treatment includes a physiotherapy program and sport modification. Twisting and cutting sports should be avoided for at least 12 wk. Some small, stable meniscal tears may heal with such a conservative approach. More often, orthopedic surgery is required. Possible operative interventions include partial meniscectomy or meniscal repair using various techniques. Meniscal repair (rather than resection as in adults) has been found to be successful in 75–100% of patients under the age of 30 (20–22). Kocher et al. (16) reviewed several studies that suggest the increased healing potential of meniscal repairs in this population may be caused by young age, characteristics of the tear, timing of operative intervention, and concomitant ACL reconstruction. Postoperative rehabilitation is more extensive than the nonoperative protocol and includes a period of protected ROM immediately after the surgery. Return to play can be expected by the 3-mo mark in isolated meniscal repairs with an uncomplicated postoperative course.

Collateral Ligament Injuries

Injuries to the collateral ligaments occur as a result of valgus or varus forces at the level of the knee. A valgus force to the lateral aspect of the knee may result in injury to the MCL. Less often, a varus force applied to the medial aspect of the knee may injure the LCL. MCL injuries may occur in isolation; however, an isolated injury of the LCL is unusual, and concurrent injury to the popliteus or arcuate complex should be considered (12). Injury to the ACL and MM can occur in conjunction with MCL injury, especially in cases with a rotational component to the insulting force. Grading of collateral ligament injury is outlined in Table 11.1 (23).

Clinical Examination

The patient will be tender along the length of the affected collateral ligament. Stress testing in 30 degrees of flexion will produce pain and in more severe injuries, instability. If instability is evident in full extension, specifically with varus loading, injury to the posterior capsule should be considered in addition to the LCL. Isolated collateral ligament injury produces pain and instability only in flexion. With complete avulsions of the MCL,

TABLE 11.1. Grading of MCL injuries.

Grade 1	microscopic disruption of collagen fibers, no laxity; pain with stress testing, but no laxity
Grade 2	macroscopic partial tearing of the ligament, <1 cm opening with stress testing
Grade 3	complete disruption of collagen fibers, >1 cm laxity with stress testing

Sources: Mintzer et al., 1988; Diduch et al., 2005.

an osseous fragment at the site of origin of the MCL on the femur may be evident on x-ray.

Management

Treatment of isolated collateral injuries is conservative and consists of rest and cryotherapy. If needed for comfort, a double-hinged knee brace that allows for early range of motion may be used. Physiotherapy may be helpful in maintaining strength and range of motion during ligamentous healing. Return to play is usual in 4–6 wk for grade 1 sprains, 8 wk for grade 2 sprains, and up to 12 wk for grade 3 sprains (Table 11.1). A small amount of ligamentous laxity may persist, and athletes may wear the hinged brace for the first 6 mo after returning to play.

Tibial Tubercle Avulsion Fracture

Tibial tubercle avulsion fractures are uncommon injuries that typically occur in well-developed adolescent male athletes nearing the end of their growth (ages 13–16) as the tibial apophysis is closing (24,25). These injuries make up less than 3% of all proximal tibial fractures (26) and less than 1% of all physeal injuries. Only 168 cases have been reported in the literature since this injury's first description in 1853 (24).

This injury happens by one of two mechanisms: a) active knee extension through a strong quadriceps contraction, such as with aggressive jumping, or b) passive knee flexion against a contracting quadriceps muscle group, as in landing after a jump from a height. Both of these mechanisms generate enough force for the strong quadriceps to overcome the strength of the fusing tibial tubercle and result in an avulsion of this fragment. Tibial tubercle avulsions most commonly occur in athletes playing basketball (24). Although no cause–effect relationship has been found, there is speculation that OSD may play a role in the occurrence of tibial tubercle avulsion fractures (24,25,27). These fractures were originally classified with the Watson–Jones classification system (28), which was later modified by Ogden et al. (29) (Table 11.2).

TABLE 11.2. Tibial tubercle avulsion fractures.

Type 1	Fracture distal to the junction of the ossification center of the proximal tibial epiphysis and tuberosity
Type 2	Fracture with extension to the junction of the proximal tibial physis
Type 3	Fracture extends into the joint through the proximal tibial epiphysis with displacement of the fracture fragment
Type 4	Fracture extension transversely through the proximal tibial physis with displacement of the fracture fragment

Each of these types is further subdivided into A (noncomminuted) and B (comminuted). *Source:* Adapted from Chow SP, Lam JJ, Leong JC. Fracture of the tibial tubercle in the adolescent. J Bone Joint Surg Br 1990;72(2):231–234. Reproduced with permission and copyright of the British Editorial Society of Bone and Joint Surgery.

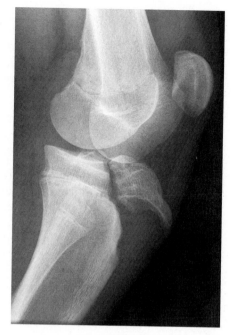

FIGURE 11.11. Type 3 tibial tubercle avulsion fracture. Note extension of fracture through the physis and into the articular surface. Displacement of the fragment is also present.

Clinical Examination

The physical examination reveals a swollen, tender bony deformity at the site of the tibial tubercle. Depending on the degree of disruption, there may be evidence of a superiorly displaced patella. The knee is often held in the position of comfort, at approximately 30 degrees of flexion. If an effusion or hemarthrosis is present, it suggests the presence of an associated injury (ACL or meniscus) or a more severe injury with extension into the joint. The patient will be unable to actively extend the knee secondary to the interruption in the quadriceps mechanism.

Diagnosis is confirmed with knee x-rays. The lateral view (Figure 11.11) is helpful in classification of the injury (Table 11.2). Often patella alta will also be evident on the lateral view.

Management

Management of tibial tubercle avulsion fractures should be guided by an orthopedic surgeon. Type 1 fractures may be treated conservatively with a cylindrical cast for 2–6 wk. Types 2–4 are treated with open reduction with internal fixation (30). Weekly plain films are suggested during recovery to monitor displacement of the reduced fragment (25).

If operative intervention has been necessary, resistance training may begin 6 wk after the initial injury in an isolated tibial tubercle avulsion fracture. Patients with types 1 and 2 injuries can often return to activities in 2 mo; those with types 3 and 4 fractures need 4–6 mo to return to activities demanding a high quadriceps load (25). As with all other injuries, full joint range of motion and full muscle strength must be attained before return to play. A graded return to play is recommended.

Chronic Injuries

Patellofemoral Pain Syndrome

Patellofemoral pain syndrome is associated with activities that load the patellofemoral joint in the anterior–posterior direction. The young athlete with patellofemoral pain syndrome complains of chronic vague anterior knee pain that may limit activity. Pain is aggravated with activity engaging the quadriceps. The pain decreases with rest; however, patients may complain of a vague ache or stiffness after prolonged sitting (car ride, sitting in a movie theater). This is referred to as the theater sign. There is no true swelling, locking or giving way; however, some patients will experience impending giving way or a minor sense of instability.

Clinical Examination

The physical examination may reveal varying degrees of malalignment of the lower extremity, including internal tibial torsion, genu valgum, and pes planus. Increased Q-angle is also often implicated in this diagnosis, although its significance has been debated (31). The knee maintains full range of motion, and there is no effusion. The patella may be tender to palpation. All provocative ligamentous testing is within normal limits. Imaging is not usually indicated unless the diagnosis is in question.

Management

The first line treatment for patellofemoral pain is often physiotherapy. Crossley et al. performed a systematic review of various interventions for patellofemoral pain syndrome and found that pain was reduced with the implementation of physiotherapy; symptoms worsened when no therapy was implemented (32). This paper found there was a paucity of evidence to support patellofemoral orthoses, taping, therapeutic modalities, chiropractic manipulation, and acupuncture in the treatment of patellofemoral pain syndrome. Despite the lack of evidence, many practitioners have found that some patients do benefit from these interventions. It is suggested that these interventions be recommended to patients on an individual basis.

Return to play is based on patient symptoms. A period of relative rest from the offending activity may be helpful in the alleviation of symptoms. If an athlete is experiencing low levels of pain with activity, without increases from day to day, continuation in the sport is allowed during the rehabilitation process. When the patient's pain has subsided sufficiently to allow full participation, return to play is encouraged.

Subluxing Patella

The subluxing patella is a result of a variety of factors that lead to lateral tracking of the patella in the femoral groove during knee flexion and extension, resulting in vague complaints of instability, giving way and anterior knee pain. Several factors may predispose an athlete to patellar subluxation. Hinton and Sharma have divided these factors into those of the host, agent, and environment (7). Host factors include the rapid growth of adolescence that induces muscular tightness in an individual who still has the ligamentous laxity of childhood. Suggested but not proven host factors include patella alta, increased Q angle, increased femoral anteversion, excessive midfoot pronation, lateral facet dominance, deficient lateral trochlea, vertical VMO insertion and ITB tightness (7). The offending agent may be macrotrauma (plant of a lower extremity with subsequent internal rotation and knee valgus) or repetitive microtrauma, such as the repetitive whip kick used in the breaststroke. Environmental factors include the frequency of exposure to the micro- or macrotrauma, the accuracy of previous diagnoses, effectiveness of rehabilitation, and the amount of general lower extremity conditioning (7).

Clinical Examination

The lower extremity is assessed looking for evidence of malalignment (valgus, angular deformities, increased Q angle, pes planus). Patellar tracking during passive and active knee extension shows lateral movement (J-sign). Patellar apprehension is present, and tightness may be appreciated when trying to lift the lateral edge of the patella with the patient lying prone (decreased patellar tilt). Decreased bulk of the VMO compared with the vastus lateralis may be evident. There should be no effusion and ligamentous stability should be intact. The degree of generalized ligamentous laxity of the patient should also be assessed.

AP, lateral and skyline (20–30 degree knee flexion) views are helpful in the evaluation of patellar subluxation (Figure 11.12). Patella alta can be assessed on the lateral view using the method of Koshino (33) for children and the Blackburn–Peel method for adolescents (34). The skyline view is used to assess the degree to which the patella sits in the trochlear groove, as well as the amount of "tilt" present in the lie of the patella.

Management

Identification of the primary offending agent (host, environment, agent) is essential to appropriately focus the management plan. The mainstay of conservative management is physiotherapy emphasizing the restoration of

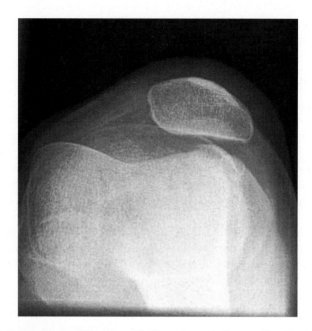

FIGURE 11.12. Patellar subluxation. Skyline view of the patella showing extreme lateral placement of the patella within the femoral groove.

balance between medial and lateral forces acting on the patella. A quadriceps-strengthening program with this focus is generally helpful within 8–12 wk in a compliant patient. Sound evidence is lacking to support the routine use of knee orthoses, however, some physicians have found the use of a J-brace to be of subjective benefit to some patients.

An initial period of rest from offending activity is helpful while the therapy program is initiated. Once the athlete is pain-free, return to play is allowed in a graduated approach. If conservative therapy fails, referral to an orthopedic surgeon for assessment of surgical intervention is appropriate.

Iliotibial Band Friction Syndrome

With flexion and extension of the knee, the ITB slides anteriorly and posteriorly over the bony prominence of the lateral femoral condyle when the knee is at 20–30 degrees of flexion. Repeated excessive movement of this band over the femoral condyle causes injury to the tendon, which manifests in pain and tenderness over the lateral aspect of the knee. This pain may be secondary to degenerative changes in the ITB or inflammatory changes in the associated bursa (35). In addition to repetitive flexion and extension of the knee (which may be seen with increases in training load), risk factors may include genu varum, a prominent lateral condyle, foot pronation, and internal tibial torsion (36). It has also recently been proposed that hip abductor weakness may increase thigh adduction and therefore lead to increased tension and friction of the ITB (37). Aggravating factors include prolonged activity, such as biking or running, particularly downhill running or running on the same side of the street.

Clinical Examination

The patient's pain can often be reproduced by palpating the lateral femoral condyle as the patient's knee is moved through a 20–30 degree arc of flexion. A snapping sensation may be appreciated. Patients will often have a positive Ober's test. Imaging is seldom necessary if the history and physical findings are consistent. If confirmation is needed, ultrasound or MRI may be helpful (36).

Management

Conservative management is usually successful in young athletes with ITB friction syndrome. Control of pain and inflammation may be necessary with ice and nonsteriodal antiinflammatory drugs (38). Management should include a period of relative rest, as well as modification of training errors, such as stride length, hills, cant of the training surface, and height of the cycle seat. A physiotherapy program emphasizing gluteal strengthening and flexibility is the mainstay of treatment. If symptoms are persistent, an injection of steroid into the associated bursa may help. Caution is advised when using this procedure in children. In rare refractory cases, where conservative management has failed, orthopedic consultation is helpful to assess the need for surgical intervention.

Sindig–Larsen–Johansson Disease

Sindig–Larsen–Johansson disease (SLJD) is a traction apophysitis of the inferior patellar pole, resulting in insidious onset of anterior knee pain localized to the inferior patellar pole. Pain is aggravated by running and jumping. The persistent traction of the quadriceps–patellar tendon unit on the immature inferior patellar pole leads to varying degrees of calcification and ossification of this apophysis. A classification system was proposed by Medlar and Lyne (39) (Table 11.3). SLJD can present concurrently with OSD and patellar tendonitis. The condition is common in growing athletes, particularly boys between the ages of 10–12 yr. Occasionally, the pain may be located at the superior poles of the patella.

Clinical Examination

Examination of the knee will reveal point tenderness at the inferior patellar pole (or the superior patellar poles if these are involved). There may be

TABLE 11.3. Classification system of Sindig–Larsen–Johansson syndrome.

Stage 1	Normal patella on roentgenograms
Stage 2	Irregular calcification at the inferior patellar pole
Stage 3	Progressive coalition of this calcification
Stage 4 A	Incorporation of the calcification within the patella
B	Calcific mass remains separate from the main body of the patella

Source: Medlar and Lyne, 1978. Reprinted with permission of The Journal of Bone and Joint Surgery, Inc.

pain with active resisted knee extension and passive knee flexion. The remainder of the knee examination is within normal limits. Knee x-rays, particularly a lateral film, may be normal or they may show varying degrees of ossification and calcification of the inferior patellar pole (Figure 11.13).

Management

The natural history of this condition is spontaneous resolution of symptoms. The resolution of symptoms can be expedited, however, by a few simple interventions. Moderation of the aggravating activity is essential. Ice and antiinflammatories may help with reduction in pain and inflammation. Physiotherapy consisting of a series of strengthening and flexibility exercises can promote healing and help prevent recurrence of symptoms once normal activities have resumed.

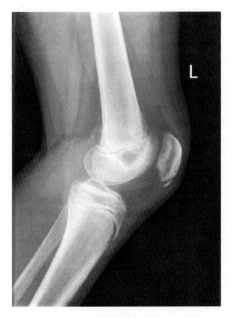

FIGURE 11.13. Plain film of SLJD. Lateral plain film showing fragmented ossification of the inferior patellar pole in SLJD.

Osgood–Schlatter Disease

Osgood–Schlatter disease is a common cause of knee pain in the adolescent athlete involved in running or jumping sports. This injury manifests as pain and tenderness at the site of insertion of the patellar tendon into the tibial tubercle, usually occurring during a growth spurt. Symptoms are the result of minor avulsions at the junction of the patellar tendon and the tibial tubercle. These avulsions are secondary to the forces of the patellar tendon when it overcomes the strength of the growing bone at the tibial tubercle apophysis. Repeated attempts at bony repair result in a callous of varying size at the site of the tibial tubercle. Pain that is more prominent in the patellar tendon rather than the bony prominence would be consistent with patellar tendonitis (jumper's knee) rather than OSD. Aggravating and alleviating factors are similar to those of SLJD. Management of these two conditions is similar.

The condition was described in 1903 by both Osgood (40) and Schlatter (41). Kujala confirmed that this condition is more common in athletes, finding an incidence of 21% in a group of adolescent athletes compared with 4.5% in an age-matched, nonathletic group (42). Athletes are affected during their adolescent growth spurt, at 11–13 yr of age for girls and 12–15 yr of age for boys. Traditionally, OSD is more common in boys, but the increase in sport participation in girls has led to an increase in incidence of this disease in females (30). The natural history of the condition is improvement with time (43). However, some adults are left with minor symptoms, including the inability to kneel for prolonged periods. Complications of this condition are minimal and consist mainly of the nonunion of a tibial tubercle fragment/ossicle resulting in persistent pain.

Clinical Examination

Physical examination often reveals a prominent tibial tubercle that is tender to palpation. This tenderness may extend proximally into the patellar tendon. There may also be mild edema in this area. There is pain with active resisted extension of the knee and with passive flexion of the knee as the quadriceps are stretched. Lateral x-rays of the knee show increased fragmentation of the tibial tubercle or separation of these fragments (Figure 11.14). There may also be soft tissue edema anterior to the tibial tubercle, thickening of the patellar tendon, and loss of the sharp inferior angle of the infrapatellar fat pad (42).

Management

Because of the self-limiting nature of the disease, the outcome is universally good. Recovery may be expedited by a relative reduction in the frequency or duration of offending activities, such as running, jumping, squatting, and kneeling. Ice massage of the tibial tubercle, along with nonsteriodal

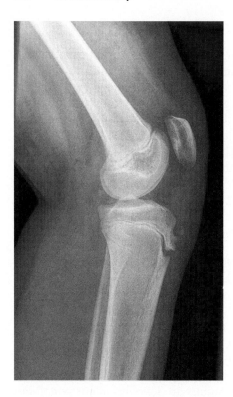

FIGURE11.14. Osgood–SchlatterDisease. Note the fragmented ossification of the tibial tubercle and thickened soft tissue anterior to the tibial tubercle.

antiinflammatory drugs, is often helpful with reduction of pain and inflammation. A physiotherapy program emphasizing quadriceps and hamstring flexibility may be beneficial as well. Immobilization is generally not recommended in the management of OSD. Although the pain associated with OSD is often reduced with these treatments, the bony deformity of the tibial tubercle will persist to varying degrees in many patients. Occasionally, pain will persist despite compliance with the treatment program. In these patients, the presence of a nonunited ossicle should be sought. Excision of a symptomatic ossicle will often result in prompt relief of symptoms (44).

Juvenile Osteochondritis Dissecans

Osteochondritis dissecans is a lesion of bone and articular cartilage of uncertain etiology that results in delamination of subchondral bone with or without articular cartilage mantle involvement (45). The etiology of this lesion remains uncertain. Possible etiologies have included trauma, ischemia, and genetics (46). In less advanced lesions, the affected area remains continuous with its origin. In more severe cases, the damaged bone and cartilage may partially or completely separate from their origin, resulting in irregularity of the articular surface or even a loose body within the joint.

TABLE 11.4. Classification system of osteochondritis dissecans.

Stage 0	No symptoms
Stage 1	Intermittent pain and swelling related to activity
Stage 2	Persistent pain and swelling without mechanical symptoms
Stage 3	Mechanical symptoms other than locking
Stage 4	Frank locking of the knee

Source: Litchman et al., 1988.

The lesions typically present in active adolescents, more often in males than females (3:1 or 4:1). Linden reported less variability between the sexes, with an incidence of 19 per 100,000 in females and 29 per 100,000 in males (47).

It has been reported that juvenile osteochondritis dissecans (JOCD) (OCD in athletes with open physes) has more potential to heal than the adult osteochondral lesion with conservative management (46–48). JOCD lesions are most commonly located in the lateral, non–weight bearing portion of the medial femoral condyle (51–72%), but can also be located on the lateral femoral condyle (17–20%) and the articular surface of the patella (7–15%) (48,49). OCD is often unilateral, although it can be bilateral. Litchman (50) proposed a staging system based on clinical presentation (Table 11.4).

Adolescent athletes with JOCD often present with a chronic (several months) history of vague anterior knee pain aggravated by activity. They may complain of knee swelling after activity. Complaints of locking may be present if there is an intraarticular loose body. Hefti reported that one third of patients had little or no pain at presentation (48). A history of trauma may be reported in 40–60% of cases (51).

Clinical Examination

The physical examination often reveals a limp secondary to pain or stiffness. Tenderness to palpation of the affected bony surface (femoral condyles, articular surface of patella) and a small effusion may be all that are present on the examination of the knee. X-rays of the knee, including AP, lateral, and tunnel (notch) views, will usually reveal the lesion (Figure 11.15). The tunnel view allows for better visualization of the posterior two thirds of the femoral condyle, where many OCD lesions are found (52). This area is poorly visualized on the standard AP film, and therefore an AP film interpreted as normal may be falsely reassuring (Figure 11.16). JOCD lesions can often be seen on the lateral view, but can be subtle and easily overlooked.

Technetium bone scintigraphy has also been used in the evaluation of JOCD. Cahill proposed the use of bone scintigraphy in both the diagnosis and management of JOCD (53,54). Regional bloodflow is reflected in the

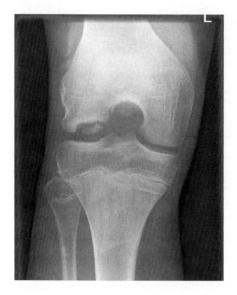

FIGURE 11.15. Notch view of OCD. Note significant fragmentation of the advanced lesion on the medial aspect of the lateral femoral condyle. This lesion is obvious, and the articular surface is clearly disrupted.

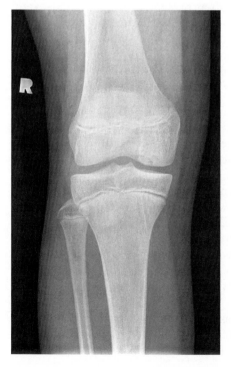

FIGURE 11.16. OCD as seen on AP plain films. Note the subtle lucency on the lateral aspect of the medial femoral condyle. Many lesions can be even more subtle.

degree of osseous uptake on bone scan. Lesions with increased uptake were shown to have increased potential for healing with conservative management. Cahill proposed regular bone scans at 6–8 wk intervals to assess the stage and healing of the lesion (53).

MRI can be helpful in the evaluation of JOCD. MRI helps to determine the size of the lesion and whether the cartilage overlying the lesion is intact, which in turn determines stability of the lesion. Unstable lesions are those that have separated themselves from their base. Stable lesions and small lesions have better healing potential. Lesions with intact cartilage improved with conservative treatment, regardless of extensive subchondral bone changes evident on MRI (55). O'Connor reviewed the interpretation of signal change at the site of JOCD lesions imaged by MRI and reported increased prediction of stability if the high signal line on the T2 weighted image did not breach the articular cartilage on the T1 weighted image (56).

Management

The primary goals in the management of JOCD include symptom relief, maintaining or restoring the integrity of the articular cartilage surface, and the prevention of the development of arthritis. Wall indicates that because 50–94% of stable JOCD lesions heal with conservative management, a 3–6 mo trial of nonoperative therapy should be initiated (46). Hefti has shown that when these lesions are initially treated operatively, a worse outcome can be expected (48). Several options for conservative treatment have been recommended with variable success rates. Most authors recommend a period of protected weight bearing with a removable knee immobilizer to allow for intermittent controlled knee range of motion (51). Wall, however, prefers casting to decrease the likelihood of noncompliance (46). Regardless of type of immobilization and protected weight bearing, this intervention is necessary for at least 8–12 wk, and sometimes up to 1 yr, depending on the amount of healing evident on either plain films, bone scan or MRI. In six patients with open physes, Paletta was able to show that increased uptake on bone scan was positively correlated with healing with conservative management (57). Cahill proposed that if three consecutive bone scans showed no improvement, then it was unlikely that the lesion would heal spontaneously, and surgical intervention would be appropriate (53).

Once significant reossification has been documented, a gradual increase in weight bearing and return to sport is implemented. Physiotherapy is essential in regaining the strength lost from deconditioning and immobilization during the healing phase.

If healing is not documented after 6 mo of conservative treatment, operative intervention may be necessary. There are several options for operative intervention, including arthroscopic drilling and fixation, abrasion chondroplasty and microfracture, allograft, osteochondral autograft transplantation, and autologous chondrocyte transplantation (51).

Plicae

Plicae are an uncommon cause of knee pain in the adolescent athlete. A plica is a fetal remnant of mesenchymal tissue, initially formed as the knee joint was dividing into its various compartments. It has been estimated that 20% of the adult population has asymptomatic persistent synovial plica (58,59). Pain is experienced in the anterior aspect of the knee when the plica becomes inflamed. This may result from a direct contact injury (hit to the knee in the area of the plica). The plica may also become inflamed as it bowstrings across the medial femoral condyle in knee flexion, causing painful snapping (60). During childhood this tissue glides uneventfully over the condyle. During the adolescent growth spurt, the imbalances in growth increase the tension of this band as it crosses over the condyle. With the increase in tension, there is an increase in friction, which results in inflammation, fibrosis, and hypertrophy of the plica. This is amplified with repetitive running and jumping (30). Although there can be up to four plica within the knee joint (infrapatellar, suprapatellar, medial patellar, and lateral patellar), it is the medial patellar plica that is most commonly implicated in the painful plica syndrome.

Clinical Examination

The physical examination may contain little in the way of positive findings. There may be pain to direct palpation of the plica (one fingerbreadth medial to the medial border of the patella). A popping may be palpated in the medial compartment as the knee ranges from 30–60 degrees of flexion. Occasionally, the band itself is palpable. Classically, there is no effusion. This may be helpful in distinguishing between the pain from an inflamed plica and a torn meniscus. Imaging is not helpful.

Management

The management of an inflamed plica begins with identification of any training errors and modifying training accordingly. Relative rest will help decrease pain. Physiotherapy aids in the improvement of balance of strength and flexibility. Antiinflammatories such as ice and ibuprofen are helpful in controlling both pain and inflammation (61). Although Rovere and Adair found some benefit to steroid injection into the inflamed plica (62), this method of treatment is uncommonly used. If conservative therapy fails and other diagnoses have been ruled out, surgical resection of the plica may be necessary.

Congenital

Discoid meniscus

The discoid meniscus is a congenital variation in the shape of the meniscus, most often the LM. The discoid meniscus does not have the C-shaped concavity found in the normal meniscus; rather, it is shaped like a disk, thicker centrally. Kelly and Green have summarized the proposed theories on the origin of the discoid meniscus, which culminate in the current theory of the discoid meniscus as a congenital anatomic variant (63). The incidence of discoid meniscus has been noted to be up to 17%, depending on the population studied (63). It can occur bilaterally in up to 20% of cases (64). The discoid meniscus is most often characterized using the Watanabe classification system (Table 11.5) (65). Types 1 and 2 tend to be asymptomatic and are discovered incidentally. Type 3 is thought to produce the "snapping knee" syndrome. Kocher et al. proposed a classification system based on the type of discoid (complete vs. incomplete), the presence of peripheral rim stability (stable or unstable), and the associated tear of the meniscus (16).

A symptomatic discoid meniscus may present with a history of painless palpable or audible snapping (the snapping knee syndrome). Symptoms are most likely to appear after the discoid meniscus has been injured. Once torn, symptoms on presentation include pain, locking, catching, and decreased range of motion.

Clinical Examination

The physical examination reveals an effusion, decreased range of motion with pain at extremes of range, and positive provocative testing with the McMurray and Apley tests. Plain films may show subtle indications of a discoid LM, including a widened lateral joint line (Figure 11.17), calcification of the LM, squaring of the lateral femoral condyle, cupping of the lateral tibial plateau, hypoplasia of the tibial eminence and elevation of the fibular head. Discoid menisci can be identified by MRI (Figure 11.18). Although the sensitivity for detection is low, the positive predictive value is high (19).

Management

Asymptomatic discoid menisci identified incidentally require no further treatment. The symptomatic discoid meniscus necessitates referral to a pediatric orthopedic surgeon.

TABLE 11.5. Classification system of discoid meniscus.

Type 1	Complete discoid meniscus with intact posterior tibial attachment
Type 2	Incomplete discoid meniscus with intact posterior tibial attachment
Type 3	"Wrisburg ligament type"—complete or incomplete discoid meniscus lacking posterior tibial attachment

Source: Watanabe et al., 1969.

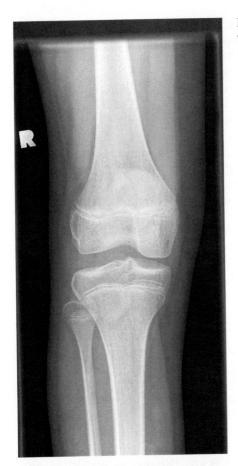

FIGURE 11.17. Discoid meniscus. Note widening of the lateral joint space.

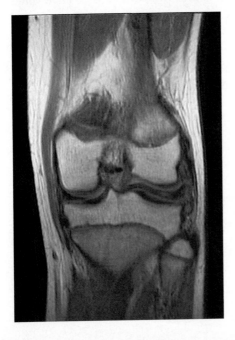

FIGURE 11.18. MRI of discoid LM. Note the disc shape of the LM compared with the concave shape of the MM.

Prevention

Although not all injuries can be prevented, a few guidelines may be helpful in preventing some injuries. It is helpful for athletes to maintain a general level of fitness year round. Many sports will have an off season, which the athlete can use to rest the muscles used repetitively during the competitive season. Participation in other sports during the off season is also helpful in achieving global strength and fitness. No specific exercises have been shown to consistently reduce the incidence of any particular knee injury; however, athletes should be encouraged to continue a year round general strength and conditioning program that is complimentary to their chosen sport.

Sport safety is essential in reducing the incidence of injuries to athletes. All recommended protective gear should be worn and "courtside rules of etiquette" should be followed. Surfaces and sporting equipment should be kept well maintained and in accordance with safety regulations.

Return to Play Guidelines

Specific return to play guidelines are discussed above in the context of each injury. In general, athletes returning to sport should have regained a baseline level of conditioning that will allow them to begin to participate in practices and drills. The treating therapist should progress the athlete from general strengthening and conditioning to sport-specific rehabilitation. Once the athlete has shown proficiency with these interventions, graded return to play can be initiated and supervised by the treating therapist. At no point should participation increase pain or dysfunction. All recommended braces and supports should be used until the treating therapist or physician has advised the athlete that their use may be discontinued.

Clinical Pearls

- Always compare the injured side with the uninjured side to gain an accurate appreciation for what is normal for each patient.
- The presence of a knee effusion in a child is always significant. Its presence often indicates intraarticular pathology and warrants investigation until a diagnosis is obtained.
- Quadriceps atrophy begins immediately after a significant knee injury and can be a subtle finding of a significant knee injury.
- In the absence of physical exam findings at the knee in a young athlete with knee pain, the hip must be examined and investigated as a source of pathology leading to pain referred to the knee.

- Multiple joint involvement, fevers, systemic symptoms, and night pain suggest nonmechanical causes of knee pain and should be investigated further.
- Often, an injured athlete will be able to continue participation/training in some aspect of their sport while rehabilitating an injury. When possible, this continued participation is important for the athlete's skill development and psychological well being. When a physician is unfamiliar with a sport, the coach or therapist may be helpful in determining which areas of the sport may be appropriate to continue through rehabilitation of an injury.
- Although most injuries are not career ending, caregivers must remember that these athletes are children and with proper management, can have a lifetime of athletic participation ahead of them.

References

1. Public Health Agency of Canada Injury Surveillance Online. Canadian Hospitals Injury Reporting and Prevention Program (CHIRPP). Distribution of all body parts touched by the injury. http://dsol-smed.phac-aspc.gc.ca/dsol-smed/issb/chirpp/Final%20BdyPrt.xls (accessed December 22, 2006).
2. Bernhardt DT. Knee and leg injuries. In: Birrer RB, Griesemer BA, Cataletto MB, eds. Pediatric Sports Medicine for Primary Care. Philadelphia: Lippincott, Williams &Wilkins; 2002.
3. Davids JR. Common orthopedic problems II. Pediatr Clin N Am 1996;43(5): 1067–1090.
4. Fithian DC, Paxton EW, Cohen AB. Indications in the treatment of patellar instability. J Knee Surg 2004;17(1)47–56.
5. Stanitski, CL. Patellar instability in the school age athlete. In: Dilworth Cannon W, ed. AAOS Instructional Course Lectures. Vol. 47. Rosemont, Ill.: American Academy of Orthepedic Surgeons; 1998.
6. Virolainen H, Visure T, Kuseela T. Acute dislocations of the patella: MR findings. Radiology 1993;189:243–246.
7. Hinton RY, and Sharma KM. Acute and recurrent patellar instability in the young athlete. Orthop Clin North Am 2003;34:385–396.
8. Maenpaa H, Lehto MU. Patellar dislocation. The long term results of nonoperated managements in 100 patients. Am J Sports Med 1997;25: 213–217.
9. Mikku R, Nietoscaara Y, Kallio PE, Aalto K, Michelsson JE. Operative versus closed treatment of primary dislocation of the patella: similar 2-year results in 125 randomized patients. Acta Orthop Scand 1997;68:419–423.
10. Andrade A, Thomas N. Randomized comparison of operative vs. non operative treatment following first time patellar dislocation. Presented at: The European Society of Sports Traumatology, Knee Surgery and Arthroscopy; April 2002; Rome, Italy.
11. Bales CP, Joseph HG, Moorman CT. Anterior cruciate ligament injuries in children with open physes. Am J Sport Med 2004;32(8):1978–85.

12. DeLee JC. Ligamentous injury of the knee. In: Stanitski CL, DeLee JC, Drez D, eds. Pediatric and Adolescent Sports Medicine. Vol. 3. Philadelphia: WB Saunders; 1994:406–432.

13. Prince JS, Laor T, Bean JA. MRI of anterior cruciate ligament injuries and associated findings in the pediatric knee: changes with skeletal maturation. AJR 2005;185:756–62.

14. Huston LJ, Greenfield ML, Wojtys EM. Anterior cruciate ligament injuries in the female athlete: potential risk factors. Clin Orthop Rel Res 2000;372:50–63.

15. Kocher MS, Garg S, Micheli LJ. Physeal sparing reconstruction of the anterior cruciate ligament in skeletally immature prepubescent children and adolescents. J Bone Joint Surg 2005;87A(11):2371–2379.

16. Kocher MS, Klingele K, Rassman SO. Meniscal disorders: Normal, discoid and cysts. Orthop Clin N Am 2003;34:329–340.

17. Kocher, MS, Micheli LJ. The pediatric knee: evaluation and treatment. In: Insall JN, Scott WN, eds. Surgery of the knee. 3rd ed. New York: Churchill-Livingstone; 2001:1356–1397.

18. Andrish JT. Meniscal injuries in children and adolescents. J Am Acad Orthop Surg 1996;4:231–237.

19. Kocher MS, Di Canzio J, Zurakowski D, Micheli LJ. Diagnostic performance of clinical examination and selective magnetic resonance images in the evaluation of intra-articular knee disorders in children and adolescents. Am J Sports Med 2001;29:292–296.

20. Mintzer CM, Richmond JC, Taylor J. Meniscal repair in the young athlete. Am J Sport Med 1988;26:630–633.

21. Noyes FR, Barber-Westin SD. Arthroscopic repair of meniscal tears that extend into the vascular zone in patients younger than twenty years of age. Am J Sports Med 2002;30:589–600.

22. Rubman MH, Noyes FR, Barber-Westin SD. Arthroscopic repair of meniscal tears that extend into the avascular zone: a review of 198 single and complex tears. Am J Sports Med 1998;26:87–95.

23. Diduch D, Scuderi GR, Scot WN. Knee Injuries. In: Scuderi GR, McCann PD, eds. Sports Medicine: A Comprehensive Approach. 2nd ed. Philadelphia: Elsevier Mosby; 2005:346–387.

24. Mosier SM, Stanitski CL. Acute tibial tubercle avulsion fractures. J Pediatr Orthop 2004;24(2):181–184.

25. McKoy BE, Stanitski CL. Acute tibial tubercle avulsion fracture. Orthop Clin N Am. 2003;34:397–403.

26. Hand WL, Hand CR, Dunn AW. Avulsion fractures of the tibial tubercle. J Bone Joint Surg Am 1971;53(8):1579–1583.

27. Stanitski CL. Acute tibial tubercle avulsion fracture. In: Stanitski CL, DeLee JC, Drez D, eds. Pediatric and Adolescent Sports Medicine. Vol. 3. Philadelphia: WB Saunders; 1994:329–334.

28. Watson-Jones R. Fractures and Joint Injuries. 5th ed. Baltimore: Williams and Wilkins; 1976.

29. Ogden JA, Tross RB, Murphy MJ. Fractures of the tibial tuberosity in adolescents. J Bone Joint Surg Am Mar 1980;62(2):205–215.

30. Duri ZAA, Patel DV, Aichroth PM. The immature athlete. Clin Sports Med 2002;21(3):461–482.

31. Fairbank JC, Pynsent PB, van Poortvliet JA, Phillips H. Mechanical factors in the incidence of knee pain in adolescents and young adults. J Bone Joint Surg 1984;66B(5):685–693.

32. Crossley K, Bennell K, Green S, McConnell J. A systematic review of physical interventions for patellofemoral pain syndrome. Clin J Sport Med 2001;11:103–110.

33. Koshino T, Sugimoto K. New measurement of patellar height in the knees of children using the epiphyseal line midpoint. J Pediatr Orthop 1989;9(2):216–218.

34. Blackburn JS, Peel TYE. A new method of measuring patellar height. J Bone Joint Surg 1977;59B(2):241–242.

35. Panni AS, Biedirt RN, Maffulli N, Tartarone M, Romanini E. Overuse injuries of the extensor mechanism in athletes. Clin Sports Med 2002:21(3);483–498.

36. Safran MR, Fu FH. Uncommon causes of knee pain in the athlete. Orthop Clin N Am. 1995;26(3)547–559.

37. Fredericson M, Cookingham CL, Chaudhari AM, et al. Hip abductor weakness in distance runners with iliotibial band friction syndrome. Clin J Sport Med 2000;10(3):169–175.

38. Fyfe I, Stanish WD. The use of eccentric training and stretching in the treatment and prevention of tendon injuries. Clin Sports Med 1992;11(3):601–624.

39. Medlar RD, Lyne ED. Sinding-Larsen-Johansson disease. J Bone Joint Surg 1978;60A:1112–1116.

40. Osgood RB. Lesions of the tibial tubercle occurring during adolescence. Boston Med Surg J 1903;148:114–117.

41. Schlatter C. Verletzungen des schnabelforminogen fortsatzes der oberen tibi-aepiphyse. Beitre Klin Chir Tubing 1903;38:874–878.

42. Kujala UM, Kvist M, Heinonen O. Osgood Schlatter's disease in adolescent athletes: retrospective study of incidence and duration. Am J Sports Med 1985;13:236–241.

43. Krause BL, Williams JP, Catteral A. Natural history of Osgood Schlatter's disease. J Pediatr Orthop 1990;10:65–69.

44. Mital MA, Matza RA, Cohen J. The so-called unresolved Osgood Schlatter lesion. Clin Orthop 1993;289:202–204.

45. Stanitski CL. Osteochondritis dissecans of the knee. In: Stanitski CL, DeLee JC, Drez D, eds. Pediatric and Adolescent Sports Medicine Vol. 3. Philadelphia: W.B. Saunders; 1994:387.

46. Wall E, Von Stein D. Juvenile osteochondritis dissecans. Orthop Clin N Am 2003;(34):341–353.

47. Linden B. The incidence of osteochondritis dissecans in the condyles of the femur. Acta Orthop Scand 1976;47:664–667.

48. Hefti F, et al. Osteochondritis dissecans: a multicenter study of the European Pediatric Orthopedic Society. J Pediatr Orthop B 1999;8(4):231–45.

49. Carroll NC, Mubarack SJ. Juvenile osteochondritis dissecans of the knee. J Bone Joint Surg 1977;59B:506.

50. Litchman HM, McCullough RW, Gandsman EJ, et al. Computerized bloodflow analysis for decision making in the treatment of osteochondritis dissecans. J Pediatr Orthop 1988;8:208–212.

51. Cain EL, Clancy WG. Treatment algorithm for osteochondral injuries of the knee. Clin Sport Med 2001;20(2):321–342.

52. Milgram JW. Radiological and pathological manifestations of osteochondritis dissecans of the distal femur. Radiology 1978;126(2):305–311.
53. Cahill BR, Berg BC. 99m-Technetium phosphate compound joint scintigraphy in the management of juvenile OCD of the femoral condyles. Am J Sports Med 1983;11(5):329–335.
54. Cahill BR, Phillips MR, Navarro R. The results of conservative management of juvenile osteochondritis dissecans using joint scintigraphy. A prospective study. Am J Sports Med 1989;17(5):601–605.
55. Hughes JA, Cook JV, Churchill MA, Warren ME. Juvenile osteochondritis dissecans: a 5-year review of the natural history using clinical and MRI evaluation. Pediatr Radiol 2003;33:410–417.
56. O'Connor MA, Palaniappan M, Khan N, Bruce CE. Osteochondritis dissecans of the knee in children. J Bone Joint Surg 2002;84B:259–262.
57. Paletta GA, Bednarz PA, Stanitiski CL, et al. The prognostic value of quantitative bone scan in knee ostechondritis dissecans. Am J Sport Med 1998;26(1): 7–14.
58. King JB, Cook, JL, Khan KM, Maffulli N. Patellar tendinopathy. Sports Medicine Arthrosc Rev 2000;8:86–95.
59. Testa V, Capasso G, Maffulli N, et al. Ultrasound guided percutaneous longitudinal tenotomy for the management of patellar tendinopathy. Med Sci Sports Excer 1999;31(11):1509–1515.
60. Ferretti A, Ippolito E, Mariani PP, et al. Jumper's knee. Am J Sports Med. 1983;11:58–62.
61. Stanitski CL. Plica. In: Stanitski CL, DeLee JC, Drez D, eds. Pediatric and Adolescent Sports Medicine. Vol. 3. Philadelphia: WB Saunders; 1994:317–319.
62. Rovere GD, Adair D. Medial synovial shelf plica syndrome; treatment by intraplical steroid injection. Am J Sports Med 1985; 13:383.
63. Kelly BT, Green DW. Discoid lateral meniscus in children. Curr Opin Pediatr 2002;14:54–61.
64. Bellier G, Dupont JY, Larrin M, et al. Lateral discoid menisci in children. Arthroscopy 1989;5:52–56.
65. Watanabe M, Takada S, Ikeuchi H. Atlas of arthroscopy. Tokyo: Igaku–Shoin; 1969.

12
Lower Leg Injuries

Angela D. Smith

Lower leg pain rarely occurs from the usual activities of daily living of children and adolescents. Nonacute, repetitive microtraumatic injuries are typically related to running and jumping associated with sports. Pain in the tibia or fibula not caused by acute trauma is most often associated with recurrent impact loading. Training errors and inappropriate equipment are often causative factors. In addition, lower leg injuries caused by acute trauma that is *unrelated* to sport may impact the young athlete's ability to participate in desired activities.

The symptom of lower leg pain, particularly when unilateral, must prompt consideration of diagnoses such as benign or malignant neoplasm, acute or chronic infection, and metabolic bone disease. The diagnosis may not be apparent from the history and physical examination alone. If a problem such as neoplasm or infection is found, choosing one particular treatment method over another may allow a young athlete to successfully return to sport sooner.

A recently published review includes excellent algorithms for developing a differential diagnosis for an athlete's lower leg pain, and most of that information applies to child and adolescent athletes (1). This chapter outlines lower leg injuries with specific attention to the young athlete, addressing methods for the most rapid, yet safe, return to activity. Few references in the literature specifically address the lower leg injuries of young athletes. Therefore, many of the concepts and much of the literature referenced in this chapter are derived from studies of adults, in addition to the clinical experience of the author and sports medicine colleagues. As best as possible, the database demographics and level of evidence for a given study will be identified.

Anatomy

The bones of the lower leg are the tibia and fibula, each covered by only a thin layer of skin and subcutaneous tissue in some areas (Figure 12.1).

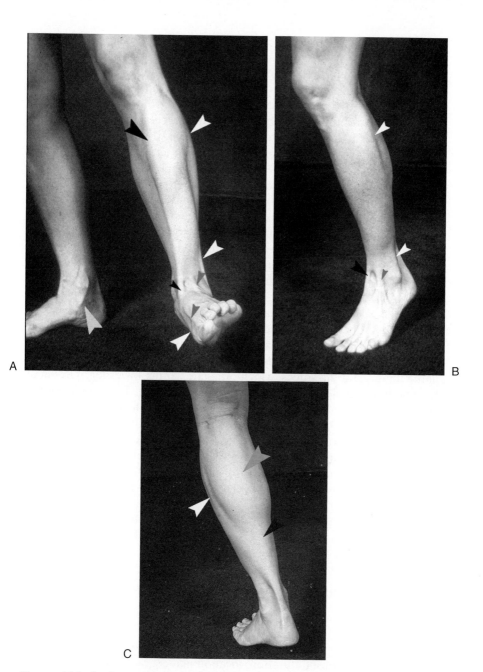

FIGURE 12.1. Surface anatomy. **(A and B)** The anterior tibial muscle and tendon (black arrows) and the toe extensors (dark gray arrows) dorsiflex the ankle. The peroneus longus (white arrows) courses down the lateral leg and foot, then deep across the plantar aspect of the foot to insert at the first metatarsal. It everts the foot and depresses the first metatarsal. The dark gray arrows indicate the long toe extensors. The light gray arrows indicate the right foot posterior tibial tendon that inserts into the prominent medial navicular bone. **(C)** The two heads of the gastrocnemius (gray arrow) are superficial to the soleus muscle (white arrow). The black arrow indicates roughly the center of the long musculotendinous junction of the triceps surae/Achilles tendon unit.

Although almost all the muscles that control knee motion insert onto the proximal tibia and fibula, their muscle bellies are in the thigh. Most lower leg muscles control only ankle and foot motion, but the gastrocnemius muscle also flexes the knee. The greater total excursion of the gastrocnemius makes it the most likely lower leg muscle to be strained.

The anterior compartment contains the tibialis anterior, extensor hallucis longus, extensor digitorum longus, and peroneus tertius muscles. These muscles are primarily dorsiflexors. The deep peroneal nerve supplies these muscles and is the sensory nerve for the dorsal web space between the first and second toes. The lateral compartment contains the peroneus longus and brevis muscles, the most important evertors of the foot. Also in the lateral compartment is the superficial peroneal nerve, which is sensory. The peroneal nerve divides into the deep and superficial peroneal nerves at the level of the fibular head where it is quite superficial, tented across the bone. Near the midpoint of the lower leg, the superficial peroneal nerve pierces the lateral fascia of the lateral compartment to continue to the lateral ankle subcutaneously before branching and supplying sensation to the lateral foot distally. The superficial posterior compartment muscles include the medial and lateral heads of the gastrocnemius, which originate on the femur, and the soleus, which originates in the lower leg. The small, thin plantaris muscle also resides in this compartment. The deep posterior compartment contains the tibialis posterior, flexor hallucis longus, and flexor digitorum longus muscles. There may be a variable "fifth" compartment, a subcompartment of the deep posterior compartment, related to variation of the fibular attachment of the flexor digitorum longus (2).

The popliteal artery bifurcates at or just below the popliteal fossa, into the anterior and posterior tibial arteries. The anterior tibial artery courses through the anterior compartment, palpable as the dorsalis pedis pulse. The posterior tibial artery courses through the deep posterior compartment, which is palpable adjacent to the medial malleolus. The large saphenous vein is superficial over the distal medial leg.

Clinical Evaluation

History

The differential diagnosis of lower leg problems is narrowed by determining the mechanism of onset, duration, location and character of the pain. The timing of the pain, when it occurs in relation to different activities and whether it then resolves or recurs during the same activity, further indicates the most likely diagnosis (Table 12.1).

Young athletes who sustain repeated injuries may have an underlying systemic disorder, such as Ehlers–Danlos or osteogenesis imperfecta. Their injuries may be related to a psychological disorder, such as depression or anorexia nervosa. A young athlete who no longer finds a sport exciting may

TABLE 12.1. Key history details in lower leg injuries.

	Exertional compartment syndrome	Stress fracture	Posteromedial tibial stress syndrome	Tendon overuse injury
Pain Location	Large area, muscle	Focal, bone	Longitudinal, along much of posteromedial border of tibia	Tendon, possibly musculotendinous junction
Pain Character	"Dead," "numb," weak	Sharp, stabbing, boring, like toothache	Sharp or dull	Burning, stabbing, searing with radiation into muscle
Timing	Resolves within minutes after stopping activity, but may remain "sore"	Worse as activity continues; improves with rest	Persists long after activity, may decrease during activity	Pain with any use of the structure, persistently tender
Typical Location	Anterior compartment, anterolateral leg	Small, defined area of anterior tibia, distal fibula	Central and distal posteromedial tibia	Tendon, musculotendinous junction, usually Achilles

even need an excuse to bow out of a sport without losing esteem in the eyes of parents or friends. Those caring for children and adolescents need to be sensitive to subtle signs from the athlete and the parent, not simply care for the physical injury blind to the psychosocial context. Red flags may include overbearing parents who answer all the questions that are addressed to the athlete, an athlete avoiding eye contact, unusual constellations of symptoms and physical findings, excessive leanness or obesity, and loss of regular menses for young female athletes.

Physical Examination

The physical examination of the injured lower leg includes observation of the legs, both still and in motion. Abnormal color of the entire lower leg may indicate actual or incipient reflex sympathetic dystrophy. Muscles should be symmetric side to side. They should also be proportional within the limb. Very slender lower legs and heavily muscled thighs may simply reflect normal heredity, but such proportions may also suggest a diagnosis of progressive peroneal muscular atrophy. Even the foot shape should have relative bilateral symmetry. If the normal right forefoot appears filled out but the injured left foot looks flat like a pancake, the intrinsic muscles are probably atrophied.

Walking and running gait should be observed, followed by jumping on two feet and jumping up from a full squatting position. Tiny steps on tiptoes or heels, with the knees fully extended, may readily show lack of muscular symmetry or subtle strength deficits of the intrinsic muscles of the feet. Successfully hopping repeatedly on one foot without any functional angular or rotational problem usually indicates satisfactory balance and coordination, as well as good strength of the lower extremity kinetic chain. The athlete who hops with knees medial to the second toes, with apparent hip internal rotation, knee valgus, and excessive hindfoot pronation, is not prepared to return safely to unrestricted jumping, cutting, and pivoting sports. These findings often indicate weakness of the hip external rotators, subtalar joint invertors, and, often, evertors and foot intrinsics.

Palpation of the lower leg includes the subcutaneous portions of the tibia and fibula, as well as the muscles and tendons. Irregularities of the subcutaneous tissue and skin may be apparent. Palpation also includes checking for pitting edema and unusual skin texture (which may suggest hypothyroidism, for example), as well as noting skin temperature.

Range of motion of the foot and ankle joints may be limited. A cavus foot is usually somewhat rigid even when the young athlete is otherwise hypermobile. Limited subtalar joint inversion suggests tarsal coalition, which is more readily apparent if the athlete has just completed a short jog in the hall. Ligament injury may cause excessive proximal or distal tibiofibular mobility.

Muscle strength is tested functionally with the maneuvers above, but manual resistance can also be useful. One simple test to assess for complete strength rehabilitation of the peroneal muscles is resisted manual muscle testing.

Calf muscle flexibility is checked by passively dorsiflexing the athlete's ankle with the knee extended and the hindfoot held in varus. In this position, the young athlete's ankle should typically dorsiflex 10 degrees above neutral.

Acute Injuries

Acute Fracture

Acute fractures of the tibial or fibular shaft may occur from an athlete's collision with another athlete or with an object, or simply from a bending or rotational force, such as cutting on a planted foot or catching a ski edge. Initial treatment for an athlete is no different from any other child and involves splinting the limb without circumferential or other material that would constrict the limb as it swells. Because the entire tibial shaft and the distal third of the fibula are subcutaneous, open fractures in this setting are not unusual. A moist, sterile dressing, if available, should be applied to the open area. Transport to an appropriate facility for imaging and treatment should not be delayed.

Tibia fractures may lead to acute compartment syndrome, and more than one of the lower leg compartments may be involved. Often, the earliest sign of compartment syndrome is pain in the lower leg when the involved muscle is passively stretched. By the time the patient experiences actual change of sensation, circulation, or motor function, there may already be some permanent loss of muscle. Measurement of compartment pressure is indicated if there is clinical suspicion of compartment syndrome, or if the patient is unable to adequately feel pain and communicate a response to pain.

Among adolescents, particularly those nearing tibial growth plate closure, rigid internal fixation has long been considered for athletes with tibial fractures. This allows them to begin rehabilitation very early in the healing process, so they may be able to return to full activity weeks earlier than they would if treated with cast immobilization. In recent years, there has been a trend toward the use of flexible nails, internal plate fixation, or external fixation devices for long bone fractures even in younger children. These procedures may speed the return to sport for a child, but the difference relative to treatment by cast immobilization is probably small. In general, when treating young athletes we recommend using functional bracing rather than rigid cast immobilization as soon as is reasonable during fracture healing. The role of bone growth stimulating substances and devices has not yet been adequately studied in children and adolescents, but will likely play a role in the near future.

Muscle Strain/Peroneal Tendon Subluxation

Triceps Surae

Calf muscle strains occur rarely among children, but somewhat more often among adolescent athletes. The athlete with an acute strain of the triceps surae often reports some preexisting, dull pain related to sport activity. A sudden contraction, usually an eccentric contraction, may result in tearing of the muscle. An area of swelling, often described by the patient as a "knot" may be accompanied by ecchymosis. The discoloration of the skin often doesn't appear for several days, however, until blood breakdown products dissect to the surface. Unilateral strain must be differentiated from deep venous thrombosis, as passive stretch of the calf muscles may cause pain with either entity.

Treatment is generally rest until the pain and swelling have resolved. Use of a heel lift may decrease symptoms, but often, a removable boot is needed to allow easy and relatively painless ambulation. If the strain is severe, crutch ambulation may be required, but early weight bearing (partial weight bearing as tolerated) is encouraged to decrease disuse atrophy of the entire lower extremity.

Peroneals (with Ankle Sprain)

In an inversion injury such as a lateral ankle sprain, the peroneal muscles may contract in an effort to stop the inversion. This eccentric contraction can lead to peroneal muscle strain or peroneal tendon subluxation. A single injury may result in all three: significant anterolateral ankle sprain, anterior subluxation of the peroneal tendons, and peroneal muscle strain. Recovery in this situation is significantly prolonged compared with a simple, mild ankle sprain. Early recognition of this more complex injury can help the athlete prepare emotionally for the typically longer recovery time, as well as allow better planning for future training opportunities and competitive events.

In most cases, treatment is similar to that of the more typical isolated ankle sprain: cold therapy, elevation, and functional immobilization, with early range of motion and strengthening as tolerated. However, when there is peroneal injury, the athlete is much more likely to require the use of an air stirrup brace that reaches proximally almost to the knee, or even a removable walking boot. We prefer the removable boot to a rigid cast so that the athlete and those providing the medical care can monitor the progress more easily and more frequently, and allow the most rapid progression through the rehabilitation process that is safely possible.

Achilles Tendon Rupture

Achilles tendon rupture, which is relatively common among adult athletes, is virtually unheard of among healthy children, the first case just recently having been reported (3). It is rare among adolescents, but does occur, particularly in older adolescence. The author is not aware of any studies specifically comparing treatment options for Achilles tendon ruptures in children or adolescents.

Contusions

Bone Bruise

Shins are frequent sites of bumps and bruises. Because the tibia has only a thin layer of subcutaneous fat over it, blunt trauma may cause a significant bone contusion with subperiosteal bleeding. The resulting fusiform mass may appear frightening to the athlete and parents. The erythema and induration may even suggest subacute osteomyelitis, which typically occurs in a metaphyseal region a few days after blunt trauma that alters the local intraosseous circulation (Figure 12.2). The subcutaneous or subperiosteal mass may persist for months before finally remodeling away. There may be associated focal fat necrosis that causes the appearance of a dent in the contour of the lower leg. This change in contour usually persists.

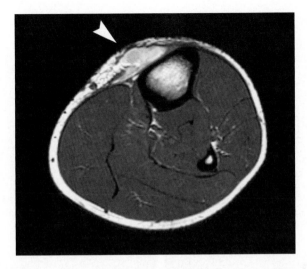

FIGURE 12.2. A 15-yr-old baseball player slid into home base, striking his proximal medial shin against the catcher's shin guard. The game was almost over, and 4 d later at the next scheduled game he was able to play a full game as catcher himself. However, by the end of the game he had significant pain, and it was so much worse the following day that he stopped all training. Ten days after the injury, he had exquisite tenderness of the entire tibia, with moderate induration of the deep soft tissues over the medial border of the tibia, surrounding a long, healing superficial abrasion. He had moderately tender enlarged lymph nodes in the left inguinal region, larger than on the right. He was afebrile. Laboratory studies and plain x-rays were unremarkable. An MRI scan showed a subcutaneous fluid collection consistent with resolving hematoma, with additional subcutaneous edema, most likely from a significant shearing injury similar to a ring avulsion or bicycle spoke injury.

Saphenous Vein Hematoma/Occlusion

Blunt trauma to the saphenous vein, especially in its distal course over the distal third of the tibia, may also result in an area of tenderness and swelling, but it may be slightly mobile relative to the tibia, unlike the subperiosteal hematoma. The saphenous vein usually recanalizes within 1–2 wk, but swelling and tenderness may persist many weeks longer.

Chronic Injuries

Many lower leg injuries result from training errors. A sudden increase in training time or intensity, adding hill running or intervals, and changing footgear or training surface are some of the most common etiologies for nonacute injuries to the lower legs. Changes in technique, such as increasing

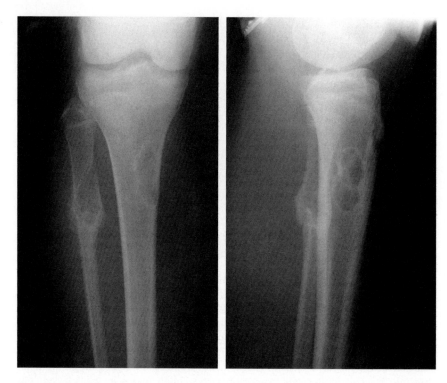

FIGURE 12.3. The healing stress fracture through the large fibular nonossifying fibroma was symptomatic. The smaller nonossifying fibroma in the tibia was not.

the running stride length or the approach to the gymnastics vault spring-board, also change the forces applied to the lower leg in sport.

Athletes and coaches alike may not realize that return to activity after an injury or illness requires gradual, progressive reconditioning. Without the progressive approach in returning to a sport that includes running or jumping, lower leg injury is more likely to occur. Complete rehabilitation of any injury is important before safe return to unrestricted activity. This includes restoration of muscle symmetry, flexibility, quickness, and endurance.

More unusual etiologies of lower leg pain, such as neoplasm or infection, must be ruled out, particularly if symptoms are unilateral (Figure 12.3). Metabolic bone disease may weaken the long bone structure, leading to stress fracture. Inadequate nutrition, especially inadequate energy intake, may disrupt the normal, daily bone healing that allows the bone to adapt to training stress rather than fracture.

Recurrent Exertional Compartment Syndrome

Recurrent (also called chronic) exertional compartment syndrome causes aching or cramping pain, or a sensation of severe heaviness, in one or more lower leg compartments. Between episodes, the athlete feels normal or has only slight discomfort. The anterior compartment is often involved. Some young athletes experience compartment syndrome symptoms in both the anterior and lateral compartments, but lateral compartment involvement among children and adolescents seems to occur much less often than anterior compartment syndrome.

Symptoms are more often bilateral than unilateral, usually involving the same compartment in each leg. Pain begins soon after onset of the exacerbating activity. Onset of symptoms may not occur until a certain level of activity intensity is reached, such as running at a certain speed. A change in stride length may alter the running biomechanics sufficiently to increase or, rarely, to decrease symptoms. Athletes with recurrent anterior compartment syndrome complain of pain in the front of the shin, described as aching, burning, heavy, or tense. They may notice foot slapping as the muscle function decreases. A few athletes may appreciate numbness in the dorsal web space between the first and second toes, the sensory distribution of the deep peroneal nerve. Symptoms of superficial and/or deep posterior exertional compartment syndrome may initially be posterior or posteromedial leg pain. However, the young athlete may report numbness spreading across the plantar surface of the foot as the first symptom.

It is often possible to reproduce anterior compartment syndrome symptoms in the office with repeated, resisted ankle dorsiflexion. While the examiner applies manual resistance, the athlete's ability to dorsiflex decreases within a minute or so, as the pain increases. The affected muscle compartment becomes taut and tender. First dorsal web space sensation may decrease. This can be a simple screening test for exertional compartment syndrome.

If definitive diagnosis is required, particularly if surgical compartment release is under consideration, formal compartmental pressure measurements should be performed. Often, the best test involves having the athlete perform the exacerbating activity and measuring the pressure immediately after activity stops. At least anterior and posterior/deep posterior pressures should be checked, as both may be elevated although the athlete only appreciates pain in one. Pressure measurements may be repeated 15 min later to monitor whether the pressure returns to normal range. Surgeons who studied 23 adolescents suggest using the following intracompartmental pressure (ICP) criteria for consideration of fasciotomy: baseline ICP (at rest) >10 mm Hg, >20 mm Hg 1 min after stopping exercise, >20 mm Hg 5 min later, and >15 min to achieve ICP normalization (4).

Although several theories have been published, the etiology of recurrent exertional compartment syndrome is not yet clear. Physicians who care for many young athletes with this condition have noted that it rarely occurs among athletes with gracile, slender builds. More commonly, these patients are mesomorphic, with well-developed, sturdy, and relatively bulky muscles (Figure 12.4). Female adolescent athletes seem much more likely to develop

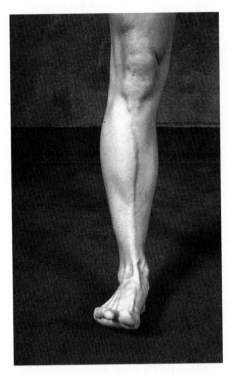

FIGURE 12.4. The muscular build of a young woman afflicted with bilateral recurrent exertional anterior compartment syndrome.

exertional compartment syndrome than their male peers. Although typically a problem of runners and jumpers, lower leg exertional compartment syndrome may even occur in swimmers.

An interesting observation is that some very muscular girls, especially those playing running sports such as soccer, field hockey, and lacrosse, seem more prone than other groups to suffer from both anterior exertional compartment syndrome and midshaft anterior tibial stress fracture. Both of these problems in this group seem more difficult to treat successfully than other athletes. It is also interesting that exertional compartment syndrome is almost unheard of among prepubertal children.

Early investigators of this problem surmised the pain was related to muscle ischemia, as the enlarging muscle pushed against its enveloping fascia to the extent that venous drainage, and then arterial inflow, were diminished. However, several studies using radionuclide bone scans or magnetic resonance imaging have not found ischemia, although one study did note improved perfusion of the compartment after compartment release in adults tested with thallium SPECT imaging (5). An ultrasound study of anterior tibial muscle "size" of adult chronic exertional compartment syndrome patients found that their muscle size increased 8% with an isometric exercise protocol, no different from the control group (6). The patients developed pain, but had no greater muscle volume increase, suggesting that the theory of excessively tight fascia surrounding the compartment may be flawed. The hypothesis that the pain is caused by ischemia has also been challenged by scintigraphic study (7,8) and magnetic resonance imaging (8) that show no perfusion difference. However, the magnetic resonance imaging (MRI) study did show that four of the five patients with both typical symptoms and elevated pressures took longer than those in the other groups for the blood flow to return to normal after exercise ceased (8).

An unusual cause of lower leg pain that mimics exertional compartment syndrome is an accessory soleus muscle (9). A painful muscular bulge distal to the normal soleus contour may be visible and palpable after activity such as running. Magnetic resonance imaging shows normal muscle. If the athlete cannot participate in activities because of the pain, surgical resection may be considered and typically leads to resolution of symptoms (9).

Plain x-rays are important to rule out other causes of lower leg pain. Routine MRI does not show findings specific for recurrent compartment syndrome.

Nonoperative treatment is generally unsuccessful unless the athlete decreases activity or changes sport. Stretching the antagonist muscle groups has been suggested but has not generally proved helpful. Altering footwear, using customized shoe inserts, or changing technique may provide relief.

Stress Fracture/Stress Reaction

Growing children and adolescents undergo remarkable changes in the tibia and fibula, especially if they participate in sports at an intense level. Each long bone must lengthen, widen, and nearly constantly remodel its shape. The growing bone adapts to the forces applied to it. Bone generally adapts effectively to these loads. However, if too large a force is applied too frequently, new bone formation and remodeling cannot match the level of recurrent stress and microscopic injury, and stress reaction or stress fracture occurs.

A study of 11–17 year old girls, part of a longitudinal health study carried out by written questionnaire, found that girls who participated in moderate to vigorous activity 16 or more hours per week were almost twice as likely to sustain stress fractures as girls who did less than 4h per week of moderate to vigorous activity. Of 5,461 girls, approximately 3% reported having sustained a stress fracture. Each hour per week of high impact activity increased the chances of stress fracture (10). These findings must be interpreted with caution, however. The girls' mothers were questioned only once about whether the daughter had ever had a stress fracture, and stress fracture was not further defined. In addition to the validity issues related to a study based on recall, over 2% of the 11- and 12-yr-old girls were reported as having had stress fractures. This finding suggests either a methodological flaw or that the mothers considered calcaneal apophysitis or other similar common injuries to be stress fractures. No other study has found such a high incidence of stress fractures among a similar group of preteen girls.

The young athlete may experience soft tissue symptoms related to a new or increased activity. If appropriate action to decrease the loading is not taken, the soft tissues may fail, followed by bony failure, resulting in a stress fracture. For example, among figure skaters in a longitudinal injury study, we found several instances of posterior tibial tendonitis followed a week or two later by distal medial tibial stress reaction or stress fracture, and others of peroneal tenderness soon followed by fibular fracture (11). As a result of this finding, we began treating these skaters' tendon injuries earlier and more aggressively with rest and protection before development of a stress fracture, followed by altering the biomechanics of the boot/leg interface and their skating technique as appropriate.

The typical history of a young athlete with a lower leg stress fracture is increasing, focal pain made worse with activity. In the early stages (stress reaction), the pain resolves within minutes after stopping the aggravating activity. In later stages, when a stress fracture is apparent by imaging techniques, aching or throbbing pain may still be present even the morning after the aggravating activity. However, lower leg stress fractures may be asymptomatic, found serendipitously (usually healed) on imaging studies done for symptoms at another site. There is often a logical reason for the stress fracture, such as significant training error as discussed earlier. Nutritional and menstrual history may include significant abnormalities.

Physical findings include focal tenderness and palpable deep swelling or callus. The location of the injury may be related to the sport equipment. For ballet dancers, fibular stress fractures occur at the level of transversely tied ribbons, and for skaters this level is near the boot top. Although equipment has been implicated in these fibular stress fractures, they also tend to occur at this level in other running or jumping athletes who wear low-top shoes or are barefoot.

On plain x-ray, a stress fracture can be diagnosed if an actual fracture line is apparent or if periosteal new bone has formed (Figures 12.5 and 12.6). These x-ray findings rarely appear sooner than 10–14 d after onset of symptoms. Radionuclide bone scan or MRI may show evidence of a stress fracture only a few days after the onset of symptoms. There is often inconsistency among radiologists in the diagnosis of stress fracture. Using bone scans, Jones and his colleagues considered four grades of stress injury, based on what percentage of the cross-sectional area of the bone showed increased uptake (12). An MRI classification of stress fractures is also available (13). One useful criterion for enhancing consistency is to define stress reaction as incomplete stress fracture, with fewer disrupted trabeculae across only a portion of the bone diameter. In contrast, a stress fracture either has a fracture line clearly visible on plain x-ray, MRI, or computed tomography (CT), or a bone scan shows significantly increased uptake

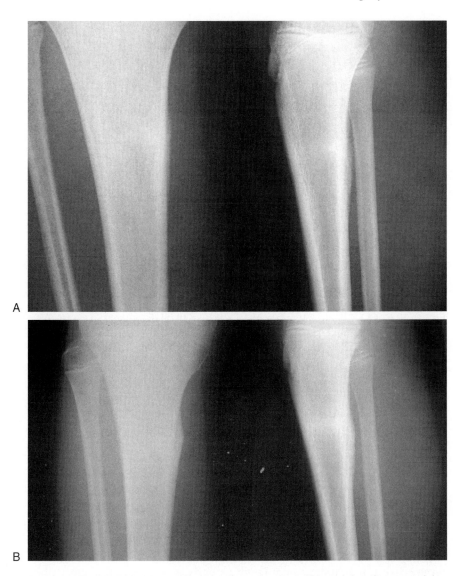

FIGURE 12.5. **(A)** This 14-yr-old soccer player increased his training time, practicing corner kicks repeatedly, kicking the ball with the medial foot. One month later, he had persistent pain in the upper medial shin. Anteroposterior and lateral plain films show periosteal new bone formation just distal to the metaphyseal–diaphyseal junction of the tibia. **(B)** One month later, he was asymptomatic, with mature healing callus on AP and lateral x-rays.

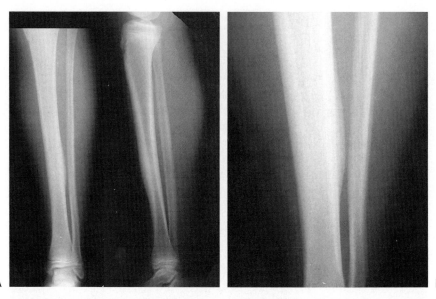

A   B

FIGURE 12.6. **(A)** AP and lateral x-rays of a healed tibial diaphyseal stress fracture, showing markedly thickened cortex. **(B)** Magnified view of the AP x-ray.

through most or all of the cross-section of a long bone. Recent information suggests that if plain x-rays are negative, the most sensitive and accurate study to diagnose a tibial stress fracture is an MRI (14).

Nonoperative treatment of lower leg stress fracture is usually successful. The athlete's first goal should be to become pain-free as rapidly as possible. If the athlete has reported the injury after only a few days of pain, the problem is likely stress reaction, and a few days of rest from the specific, aggravating activities may be all that is needed to regain pain-free status. More prolonged symptoms typically require immobilization. Removable devices are used if possible to allow maintenance of range of motion and easy, frequent examination by the athlete and medical personnel, so that progressive rehabilitation may begin as early as possible. For most tibial stress fractures, a well-fitted removable walking boot is effective. For fibular stress fractures at or distal to the midshaft level (as almost all are), a long air stirrup brace that extends proximally, almost to the knee, is effective in treating the fracture, while allowing normal ankle motion. This decreases muscle atrophy compared with a completely immobilizing device.

The second treatment phase includes strengthening and flexibility exercises. The athlete must remain pain-free during both the therapeutic exercise program and the progressive resumption of sport activity.

The use of adjunct bone stimulation, either electrical stimulation or low-dose pulsed ultrasound, may occasionally be considered when even a slight decrease in healing time is critical to the athlete. Given the variability of lower leg stress fractures, carefully controlled studies of bone stimulator efficacy in treating them are unlikely in the near future. Because adolescent athletes' stress fractures generally heal rapidly, and little is known about the effectiveness of bone stimulation among growing children, the expense of stimulators is generally not warranted.

One exception is the established "black line" stress fracture of the anterior tibia. Even prolonged cast immobilization may not lead to complete healing. Tibial reaming with internal fixation has been shown to be effective, typically allowing the athlete to return to running and jumping in 2 mo or less (15). Before embarking on surgical treatment, electrical stimulation or pulsed ultrasound treatment may be considered.

Posteromedial Tibial Stress Syndrome

Activity-related pain and tenderness along much of the posteromedial border of the tibia is known by several names, including "shin splints" and periostitis. Given the anatomic location of the physical findings and the diffusely increased uptake seen on radionuclide bone scan, posteromedial tibial stress syndrome is a reasonable, descriptive name for this entity. In addition to the findings along the bone, there may be associated tenderness and swelling of the posterior tibial tendon and possibly even a painful accessory navicular. The differential diagnosis includes the much less common deep posterior compartment syndrome. Both may coexist.

Development of this syndrome most often seems related to excessive hindfoot pronation. Decreasing the pronation by improving calf flexibility, strengthening the foot and ankle, and changing shoes or their insole configuration (with or without orthotics) often markedly improves the posteromedial symptoms.

Plain x-ray is recommended to check for stress fracture, neoplasm, and infection. Radionuclide bone scan may further rule out more concerning diagnoses. The scan typically shows moderately increased uptake localized to the posteromedial border of a long portion of the distal and often even the central tibia (Figure 12.7).

The first step of treatment is careful exploration of the history of the injury to attempt to learn what changed (training error, footwear change, technique change, etc.). These factors are addressed before recommending additional changes. Further treatment recommendations include correcting abnormal gait mechanics, if present. Inadequate calf muscle flexibility causing excessive hindfoot valgus in gait is often related to rapid growth in adolescence. It can usually be reversed rapidly with calf stretching for a few minutes daily. Athletes who perform barefoot may need to strengthen the intrinsic muscles of their feet to stop the arch collapse of a flexible flat foot. Athletes who perform in shoes often return to activity more quickly simply by choosing more appropriate athletic shoes for their foot type or adding

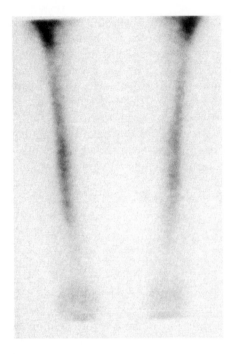

FIGURE 12.7. Diffusely increased uptake of Tc99 along nearly the entire medial border of the tibia is consistent with posteromedial tibial stress syndrome.

over-the-counter or custom arch supports. The entire lower extremity kinetic chain should be addressed, correcting poor mechanics of coupled motions, including internal hip rotation, knee valgus, and subtalar joint eversion.

Tendon Injury

There are no studies of children and young adolescents that indicate whether tendon injuries are tendinitis or tendinosis. The physical findings of tendon tenderness, bogginess, and peritendinous swelling often respond to treatment within days, suggesting the pathology is inflammation rather than significant structural change. The Achilles is involved much more frequently than the other lower leg tendons in this age group. Symptoms are often bilateral, so unilateral symptoms may prompt a more complete diagnostic work-up. Plain x-rays of the tibia/fibula, ankle and/or foot as indicated by symptoms and physical findings, are appropriate to rule out underlying bone abnormality. Nontraumatic tendon injuries of children and adolescents are generally short-lived, and further imaging such as ultrasound or MRI is rarely indicated.

Achilles

Among children and adolescents, Achilles tendon symptoms are often associated with either excessively tight or hypermobile calf muscles and heel cords. Passive ankle dorsiflexion with the knee extended and the hindfoot held in varus is usually less than 10 degrees. Paradoxically, some athletes, particularly gymnasts and dancers, have excessive ankle dorsiflexion (greater than 20 degrees). The athlete's foot configuration is often cavus, suggesting that poor shock absorption plays a role. Symptoms are related to sudden impact or force such as jumping and landing. Careful observation of the young jumping athlete with Achilles pain may show excessively abrupt and explosive plantarflexion isolated to the ankle, rather than jumping by working through the feet, then the ankles, then the knees, and on up through the kinetic chain. Similarly, landings may be poorly cushioned.

Diagnostic findings include focal tenderness and swelling. The tenderness often tracks along the broad musculotendinous junction, well into the calf.

Initial treatment is a heel lift to decrease tension on the tendon. Girls often find it easy to wear 1-inch heels, even in the house. Some young athletes feel relief with a counterforce brace or strap. Patients with severe or prolonged symptoms may need a walking boot, wearing it full-time initially and weaning out of it as symptoms improve. Unless the injury is of short duration, caused by obvious training error or direct tendon compression by equipment, more comprehensive treatment is usually needed, including correcting flexibility deficits, jumping and landing biomechanics, and foot intrinsic muscle strength.

Peroneal

Nonacute peroneal tendon injury may be related to a previous acute injury such as peroneal strain or ankle sprain. It may result from direct pressure from sport equipment. Less frequently, a young athlete with a cavus foot configuration and relatively inflexible calf muscles may chronically walk, run, and jump with hindfoot varus and develop recurrent microtraumatic injury of the peroneal tendons.

The diagnosis of peroneal tendon injury is made by physical findings of focal tenderness and swelling, and often pain with resisted eversion of the foot. The treatment includes removing any obvious causes of the injury. Therapeutic exercises include evertor strengthening and calf stretching. Occasionally, bracing is useful to decrease subtalar joint inversion. It is important to correct any faulty landing biomechanics that persist after strength is normalized.

Flexor Hallucis Longus

Flexor hallucis longus tendon injury of adolescents occurs mainly among ballet dancers and Irish dancers. Rarely, athletes in running sports may develop the problem. Injury may be related to an atypically long muscle belly that is pulled into the flexor retinaculum. The diagnosis is made by finding focal pain and swelling along the course of the tendon. There is typically pain with resisted active great toe plantarflexion, tested with the ankle both in neutral and in full plantarflexion.

Initial treatment, particularly for the young dancer, consists of correcting any faulty technique and strengthening the foot's intrinsic muscles. An in-shoe rigid or semirigid splint can decrease dorsiflexion and provide some relief, particularly for runners. Persistent symptoms in adolescents generally respond to immobilization in a walking boot. For very persistent pain and swelling, surgical release of the tendon sheath is recommended (16,17).

Ankle and Toe Dorsiflexors at the Distal Tibia

Painful swelling of the ankle and toe dorsiflexor tendons is usually caused by pressure from sports equipment, such as skating or snowboard boots. Symptoms may be initiated by a contusion. Tenosynovitis in this region may cause a surprising amount of swelling with fluctuance that must be differentiated from an abscess (Figure 12.8). Recommended treatment is to operate on the equipment, not the athlete.

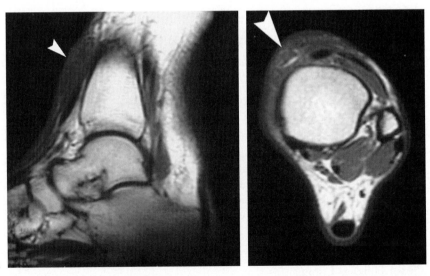

A   B

FIGURE 12.8. **(A)** A young figure skater developed painful swelling of the anterior tibial tendon sheathe, infected with staphylococcus. **(B)** The axial MRI view shows abnormal signal of the tendon itself, surrounded by excessive fluid and adjacent synovial and subcutaneous edema.

Other Causes of Lower Leg Pain

Osteoid Osteoma

Osteoid osteomas are benign tumors that have a predilection for the mid-shaft tibia region. The hallmark thickening of the surrounding cortex can mimic normal stress adaptation or a stress fracture. Possible tip-offs of osteoid osteoma include night pain that may awaken the athlete, and pain relief by nonsteroidal antiinflammatory drugs or aspirin.

Ewing's Sarcoma

The lower leg is not an unusual location for this malignant neoplasm. The history may mimic that of a typical stress fracture. Tip-offs include unilateral symptoms, aching that is incompletely relieved with rest, and circumferential swelling than seems to involve bone and deep soft tissue on palpation. Plain x-rays early in the course of the disease may show only slight periosteal new bone formation that may also mimic stress fracture. The onionskin pattern of periosteal new bone is a classic x-ray finding of Ewing's sarcoma of a long bone and should not be confused with a stress fracture.

Brodie's Abscess

The history of lower leg pain can be similar for slowly developing stress fracture, malignant or benign neoplasm, and the subacute bone infection known as Brodie's abscess. Thickened subcutaneous tissue that may appear somewhat discolored, with brawny edema, may suggest Brodie's abscess.

Osteogenesis Imperfecta or Other Metabolic Bone Disease

Bilateral, multilevel, or recurrent stress fractures should raise the suspicion of osteogenesis imperfecta, malnutrition (as in the female athlete triad), or other metabolic bone disease. Possible tip-offs of osteogenesis imperfecta include positive family history, blue sclera, and a parent with poor dentition or a hearing aid.

Reflex Sympathetic Dystrophy

Even prepubertal children may present with lower leg pain that is out of proportion to the history and the objective physical findings. They report pain that became much more severe days to weeks after a relatively minor injury, such as a contusion or twisted ankle. Even the touch of socks or bedclothes may cause severe pain and dysesthesia. The gait ranges from antalgic to bizarre, not typical of any of the usual, traumatic injuries seen in this age group.

Very early in the course of this disorder, the skin of the entire lower leg and foot can appear reddish-purple, and later significant muscle atrophy may be accompanied by color and temperature change and clammy skin. As soon as atypical skin color is noted, especially if tenderness is multifocal and does not seem to "fit" with likely mechanisms of injury, regular therapeutic exercise monitored closely by a knowledgeable physical therapist should be initiated, and the child should be checked more frequently than for the usual injury. Protection with a removable walking boot and crutches is often necessary. Cast immobilization should be avoided if there is no clear evidence of fracture that requires it. If symptoms do not respond quickly, a pain management team, including psychological counseling, may be necessary.

Management of Difficult Lower Leg Injuries

A multidisciplinary team approach is preferred when the diagnosis is difficult or unclear, or when psychosocial issues seem predominant or significant. The team may consist of the young athlete's primary physician, orthopedist and/or physiatrist, rheumatologist, physical therapist, certified athletic trainer, pain management specialist, psychologist, psychiatrist, nurse and nutritionist, depending on the patient's needs. All should interact with both the athlete and the family. The coach is a critical component. In general, even if the athlete and family have given the health care team written permission to speak directly with the coach, it's best to have a parent also involved in those discussions. The management of lower leg injuries is presented in Table 12.2 and the physical therapy prescription for lower leg injury is presented in Table 12.3.

TABLE 12.2. Management of lower leg injuries.

1. Determine why the injury happened. If symptoms are only unilateral, determine why.
2. Eliminate or change causative factors.
3. Decrease inflammation and pain; become pain-free as soon as possible, and then gradually increase activity while remaining pain-free.
4. Immobilize, use crutches as needed; rapidly decrease immobilization as healing allows.
5. Participate only with specific restrictions.
6. Rehabilitate completely.

TABLE 12.3. Physical therapy prescription for lower leg injury.

A. Typically includes
1. Active rest: do all parts of the sport and conditioning that don't aggravate the injury.
2. Correct lower extremity flexibility deficits.
3. Restore strength to normal.
4. Restore/improve proprioception and balance.
5. Modalities, taping, bracing, orthoses if indicated.

B. Pressure disorders (tendon injury, stress reaction of bone)
1. Pad or relieve tender area.
2. Alter equipment.
3. Ice massage; partial rest.

C. Adjunct nonoperative treatments
1. Ice.
2. Compressive bandage for swelling.
3. Nonsteroidal antiinflammatory drugs.
4. Brace.
5. Corticosteroid injection rarely indicated in this population.
6. Orthotic shoe inserts for angular or severe rotational malalignment, or abnormal foot biomechanics.
7. Improve footwear shock absorption.
8. Operate on the problematic equipment, not the athlete.

Prevention

Preventing lower leg injuries related to recurrent microtrauma involves the same principles as treating those injuries. Injury prevention principles include careful preparation of the young athlete to develop sufficient strength, flexibility, and endurance to meet the requirements of the sport. The athlete should gradually and progressively advance the time spent doing repetitive sport maneuvers, learning new skills at a safe rate that allows not only sufficient motor learning but also tissue adaptation.

Return to Play Guidelines

Young athletes would like a crystal ball prognosis, with specific healing times for each injury. Although such predictions can be rather accurate with most typical, acute fractures, sports injuries resulting from microtrauma are much more varied. The athletes usually understand functional goals, however.

For most injuries, the first goal is to become pain-free. With almost all lower leg injuries, as soon as the athlete is pain-free, progressively increasing rehabilitation activity may begin.

After any immobilizing devices have been discontinued, the athlete may require a protective brace, pad, or other device. Participation in conditioning or sports activity is allowed as long as:

1. The athlete does not limp.
2. Any pain that occurs during the activity is mild (no more than 2/10 on a pain scale) and resolves rapidly after stopping activity.
3. No medication or modalities are used to mask pain.
4. The athlete is able to advance in the therapeutic exercise program effectively and efficiently.

Clinical Pearls

- Lower leg injuries resulting from macrotrauma and from repeated microtrauma occur even in child athletes.
- The symptom of lower leg pain, particularly when unilateral, must prompt consideration of diagnoses such as benign or malignant neoplasm, acute or chronic infection, and metabolic bone disease.
- For young athletes, immobilization should be minimized when safely possible.
- Treatment includes full rehabilitation to normal or near normal strength, flexibility, balance, coordination, quickness, and endurance. "Normal" for a dedicated young athlete means equivalent to the uninjured side, or at the level required for the sport.

References

1. Edwards PH, Jr., Wright ML, Hartman JF. A practical approach for the differential diagnosis of chronic leg pain in the athlete. Am J Sports Med 2005;33:1241–1249.
2. Hislop M, Tierney P, Murray P, O'Brien M, Mahony N. Chronic exertional compartment syndrome: the controversial "fifth" compartment of the leg. Am J Sports Med 2003;31:770–776.
3. Eidelman M, Nachtigal A, Katzman A, Bialik V. Acute rupture of achilles tendon in a 7-year-old girl. J Pediatr Orthop B 2004;13:32–33.
4. Garcia-Mata S, Hidalgo-Ovejero A, Martinez-Grande M. Chronic exertional compartment syndrome of the legs in adolescents. J Pediatr Orthop 2001;21: 328–334.
5. Takebayashi S, Takazawa H, Sasaki R, Miki H, Soh R, Nishimura J. Chronic exertional compartment syndrome in lower legs: localization and follow-up with thallium-201 SPECT imaging. J Nucl Med 1997;38:972–976.
6. Birtles DB, Minden D, Wickes SJ, et al. Chronic exertional compartment syndrome: muscle changes with isometric exercise. Med Sci Sports Exerc 2002;34:1900–1906.

7. Trease L, van Every B, Bennell K, et al. A prospective blinded evaluation of exercise thallium-201 SPET in patients with suspected chronic exertional compartment syndrome of the leg. Eur J Nucl Med 2001;28:688–695.

8. Amendola A, Rorabeck CH, Vellett D, Vezina W, Rutt B, Nott L. The use of magnetic resonance imaging in exertional compartment syndromes. Am J Sports Med 1990;18:29–34.

9. Kouvalchouk JF, Lecocq J, Parier J, Fischer M. [The accessory soleus muscle: a report of 21 cases and a review of the literature]. Rev Chir Orthop Reparatrice Appar Mot 2005;91:232–238.

10. Loud KJ, Gordon CM, Micheli LJ, Field AE. Correlates of stress fractures among preadolescent and adolescent girls. Pediatrics 2005;115:e399–e406.

11. Smith AD. Reduction of injuries among elite figure skaters. A 4-year longitudinal study. Med Sci Sports Exerc 1991;23:151.

12. Jones BH, Harris JM, Vinh TN, Rubin C. Exercise-induced stress fractures and stress reactions of bone: epidemiology, etiology, and classification. Exerc Sport Sci Rev 1989;17:379–422.

13. Brukner P. Exercise-related lower leg pain: bone. Med Sci Sports Exerc 2000;32: S15–S26.

14. Gaeta M, Minutoli F, Scribano E, et al. CT and MR imaging findings in athletes with early tibial stress injuries: comparison with bone scintigraphy findings and emphasis on cortical abnormalities. Radiology 2005;235:553–561.

15. Varner KE, Younas SA, Lintner DM, Marymont JV. Chronic anterior midtibial stress fractures in athletes treated with reamed intramedullary nailing. Am J Sports Med 2005;33:1071–1076.

16. Kolettis GJ, Micheli LJ, Klein JD. Release of the flexor hallucis longus tendon in ballet dancers. J Bone Joint Surg Am 1996;78:1386–1390.

17. Teitz CC. Dance. In: Ireland ML, Nattiv A, eds. The Female Athlete. Philadelphia: Saunders; 2002:616.

13
Foot and Ankle Injuries

Angus M. McBryde, Jr., Mark D. Locke, and John P. Batson

Acute injuries of the ankle and nontraumatic injuries of the foot are common in the adolescent age group, particularly in running and jumping sports such as basketball, soccer, and volleyball. Although many injuries are diagnosed as sprains, skeletally immature athletes may sustain physeal injuries and growth-related injuries. To properly diagnose and manage ankle and foot injuries in growing athletes, physicians should be familiar with ankle and foot anatomy, the changes that occur with growth, and the injury patterns associated with stages of growth.

Anatomy

The ankle is an amazingly functional and durable joint (Figures 13.1–13.6). The bony anatomy is comprised of the tibia, talus, and fibula. These three bones articulate at the ankle joint and are stabilized by a number of ligaments and an interosseous syndesmosis. The tibia and fibula form a box-like mortise in which the talus rests (Figure 13.5, A and B). The tibia is the dominant weight-bearing bone in the lower leg. The medial malleolus is an extension of the tibia and provides medial bony support for the ankle mortise. The talus is wider anteriorly, providing more inherent bony stability with the ankle in dorsiflexion as opposed to plantarflexion (1). Movement at the ankle joint is primarily plantarflexion and dorsiflexion (2).

The deltoid ligament makes up the medial ankle ligamentous support (Figure 13.2). It consists of a deep layer, which runs from the medial malleolus to the talus, and a superficial layer, which originates on the medial malleolus and attaches to the medial aspect of the calcaneus. Anterior fibers attach to the talus and navicular and posterior fibers attach to the talus. The lateral ligament complex is comprised of the anterior talofibular ligament (ATFL), calcaneofibular ligament (CFL), and posterior talofibular ligament (PTFL) (Figure 13.3). The ATFL originates at the anterior aspect of the lateral malleolus and runs nearly parallel to the axis of the foot. It attaches to the talus anteriorly and is the primary ligamentous restraint to inversion stress at the ankle (3). It becomes taut with the ankle in slight plantarflexion. The ATFL is the most commonly injured ligament in the body (4). The CFL is stronger than the ATFL (4) and spans the tip of the lateral malleolus to the lateral surface of the calcaneus. The PTFL originates on the posterior tip of the lateral malleolus and attaches to the posterior talus. The high ligaments consist of the anterior inferior tibiofibular ligament, posterior inferior tibiofibular ligament, and interosseous syndesmosis.

The bones of the foot are divided into those of the hindfoot, midfoot, and forefoot (Figures 13.3 and 13.6, A–C). The talus and calcaneus make up the bones of the hindfoot (Figure 13.4). The calcaneus is the largest and strongest bone in the foot (5,6). It serves as the attachment for the Achilles tendon and as the origin of the plantar fascia. The talus and calcaneus have three articulations. This subtalar or talocalcaneal joint permits inversion and eversion of the foot (5,7). The bones of the midfoot include the cuboid, navicular, and three cuneiforms. The navicular is on the medial aspect of the foot and serves as the attachment for the posterior tibialis tendon. The forefoot is comprised of the metatarsals and their corresponding five phalanges. The great toe has a proximal and distal phalanx. The other four toes have proximal, middle, and distal phalanges. The sesamoids are two pea-sized bones in the substance of the flexor hallucis brevis tendons. They are positioned on the plantar aspect of the first metatarsalphalangeal (MTP) joint and function to increase the mechanical advantage of the flexor tendons, as well as to disperse forces with gait and stance (5,8).

Ligaments of note in the foot include the spring ligament and Lisfranc ligament (Figure 13.4). The spring, or calcaneonavicular, ligament has an important role in the stabilization of the medial arch of the foot (5,6). This ligament prevents talar head sag and medial migration commonly seen with flat foot deformity. The Lisfranc joint includes the five MTP joints and divides the foot into midfoot and forefoot. The Lisfranc, or tarsometatarsal (TMT) ligament, originates on the lateral aspect of the medial cuneiform and inserts on the medial aspect of the second metatarsal base dorsally and plantarly. This ligament is the main stabilizer of the Lisfranc complex.

Muscles of the foot and ankle can be divided into three compartments: the anterior, lateral, and posterior (6). The interosseous membrane and anterior crest of the tibia form the boundaries between these compartments (1,5). The extensor hallucis longus, extensor digitorum longus, and anterior tibialis make up the anterior compartment and primarily dorsiflex the ankle. The anterior tibialis attaches to the first cuneiform and metatarsal and inverts the foot. The lateral compartment is made up of the peroneus longus and brevis. The peroneal brevis attaches to the base of the 5th metatarsal. The longus crosses the sole of the foot to attach on the first cuneiform and base of the first metatarsal. The peroneals evert the foot. The posterior compartment has superficial and deep groups. The triceps surae is the superficial group

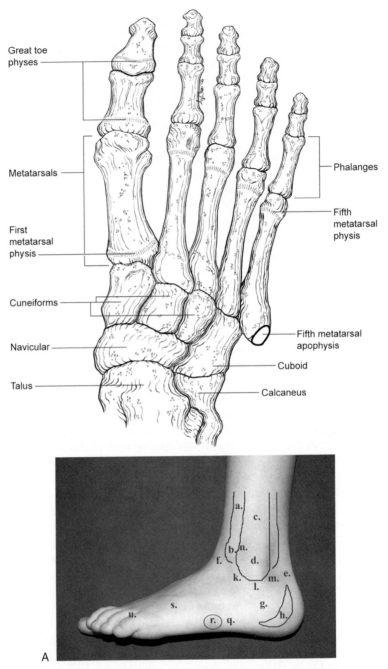

FIGURE 13.1. **(A–B)** External foot and ankle anatomy. a, tibia; b, tibia physis; c, fibula; d, fibula physis; e, Achilles tendon; f, talus; g, calcaneus; h, calcaneal apophysis; i, plantar fascia; j, deltoid ligament; k, ATFL; l, CFL; m, PTFL; n, anterior tibiofibular ligament; o, posterior tibialis tendon; p, medial navicular; q, peroneal tendon; r, 5th metatarsal apophysis; s, metatarsals; t, Lisfranc ligament; u, phalanges; v, sesamoids.

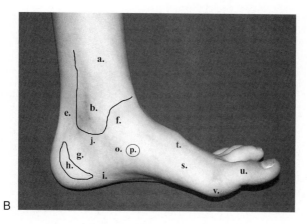

FIGURE 13.1. *Continued*

and includes the gastrocnemius, soleus, and plantaris (9). The deep compartment includes the flexor hallucis longus, flexor digitorum longus, and tibialis posterior muscles. These muscles function to plantar flex the ankle, flex the toes, and invert the foot. There are many intrinsic muscles of the foot analogous to the intrinsic muscles of the hand. The plantar fascia runs from the inferior aspect of the calcaneus to the forefoot. It has a role in support of the longitudinal arch of the foot (5).

Innervation of the lower leg, foot, and ankle is primarily supplied by the sciatic nerve (1,5). The common peroneal nerve innervates the dorsiflexors

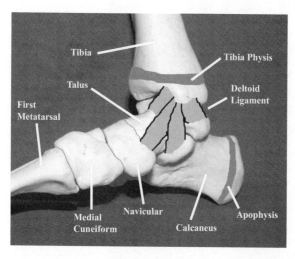

FIGURE 13.2. Medial foot and ankle bony anatomy.

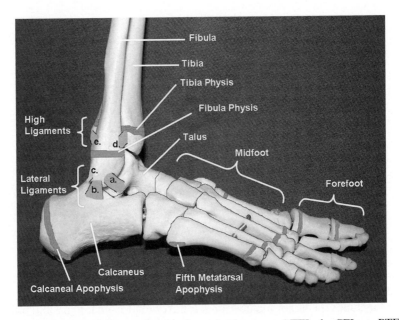

FIGURE 13.3. Lateral foot and ankle bony anatomy. a, ATFL; b, CFL; c, PTFL; d, anterior tibiofibular ligament; e, posterior tibiofibular ligament.

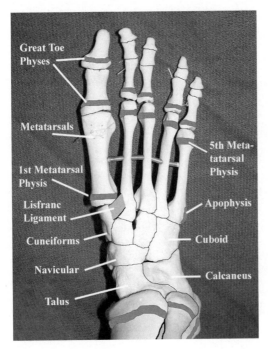

FIGURE 13.4 Dorsal foot and ankle anatomy.

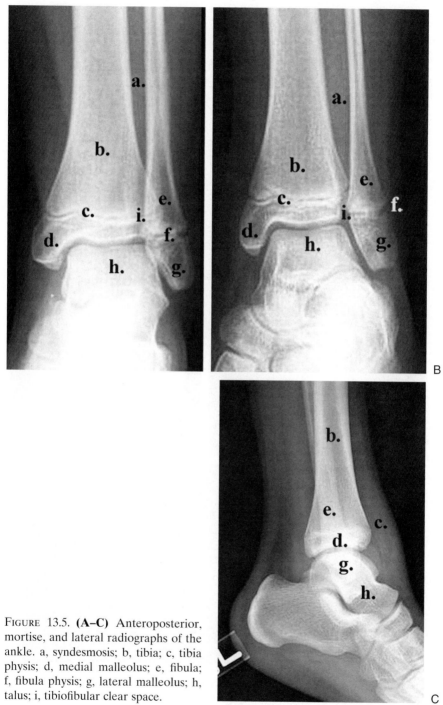

FIGURE 13.5. **(A–C)** Anteroposterior, mortise, and lateral radiographs of the ankle. a, syndesmosis; b, tibia; c, tibia physis; d, medial malleolus; e, fibula; f, fibula physis; g, lateral malleolus; h, talus; i, tibiofibular clear space.

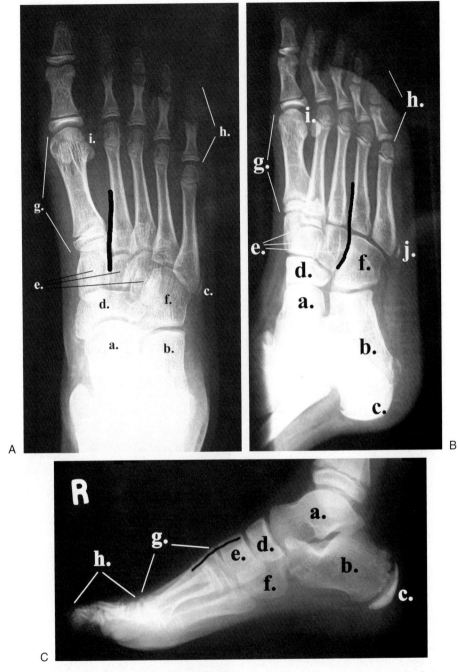

FIGURE 13.6. (**A–C**) Anteroposterior, oblique, and lateral radiographs of the foot.
a, talus; b, calcaneus; c, calcaneal physis; d, navicular; e, cuneiforms; f, cuboid;
g, metatarsals; h, phalanges; i, sesamoids; j, 5th metatarsal apophysis. The normal
relationship of the Lisfranc complex and mid foot is drawn in thick black line.

of the foot and ankle. The tibial nerve innervates the muscles of the posterior compartment of the leg and all of the intrinsic foot muscles except the extensor digitorum brevis (1). The superficial peroneal nerve innervates the peroneal muscles. The deep peroneal nerve innervates the muscles of the anterior compartment of the leg. Blood supply to the foot and ankle is derived from the popliteal artery's three branches (1,5). Venous drainage is primarily with the great saphenous vein. The majority of lymphatic flow follows the great saphenous vein to the inguinal nodes.

Clinical Evaluation

History

For acute injuries, the athlete should describe the mechanism of injury. Important information includes when the injury occurred, where it occurred, and if the athlete was able to ambulate off the field or court with or without assistance. Immediate swelling or bruising can be associated with both significant fractures and sprains. Athletes may remember hearing or feeling a "pop" or "snap" at the time of injury. A pain scale (i.e., 1–10, a pain of 1 being mild and 10 being extreme) can be utilized to describe the severity. Determining which phase of the gait cycle or what specific action causes pain is helpful. The examiner should ask if the athlete has had any prior injury to this or the opposite foot or ankle.

Chronic or overuse injuries require more questioning. A history of prior sprains or frequent injuries is helpful. Residual weakness or proprioceptive deficiency can be a potential cause of reinjury. Mechanical symptoms (snapping, clicking, or locking), or the presence of intermittent swelling can indicate conditions, such as osteochondral lesions and loose fragments in the ankle joint. Painful "snapping" or "popping" can be present with peroneal tendon subluxation. Has the athlete received any physical therapy or orthosis? Young athletes can present with conditions such as inflammatory arthritis, tumors, or infections. It is therefore important to ask about the presence of fevers, chills, weight loss, nighttime pain, rashes, as well as localized warmth or redness. Family history, such as juvenile idiopathic arthritis, tarsal coalition, or multijoint laxity, is important as well.

"Athlete" sensitive questions must be asked: What is his or her sport or position? What are the demands necessary to participate? Where is the athlete in terms of the season (beginning, middle, end)? Has there been a change in the athlete's training schedule in terms of intensity, duration, or lack of adequate rest and recovery? Is the athlete specializing in one sport and on multiple teams or simply involved in recreational activities? Which motions or movements (i.e., running, jumping, landing, or cutting) cause problems? Nutritional habits, such as hydration, overall calorie intake, and the intake of specific micronutrients (calcium, vitamin D, and other antioxidants), should be elicited, as they may play a role in the injury and the subsequent healing. Is there access to a certified athletic trainer? Is the child or adolescent an "elite" or "high demand" athlete? These young athletes and their parents will expect convenient access to care, expedient diagnosis, and rapid return to sports.

Physical Exam

The physical exam begins with a general overview of the patient in terms of development and body habitus. Body mass index, body composition, ligamentous laxity, and lower extremity alignment should be noted. Gait should also be assessed. An antalgic or "painful" gait is a gait in which the stance phase is shortened on the affected extremity. The athlete may walk "flat footed" to avoid motion at the ankle. Conversely, an ankle effusion is painful with dorsiflexion and can result in a forefoot gait. Furthermore, the athlete may "de-weight" the area of pain (i.e., in the case of a toe fracture, walking on the heel).

The foot and ankle is observed for obvious deformity, swelling, redness, or bruising. Ankle effusions are best visualized at the anterolateral aspect of the ankle. The normal hindfoot is in slight valgus when weight bearing and moves into varus with toe rise. When observing the foot from the posterior aspect, it is normal to see the 4th or 5th toe on the lateral side. Forefoot abduction can be appreciated by the "too many toes" (more than two toes present) sign.

In the nonacute setting, the athlete can attempt to walk on the toes, heels, and the lateral border of the foot. Passive and active range of motion at the ankle is approximately 10–15 degrees of dorsiflexion and 40 degrees of plantarflexion. A subtle clue to an ankle effusion is limitation or pain with passive range of motion. Subtalar motion is assessed by observing the heel move to varus with toe raise and the ability to walk on the lateral border of the foot. Subtalar motion can also be assessed by "rocking" the mid and forefoot in and out. Range of motion at the first MTP joint should be tested and compared to the opposite foot.

Immediately after an acute injury, swelling may be localized over the injured structures. With time and in the absence of ice, elevation, and compression, the swelling is often diffuse and landmarks obscured. The entire length of the tibia and fibula, the medial and lateral malleoli, and, in athletes with an immature skeleton, the tibial and fibular physes, should be palpated. Laterally, the ATFL, CFL, and PTFL, and medially, the deltoid ligament, are palpated. The anterior tibial–fibular ligament is assessed. Posteriorly, the gastrocnemius/soleus and Achilles complex are palpated. Snapping may be palpable over the lateral malleoli with peroneal subluxation when the foot is brought into dorsiflexion.

The crescent moon–shaped calcaneal physis is palpated at the superior Achilles attachment, inferiorly at the plantar fascia attachment, and centrally. The navicular bone is a helpful medial landmark. Each metatarsal should be isolated and palpated in their entirety. In the case of isolated foot trauma, particular attention should be paid to tenderness over the metatarsal growth centers. Styloid, metaphyseal–diaphyseal junction, and diaphyseal tenderness should be sought. Lastly, the MTP joints and each toe should be palpated.

Specialized tests include the anterior drawer test (Figure 13.7), which isolates injuries to the ATFL. It is performed by placing the ankle in slight plantar flexion. The tibia is stabilized with one hand and the other hand grasps the calcaneus. The calcaneus is pulled anteriorly. Excursion is assessed and compared to the opposite ankle. It is normal to have a small amount of forward excursion of the talus in the mortise (0–5 mm). The endpoint should be graded as soft or solid. A marked difference from side to side, soft endpoint, or pain with the maneuver can all indicate injury to the ATFL. The talar tilt test assesses the stability of the CFL and is performed by inverting the calcaneus with the ankle in neutral position (Figure 13.8). The test should be performed on the opposite ankle for comparison. A difference between the two can indicate an injury to the CFL. Various tests have been described for diagnosing "high" ankle sprains (injuries to the anterior tibiofibular ligament). The external rotation test is performed by stabilizing the lower leg in neutral with one hand and abducting the foot with the other hand (Figure 13.9). The squeeze test is performed by squeezing the proximal tibia and fibula together (Figure 13.10). Both tests are designed to stress the anterior tibiofibular ligament by widening the ankle mortise and are positive if the athlete experiences pain. The integrity of the Achilles tendon is assessed with the Thompson's test (Figure 13.11). In a prone or seated position, the calf is squeezed to mimic a muscle contraction. A negative test, in which the ankle passively moves into plantar flexion, is

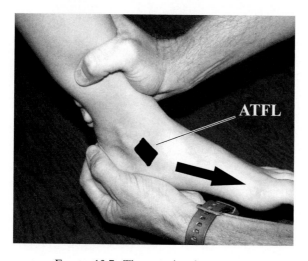

FIGURE 13.7. The anterior drawer test.

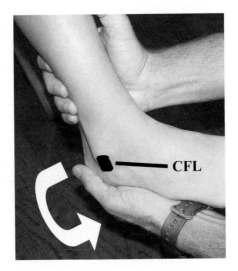

FIGURE 13.8. The calcaneal tilt test.

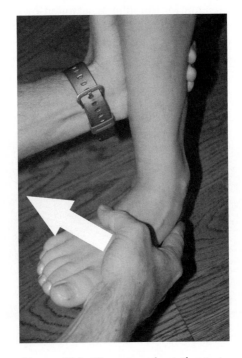

FIGURE 13.9. The external rotation test.

FIGURE 13.10. The squeeze test.

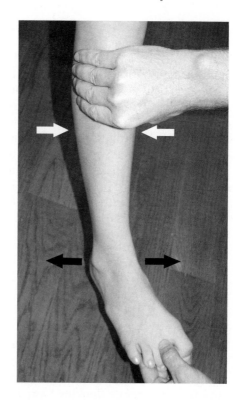

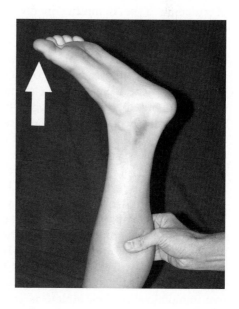

FIGURE 13.11. Thompson's test.

normal. A positive test occurs when the ankle does not move, indicating a nonfunctional Achilles tendon.

A complete exam of the foot and ankle includes a neurovascular and skin assessment. Abnormal tone involves tight hamstring or calf musculature. Pathologic tightness should be differentiated from the normal tight musculature accompanying young athletes during periods of growth. Ankle clonus can indicate an upper motor neuron abnormality. Deep tendon reflex asymmetry, differences in sensation to light touch, and strength differences should be recorded. Strength testing of the foot and ankle includes plantarflexion and dorsiflexion, as well as inversion and eversion against resistance. The vascular exam is important in the acute injury setting. Abrasions and lacerations may be present and necessitate care. Erythema may be present with injuries, infectious processes, and inflammatory conditions. Various rashes may be present with systemic conditions (i.e., psoriatic arthritis or juvenile idiopathic arthritis).

Acute Injuries

Ankle Fractures

Fractures of the ankle are very common in adolescent athletes (10–14). Physes are relatively weaker than adjacent ligaments. A good rule of thumb for members of the sports medicine team and primary care physicians is "rule out a fracture" before thinking "sprain" in athletes under 12–14 yr of age.

The Salter–Harris classification is the most commonly recognized and utilized classification system for fractures involving the physis (14,15). Type 1 injuries involve stress to the physis with or without radiographic evidence of widening. Type II injuries involve stress to the physis and a fracture exiting the metaphyseal region of the bone. In type III injuries, the fracture involves the growth center and the epiphyseal region of the bone. Type IV fractures involve both the metaphyseal region and the epiphysis. Type V injuries are crush injuries and are often only appreciated after growth arrest or deformity. The Salter–Harris classification is not only a way to describe the fracture but also provides prognostic value. Nondisplaced type I and II fractures typically do very well and rarely result in any growth disturbance or long-term problems. Type III and IV injuries involve the growth center and the articular surface. These injuries necessitate anatomic reduction and carry a high risk of growth disturbance (10,14).

Type I injuries to the distal fibula (Figure 13.12) are very common and typically occur in the same fashion as lateral ankle sprains. These are essentially clinical diagnoses with point tenderness over the distal fibular physis. A critical point to emphasize is the x-ray may or may not show any widening of the physis laterally. Type I and II Salter–Harris injuries to the distal fibula are typically treated with a short-leg cast or walking boot orthosis for 2–3 wk, and weight bearing is allowed as tolerated. After this period of relative immobilization, the athlete is given a more functional orthosis that

FIGURE 13.12. Salter–Harris type I fracture of the distal fibula with associated soft tissue swelling.

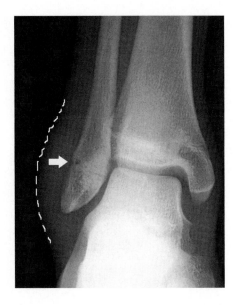

allows shoe wear and physical therapy. Type I injuries to the distal tibia are less common. Treatment is similar to lateral nondisplaced physis injuries. Because of the importance, the tibia plays in growth and weight bearing, Salter–Harris type II injuries (Figure 13.13) necessitate anatomic reduction and may require referral. More significant ankle fractures (Figure 13.14, A and B, and Figure 13.15) should be immobilized and referred to an orthopedic surgeon.

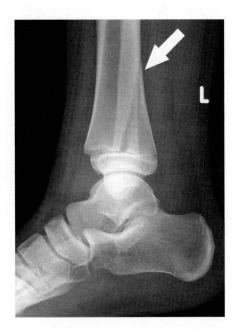

FIGURE 13.13. Salter–Harris type II fracture of the distal tibia.

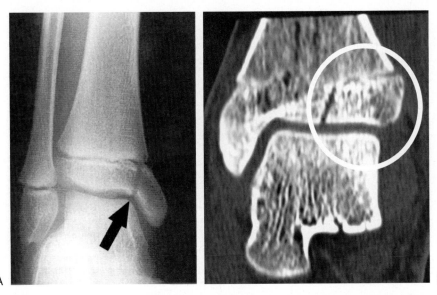

FIGURE 13.14. **(A)** Salter–Harris type III fracture of the distal tibia. **(B)** CT demonstrating a Salter–Harris type III fracture of the distal tibia.

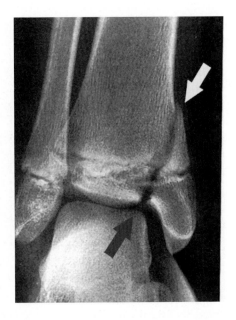

FIGURE 13.15. Salter–Harris type IV fracture of the distal tibia with displacement.

Ankle Sprains

Ankle sprains are the most common injury related to sports and recreation (3). Roughly 25,000 ankle sprains occur each day in the United States (16). Sports in which ankle sprains are common include basketball, football, soccer, and volleyball. Inversion-type injures to the lateral ligaments (ATFL, CFL, and PTFL) are most common (3,17). A "pop" may occur with the injury. The athlete may or may not be able to ambulate off the field. Swelling is primarily around and distal to the lateral malleolus. Bruising is present within the first few days and may dissect distally or proximally. The ATFL is the most common ligament involved, followed by the CFL, and the PTFL (3,4). The examiner should insure no injury has occurred to the medial structures, the anterior tibiofibular ligament, the tibiofibular syndesmosis, or the proximal fibula. Fifth metatarsal styloid fractures frequently accompany lateral ankle sprains. Stability testing (anterior drawer and calcaneal tilt tests) is often not helpful in the acute setting because of pain and guarding. Exam under anesthesia is the definitive measure for instability, but is not used in the acute setting.

Various grading scales have been described for ankle sprains. Injury to the ATFL is a grade 1 sprain, injury to the ATFL and CFL a grade 2 sprain, and injury to the ATFL, CFL, and PTFL a grade 3 sprain. A more predictive grading scale is based on the presence of pain and instability, where a grade 1 sprain is associated with pain and no instability, grade 2 with pain and slight instability, and grade 3 injury with both pain and instability. MRI findings may also allow grading based on the presence of edema or tears in the individual ligaments. The Ottawa Ankle rules (Table 13.1) were developed to help determine when radiographs of the foot or ankle are needed. Studies have shown them to have a near 100% sensitivity for detecting significant ankle and midfoot fractures (18,19). Although originally described for patients over the age of 18yr, these rules can be applied to young individuals as well (20).

TABLE 13.1. The Ottawa foot and ankle rules.

Radiographs of the foot and/or ankle are required if:
Pain or tenderness is present along the posterior edge or tip of either the lateral or medial malleolus.
Pain or tenderness at the base of the 5th metatarsal.
Pain or tenderness at the navicular.
The patient is unable to initially bear weight after the injury or take 4 consecutive steps in the office or emergency department.

Source: Reprinted with permission from Stiell IG, Greenberg GH, McKnight RD, et al. Decision rules for the use of radiography in acute ankle injuries. Refinement and prospective validation. JAMA 1993;269(9):1127–1132. Copyright ©1993, American Medical Association. All rights reserved.

In the acute setting, the ankle needs compression and splinting in the neutral position. This can be accomplished with a stirrup or posterior mold splint. At times, the athlete may be best managed in a well-molded and padded short-leg walking cast to allow ambulation without crutches. A walking boot orthotic may accomplish similar pain control and allow early physical therapy. Compression can help to reduce swelling. A horseshoe shaped soft felt pad can be placed around the lateral malleolus under taping or elastic stocking. Ice therapy helps with pain control and inflammation. Swelling requires elevation of the foot and ankle above the heart. Basic functional treatment with gentle range of motion, calf stretches, and isometric strength can begin in the subacute setting (21). Most athletes with ankle sprains can return to sports in a protective orthosis 1–2 wk after the injury. Reinjuries tend to progress more rapidly than initial injuries. The best evidence recommends aggressive physical therapy for all ankle sprains regardless of the grade, as surgery can always be performed if the athlete has problems with chronic pain or instability (3,17,22).

Two sprains deserve special mention. An injury to the deltoid ligament is not as common, and usually results from eversion/external rotation/abduction stress to the ankle (3,17). The deltoid ligament is stronger than the lateral ligaments. The ankle mortise also is more stable, from a bony standpoint, to resist eversion. Thus, a medial ankle injury generally indicates more significant trauma has occurred. The structures on the lateral aspect of the ankle may be injured and associated fractures may occur (3,17). Also, the force may extend to the syndesmosis and transmit out the proximal fibula, the so-called Maisonneuve fracture. The second injury, termed a "high" sprain, has been given more attention in recent years (23,24). This is an injury to the anterior tibiofibular ligament and proximal syndesmosis and can occur if the ankle is forced into dorsiflexion and external rotation. The squeeze test and external rotation test assess injury to the ligament and adjacent syndesmosis. With either a deltoid or high sprain, radiographs of the ankle should be obtained. Particular attention is given to the tibiofibular clear space, medial clear space, and fibular overlap (Figure 13.16) (17,22,25,26). Comparison films to the uninjured ankle may demonstrate subtle disruption of the mortise. MRI is a sensitive tool to confirm injury to the high ligaments and associated structures (24). Consideration should be given to refer suspected deltoid or high ankle sprains to a sports medicine specialist. With either injury, it is important to emphasize to the athlete a more significant sprain has occurred and it may take 6 wk or longer to rehabilitate. Athletes with disruption of the mortise or certain associated fractures often require open reduction with internal fixation.

Metatarsal Fractures

Metatarsal fractures are common injuries in the young foot. Potential mechanisms of injuries include falls from heights, axial load or twist

FIGURE 13.16. Normal mortise relationship. a–b, medial clear space; c–d, tibiofibular clear space; d–e, fibular overlap.

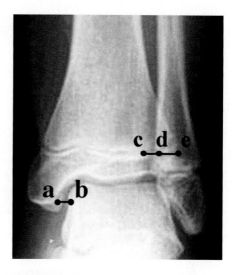

injuries to the foot, or when objects such as dumbbells or shot puts are dropped on the foot. In most cases, the athlete can pinpoint the exact location of pain. Radiograph evaluation includes an AP, lateral, and oblique view of the foot. In most cases, these injuries are treated in a wooden shoe or walking boot orthosis. An important concept is that lateral or medial displacement of the fracture is generally well tolerated and heals without consequence. Apex plantar or dorsal angulation, particularly in the metatarsal neck or heads, on the other hand, can cause future problems with shoe wear and minimal displacement or angulation is accepted. A short-leg cast with toe extension plate may be necessary for pain control in the first 1–2 wk. Weight bearing is allowed as tolerated. The fracture is generally treated a total of 4–6 wk. Some activities may be tolerated with the addition of a stiff last orthosis towards the terminal healing phase.

The fifth metatarsal bears special consideration. Middiaphyseal, neck, or head fractures are treated in a similar fashion as the aforementioned metatarsal fractures. Styloid avulsion fractures often occur with inversion injuries to the ankle. A forceful pull from the peroneal brevis tendon and/or the abductor digiti minimi, which attaches to the proximal fifth metatarsal, is thought to cause the injury (14). This fracture line in most cases runs perpendicular or oblique to the shaft of the bone (Figures 13.17 and 13.18). This is in contrast to the normal apophysis in younger athletes, which runs parallel to the metatarsal shaft (Figure 13.19). This growth center can be tender after an acute injury or with overuse. Styloid avulsion fractures are best demonstrated on the oblique or anteroposterior

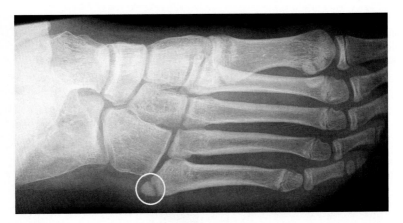

FIGURE 13.17. Fifth metatarsal styloid avulsion.

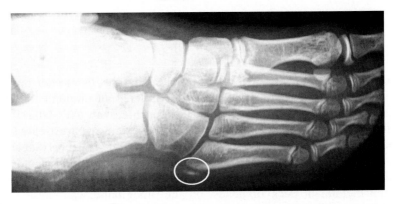

FIGURE 13.18. Lateral radiograph of the foot demonstrating the normal calcaneal apophysis (black thin arrow), unicameral bone cyst (white block arrow), an os trigonum (white circle), and a fifth metatarsal avulsion (black circle).

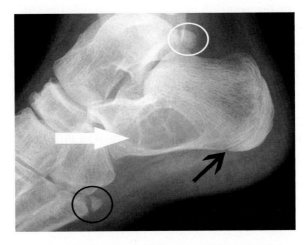

FIGURE 13.19. Normal 5th metatarsal apophysis.

Figure 13.20. Acute Jones fracture.

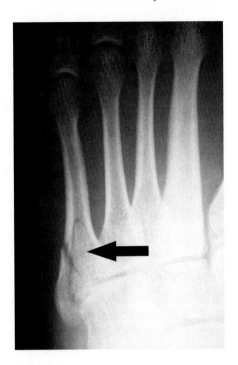

projection of the foot. These injuries are typically treated for 4–6wk in a wooden shoe, walking boot, or short-leg cast, and weight bearing is allowed. Occasionally, these fractures may go on to nonunion, but in most cases the athlete is symptom free and no long-term consequences are seen (27). Fractures that occur at the metaphyseal–diaphyseal junction (typically within 1.5cm of the tuberosity) are significant injuries (Figure 13.20). The blood supply to this area of the bone is reduced (27). These injuries (the so-called Jones fracture) often occur with an inversion and axial-load stress to the foot. Tenderness is localized distal to the styloid. The standard foot series of radiographs will confirm the fracture. These fractures require immobilization and non–weight bearing, often for 6–10wk, followed by weaning to a walking boot, provided some evidence of callous formation is present. This fracture may require a total of 12wk before advancing rehabilitation and return to sports participation. Even with compliant patients, healing may be protracted and may not occur at all. Patients committed to nonoperative management may benefit from a bone stimulator to promote healing. Recent literature favors the option of intramedullary screw placement at the time of diagnosis, with faster and more consistent healing, faster return to sport, and a lower incidence of reinjury (27–29). Refracture is a potential complication, even after intramedullary screw placement (30).

Toe Fractures

Toe fractures can occur when young athletes drop heavy items on the foot or when athletes accidentally kick a hard object. These injuries present with localized pain, swelling, and erythema. The radiograph is usually diagnostic, though in the young athlete each phalanx has a growth center, and subtle injuries may be difficult to visualize. Fortunately, most toe fractures and sprains heal without problems with simple immobilization with buddy taping and a stiff sole shoe or wooden shoe. The great toe is important for the gait cycle and balance. It therefore does require anatomic reduction and a walking boot or short leg cast with toe extension is recommended. Fractures of the distal phalanx associated with nail bed injuries are considered open fractures and require prophylactic antibiotics as well as close observation for signs of osteomyelitis (14).

Midfoot Sprains and Turf Toe

Midfoot sprains are uncommon in young athletes. These injuries involve the TMT joint, and are known as "Lisfranc sprains." Potential mechanisms include an axial load placed on the heel of a plantarflexed foot or forceful plantarflexion with a fixed forefoot, or forced abduction of the forefoot with a fixed hindfoot (10,31). The force is transmitted through the TMT joint. Such injuries have been described in football linemen, equestrian riders, and windsurfers (32,33). Tenderness is localized over the dorsum of the foot at the TMT joint. Abduction and pronation of the forefoot stress the complex and cause localized pain. Asking the individual to perform a toe raise is painful (17). Standing AP radiographs of the foot are needed. The normal relationship of the TMT complex is shown in Figure 13.6 (A–C). On the AP projection of the foot, a line drawn along the medial aspect of the second metatarsal should follow the lateral border of the medial cuneiform. On the oblique view of the foot, a line drawn down the medial border of the fourth metatarsal should line up with the medial border of the cuboid. The lateral radiograph also can demonstrate disruption of the Lisfranc ligament by showing a step-off between the metatarsal base and cuneiforms. A fracture of the proximal 2nd metatarsal should be evaluated closely for an associated Lisfranc sprain (27,34). For cases in which radiographs fail to demonstrate a suspected injury, CT is considered the best study. Bone scan and MRI have also been described as sensitive diagnostic tools (27,28,32–34). Midfoot sprains should be referred to a sports medicine specialist. Injuries without diastasis are typically treated in a short-leg cast, with weight bearing as tolerated, for 4–6 wk. Athletes with as little as 2 mm of diastasis or signs of instability require internal fixation (31,33,34). Late widening may occur, so symptoms and radiographs should be followed weekly.

Sprains of the first MTP joint are known as turf toe injuries. Usually, hyperdorsiflexion occurs with an injury to the conjoint plantar structures

(33,35). These injuries are common in football, soccer, wrestling, and dance. Artificial turf and flexible shoes have been implicated as risk factors (25). The athlete typically presents with pain localized to the first MTP joint. The pain is worse on the plantar aspect of the joint and exacerbated by dorsi-flexion of the joint. Radiographs may demonstrate a fracture or separation of the sesamoids. Typically, treatment involves immobilization of the MTP joint with a walking boot, wooden shoe, or stiff last insert. Physical therapy can reduce swelling, improve range of motion, and redevelop strength. Restrictive taping can help limit dorsiflexion of the joint and facilitate return to sport. The injury is often frustrating because of the extended healing time and inability to participate in sports.

Overuse Injuries and Chronic Pain

The Unstable Ankle

It is common to encounter the athlete with repeated ankle "sprains" or repeated episodes of their ankle "giving out." Associated injuries have been found in up to 64–77% of unstable ankles (3,35,36). Thus, every effort should be made by the examiner to diagnose any predisposing or associated conditions, such as tarsal coalition, peroneal tendon subluxation, peroneal tendonitis, impingement lesions, ankle synovitis, osteochondral pathology, as well as strength or proprioceptive deficits. Certain anatomic variants (i.e., cavus foot or hindfoot varus) have also been associated with unstable ankles (37). Joint laxity may be a result of previous injuries to the lateral ligament complex, but also can accompany medical conditions such as Down syndrome, Ehler–Danlos syndrome, and Marfan's syndrome. A flex-ible flat foot should not contribute to ankle instability unless accompanied by peroneal weakness or tendinopathy.

Anteroposterior, lateral, and mortise views of the ankle are warranted in the case of chronic pain or instability. Radiographs may reveal findings such as syndesmosis hypertrophic ossification, an osteochondral lesion, or intraarticular fragments. MRI can be helpful not only to visualize the liga-ments involved but also to rule out many associated conditions, such as tendinopathy, tendon tears, and osteochondral lesions. Any problems with the young athlete's foot should be evaluated accordingly.

The unstable ankle requires referral to a sport medicine specialist. Con-servative treatment of the unstable ankle includes physiotherapy to reduce edema, to limit range of motion, strengthen weak muscles, and improve proprioceptive deficits. Taping or bracing often allows monitored return to sports. The athlete with a weak and unstable ankle must obtain ade-quate strength and pass a functional return to sport protocol (Tables 13.2 and 13.3). Activities such as stationary biking or swimming can allow the athlete to stay physically active, while not stressing the ankle. Surgical

TABLE 13.2. Functional return to sport protocol.

1. Toe raises, both legs together: 1–3 sets, 15 repetitions
2. Toe raises, injured leg alone: 1–3 sets, 15 times each
3. Balance on the injured leg: 1–3 sets, 30 seconds in duration
4. Walk at fast pace: 1–3 times, 50 yards each
5. Jumping on both legs: 1–3 sets, 10 times each
6. Jumping on the injured leg: 1–3 sets, 10 times each
7. Easy pace straight line jog: 1–3 times, 50 yards
8. Sprint (half speed, quarter speed, and full speed): 1–3 times each, 50 yards each
9. Jog straight and gradual curves: 2–3 laps around field, court, or track

Cross-country, track, and running can gradually advance to desired distance at this point. More demanding sports (i.e., football, soccer, base and softball, tennis) need to advance to sport specific drills such as:

1. Run figure 8's (half speed, quarter speed, and full speed): 1–3 times each
2. Cross-overs-40 yards: 1–3 times to the right and left
3. Backward running (back peddling): 1–3 times, 40 yards each
4. Cutting (half speed, quarter speed, and full speed): 1–3 times
5. Sport-specific drills
6. Return to sport

Source: Reprinted from Kaft DE. Low back pain in the adolescent athlete. Pediatr Clin North Amer 2002:49(3):643–653. With permission from Elsevier.

indications include pain and instability despite 6–8 wk of dedicated physical therapy.

Osteochondritis Dissecans of the Talus

Osteochondritis dissecans (OCD) is a condition in which the articular cartilage and underlying subchondral bone is abnormal. The mean age of young athletes with an OCD lesion is 13–14 yr (14). The lesion is potentially unstable, and can separate from the body of the talus. These lesions most commonly involve the anterior-lateral or posterior-medial aspect of the talar dome (Figure 13.21) (14,17). Lateral lesions are most often the result of an acute traumatic event (13,25,38). Repetitive stress and vascular insults to the affected area are thought to be other potential causes. Chronic pain and intermittent swelling occur with OCD lesions. Detached bony or cartilaginous fragments may cause mechanical symptoms, such as locking, clicking, and catching.

The Berndt and Harty classification has been used to characterize OCD lesions and is based on the radiographic appearance (38–40). Their classification scheme describes stage I lesions as a small area of compression, stage II lesions as a separate fragment, stage III lesions as a detached but hinged fragment, and Stage IV lesions as completely detached fragments. MRI is a very sensitive and specific tool to detect OCD lesions, and it is commonly performed in suggestive cases with normal or inconclusive radiographs. In addition, MRI can help to better define the lesion's size, location,

TABLE 13.3. Specific protocol for 13-yr-old soccer player with grade 3 lateral ankle sprain.*

Goals for 3–5 Wk Postinjury
Protect healing tissue with controlled gradual stress
Minimize pain and inflammation
Retard muscle atrophy

3–4 wk
Walker boot
Progress to full weight bearing as soon as possible
Isometrics for peroneals and posttibial with limited inversion, but with Achilles stretching (elastic tubing, etc.), and home exercise program twice daily with trainer and/or therapist monitoring.
Hands-on massage and available modalities, i.e., heat, ice, ultrasound
Ongoing aerobic and closed chain work for well leg, trunk, upper body, i.e., quad and hamstring
Toe raises initially 80/20, well leg/injured leg.
Bicycle in boot

4–5 wk
Weight bearing to tolerance with taping and/or bracing except when individually monitored/hands on—only linear weight bearing
Bicycle progress to 30 a day
Increased strengthening as tolerated with inversion 75%
Mobilization protecting from stress/inversion/plantar flexion including subtalar joint
Seated (progressing to standing) balance on proprioceptive device initially blocking significant inversion and emphasizing eccentric phase in all arcs (especially peroneals)
Forward and then backward 50–75% maximal effort for 100 yards and advance if pain and limp are minimal

5–6 wk
Initiate stair climbing, controlled ankle inversion, progressive proprioceptive drills standing
Pool program good, but optional, and tape protection
Progressive linear running program with graduated agility and sport-specific moves and dribbling

Goals at 6 Wk
Full strength, power, and endurance
Monitored sports-specific activity
Easy and then advanced plyometrics
Vertical squats
Cutting activities, 45 and 90 degrees
Four corners drill
Taping and bracing for 3–4 mo with half speed, quarter speed, and full speed over 5–10 d
Return to play/sports-specific exercises, i.e., soccer, when goals are met
Full protected range of motion
Lateral moves, loaded twist 50%
Lunges/deceleration side and front
45 and 90 degree cuts
Figure 8's, backward running
Dribbling, crossovers, one-on-one half speed to full speed

*This protocol is used after 3 wk immobilization and 2 wk partial weight bearing with optional crutches, with gentle isometric bicycle in cast or boot and closed chain work on all muscle groups except the involved foot and ankle.

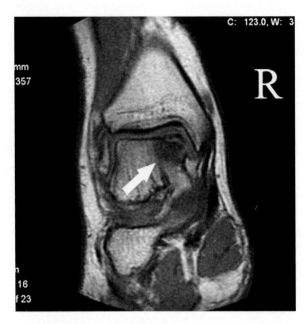

FIGURE 13.21. MRI demonstrating a medial talar osteochondral lesion.

and signs of instability such as a fluid interface between the lesion and healthy talus. Ankle arthroscopy can visualize, palpate, and grade the osteochondral defect (38,39). Grading scales based on MRI and arthroscopy findings have been proposed (41).

OCD lesions require referral to a sports medicine specialist. Skeletal immaturity is taken into consideration. Nonsurgical management is recommended for most skeletally immature athletes unless the fragment is detached (14,42). Rest and immobilization is also recommended for most stage I and II lesions and medial grade III lesions (38,39). This includes an initial period (4–6 wk) of non–weight bearing. Radiographs are repeated, and if the lesion continues to look stable and some evidence of healing is taking place the athlete is progressively advanced to protected weight bearing, as tolerated. Lateral grade III or grade IV lesions generally require operative management (38,39). Any free fragments are debrided. Drilling, microfracture, or curettage promote vascularization and healing (43). Internal fixation is considered with acute injuries and relatively large, unstable fragments (38,39). Lateral lesions generally have a better prognosis (25).

Tendonitis

Tendonitis produces pain to palpation and with active use or resisted movement of the muscle–tendon complex. These conditions in the foot and ankle are primarily overuse injuries.

Achilles tendonitis is common. It is frequent in sports, such as cross country running, track, basketball, soccer, and dance, especially in older adolescent elite athletes. Typically, the athlete has pain with activities such as toe raise, running, and jumping. The athlete usually presents with localized tenderness in the Achilles tendon. Resisted ankle plantarflexion and repeated single-leg toe raises may cause pain. The calf complex and hamstrings may have associated poor flexibility. Radiographs are not necessary. Treatment involves stretching, cryotherapy, and an antiinflammatory medication. Gel heel cups or a lift may reduce tendon stress. Steroid injections should be avoided because of the risk of tendon weakening and rupture. Older athletes are more prone to tears and tendinopathy, which often require longer and more intensive therapy.

Posterior tibialis tendonitis causes localized pain in the medial ankle or foot. There may be a recent history of an ankle sprain. The injury is common in any sport involving running, jumping, and repeated ankle plantarflexion. On physical exam, the athlete may have some localized swelling. Ankle range of motion is usually full. Tenderness is present in varying amounts from the navicular attachment to the medial malleolus, and it is proximal along the posterior medial distal tibia. Resisted ankle plantarflexion and inversion cause pain and may show weakness. A flat foot and/or an accessory navicular may be present. Radiographs are necessary if anatomic or structural abnormalities are present. Treatment involves immobilization with an ankle support, walking boot, or short leg cast. The athlete should wean to shoes with a supportive arch. An over-the-counter or custom foot orthotic can be helpful if supportive shoes are not adequate. Basic ankle therapy with an emphasis on calf stretches and strengthening the posterior tibialis should be initiated. Cryotherapy and antiinflammatory medications help as well. Chronic problems warrant referral for surgical considerations.

Peroneal tendonitis often follows a history of inversion-type sprains. A "popping" sensation may be described if the tendon is subluxing. Peroneal tendon subluxation may initiate after a forceful episode of extreme ankle dorsiflexion. This may also occur without trauma if the fibular groove is shallow. Resisted eversion of the foot and ankle cause pain, as does passive plantar flexion and inversion. Weakness may be present. Subluxation may be reproducible on physical exam by palpating the lateral malleolus and having the patient repeatedly plantarflex and dorsiflex the ankle. Radiographs of the foot and ankle should be obtained in cases of associated trauma or chronic pain. A lateral malleolus "rim" fracture is commonly seen in cases of acute peroneal subluxation (25). Treatment initially involves an ankle support. Therapy is directed at calf stretches and eversion strength. Proprioceptive work, eccentrics, cryotherapy, and other modalities are utilized. Persistent symptoms require surgical referral. Surgical options include tendinopathy resection with tubulization, split tendon repair/resection, or stabilization for instability.

Stress Fractures

Stress fractures (also known as "fatigue" fractures) occur when the stresses placed on the bone outweigh its ability to repair and remodel. Running oriented sports cause the majority of all stress fractures. These fractures occur in male and female athletes in equal numbers (44). The tibia, fibula, tarsals, and metatarsals are among the bones most often affected. Information regarding the athlete's training schedule should be obtained. Female athletes in particular with a stress fracture should be questioned about nutrition (adequate calories, calcium, and vitamin D) and their menstrual history. Athletes with recurrent stress fractures should be evaluated for conditions such as hyperthyroid and osteopenia. Biomechanical lower extremity alignment, leg length descrepancy, and other intrinsic risk factors, such as foot shape, have been associated with stress fractures (44,45). The pain with stress fractures is worse with physical activity and may occur at night. Radiographs may or may not demonstrate the fracture during the initial 3 wk. Bone scans can target early stress fractures. Most experts recommend MRI rather than bone scan to confirm the diagnosis because of its availability and specificity (44,46). Grading scales based on MRI findings have been proposed. The mainstay of treatment of stress fractures involves relative rest. Low-risk stress fractures (second metatarsal) rarely cause permanent problems. High-risk stress fractures (fifth metatarsal, navicular, and sesamoids) often require non–weight bearing treatment, and even then they may not heal sufficiently (17,47). Factors which may inhibit healing, such as tobacco, poor nutrition, and nonsteroidal antiinflammatory medications, should be discussed (48).

The second metatarsal is unique in its anatomic relationship and positioning with the tarsal bones. Motion is limited, which makes this bone prone to stress (9). Though less common, stress fractures can also occur at the 3rd and 4th metatarsal (Figure 13.22). These fractures have been described in military recruits and sports involving running and repetitive jumping. The patient is usually point tender over the fracture. Standard radiographs of the foot offer confirmation. Treatment consists of relative rest from the offending sport or activity. Activities that stimulate, but do not cause pain, are allowed. Patients may require a short-leg cast, walking boot, or crutches. These fractures are "low risk" for potential nonunion, and usually heal without permanent problems (9). The treatment time is approximately 6 wk before gradual return to sports is allowed. A semirigid orthosis with metatarsal pad may be a good transition from a walking boot orthosis. Transfer lesions with stress fracture progression across the foot must be avoided.

Stress fractures of the 5th metatarsal deserve special mention. These injuries typically occur at the metaphyseal–diaphyseal junction. It is well known, in contrast to other metatarsal stress fractures, that these injuries are prone to delayed healing, nonunion, reinjury, and chronic pain (47). These fractures are common in jumping-oriented sports, such as basketball, gymnastics, and dance. Athletes may present with the acute onset of an

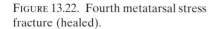
FIGURE 13.22. Fourth metatarsal stress
fracture (healed).

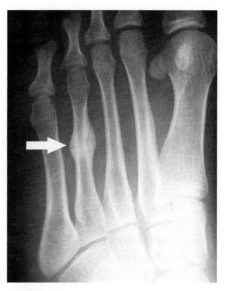

injury, but often recall intermittent and increasing pain present for weeks
prior. Tenderness is localized to the lateral border of the foot. Standard
radiographs of the foot usually confirm the diagnosis. Treatment for these
"high risk" stress fractures is controversial. Like acute Jones fractures to
this region, most experts recommend a period of 4–6 wk in a non–weight
bearing short leg cast. If evidence of healing is present on follow-up radiographs, the athlete is transitioned to a weight bearing cast for another 2–
4 wk. If clinical and radiographic evidence of healing is present, the athlete
is then placed in a walking boot and physical therapy is initiated. Return
to sports is gradually permitted at 10–12 wk. If after 6–8 wk of non–weight
bearing the fracture displays no evidence of radiographic healing, intramedullary screw placement may be warranted. A limited CT of the bone may
help to reveal the potential for healing. If nonsclerotic fracture margins are
present, a bone stimulator may be of benefit. If sclerotic margins are present,
the potential for nonoperative healing is low and surgery should be considered (44,47). Intramedullary screw placement with or without bone
grafting is recommended. Elite level athletes often undergo surgical fixation
with bone stimulation at the time of the diagnosis because of the potential
lengthy healing time.

Navicular stress fractures are another "high risk" fatigue fracture prone
to delayed healing and nonunion. As with proximal fifth metatarsal stress
fractures, these injuries are common in sports such as basketball and dance.
The athlete presents with increasing pain on the dorsum or medial aspect
of the foot. Tenderness is usually localized to the navicular "N" spot, or
medial aspect of the bone (44,47). The athlete is usually placed in a non–
weight bearing cast for 4–6 wk. If radiographic healing is present, the athlete

is advanced to a walking boot and begins physical therapy directed at calf flexibility and strength about the ankle. For cases not responding to non-operative treatment, fixation with bone grafting is considered (47).

Apophysitis

Apophysitis, or inflammation of the tendon attachment, can occur for a number of reasons. During periods of rapid growth, the physis is under stress, as there is a mismatch between the fast-growing bone and the increasingly taut musculo–tendon complex. It may be present with conditions such as juvenile idiopathic arthritis. These conditions are more common in boys and primarily a problem of the lower extremity. Athletes between the ages 8–12 yr are commonly affected.

Calcaneal apophysitis is known as Sever's disease. The calcaneal apophysis resembles a crescent moon wedged between the Achilles tendon and the plantar fascia. Young athletes often complain of pain in the heel or foot. The condition may be bilateral. The physical exam reveals tenderness at the superior and/or inferior pole of the posterior calcaneus. Other associated physical exam findings, such as elevated BMI, tight muscle–tendon complexes, and flat feet, should be noted. Occasionally, the tenderness may extend into the Achilles tendon. Radiographs are not necessary, but typically reveal the sclerotic and fragmented apophysis (Figures 13.18 and 13.23). Treatment includes rest from the activity that causes pain. Cryotherapy is

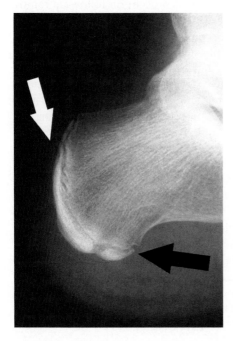

FIGURE 13.23. Normal calcaneal apophysis with attachment site of the Achilles tendon (white arrow) and origin of plantar fascia (black arrow) labeled.

helpful after physical activity. Stretching the hamstrings, calves, and foot should be done 3–4 times a day until adequate flexibility is obtained. Subsequently, the stretching should be performed at least once per day, ideally before and after physical activity. Heel cups or lifts shorten the distance from the calf to the heel, thus reducing traction stress. Shoes should be supportive in the arch and fitted appropriately. Excess body weight only adds more stress to the foot and should be avoided. Patients with continued pain warrant referral and radiographic evaluation to rule out bone cysts (Figure 13.18), tumors, and fractures. In a recent study utilizing MRI, Ogden et al. showed persistent cases resembled more of a metaphyseal stress fracture in the immature calcaneus rather than inflammation of the apophysis (49). These refractory cases required a casting protocol.

The proximal fifth metatarsal has an apophysis at the attachment of the peroneal brevis tendon. Inflammation of this apophysis is termed Islen's disease. The patient is point tender at the base of the fifth metatarsal and resisted eversion is painful. The apophysis is best visualized on the AP or oblique view of the foot (Figure 13.19). An important distinction is the apophysis runs parallel to the shaft of the diaphysis. In contrast, fractures tend to track perpendicular or oblique to the shaft of the fifth metatarsal. Treatment involves relative rest. Immobilization may be necessary with an ankle support orthosis, walking boot, or short-leg cast. Ice therapy and antiinflammatory medications also may be of benefit. Therapy is directed at calf and plantar fascia flexibility and strengthening of the peroneals. Narrow shoe wear should be avoided. The condition responds fairly quickly to treatment and rarely results in long-term pain or problems.

Anterior and Posterior Impingement

Anterior impingement refers to entrapment of anterior ankle joint structures with repetitive dorsiflexion. The condition occurs commonly in young elite level gymnasts and cheerleaders participating in repetitive high velocity tumbling. Landing "short" with tumbling and dismounts forces the ankle into maximal dorsiflexion. It has been reported in young dancers, football players, and soccer participants (43,50). The soft tissue structures that may become impinged and cause pain include the ankle synovium and/or capsule. This is usually medial or lateral and in the sulcus. Calcific deposits, spurring, and cartilage injury accrue on the tibia and talus and often precede the clinical impingement. The athlete presents with anterior ankle pain. Passive dorsiflexion reproduces the pain, and tenderness is localized. Weakness around the ankle may be appreciated, and heel cord tightness and ankle instability have been associated with the condition (43,50). A lateral projection of the ankle in maximal dorsiflexion may allow visualization of anterior talotibial bony impingement. Bony osteophytes may be present, and MRI can further visualize the inflamed structures. Treatment of the condition initially begins with avoiding the activities that exacerbate the pain, cryotherapy, and antiinflammatory medications. Gentle stretching of the heel cord and strengthening the ankle, especially plantarflexion, is recommended. A heel lift may be of benefit. Continued pain requires referral for consideration of arthroscopic debridement of the anterior soft tissue structures and any bony spurs.

Posterior ankle impingement refers to inflammation of the posterior ankle structures (bony and/or soft tissue) related to repetitive ankle plantar flexion. This is a common pain syndrome reported in young gymnasts, ballet dancers, ice skaters, and karate participants. Pain is localized to the posterior ankle. Passive and active ankle plantarflexion is painful, especially with inversion. A lateral radiograph of the ankle in extreme plantarflexion may demonstrate bony impingement. An os trigonum (Figure 13.18) may be present. MRI demonstrates the posterior soft tissue involvement or bony edema. Treatment involves relative rest, ice, antiinflammatory medications, and basic ankle therapy. An ankle support orthotic may assist by limiting plantar flexion. Chronic symptoms unresponsive to nonoperative measures undergo ankle arthroscopy and soft tissue debridement. Bony osteophytes or the os trigonum may be removed.

Sesamoiditis

Acute fractures of the sesamoids often have a preceding history of direct or indirect trauma. The sesamoids may also be subject to repetitive stress. Athletes present with the gradual onset of activity-related pain localized to the plantar surface of the 1st MTP joint. The examiner should localize the pain to the tibial or fibular sesamoid. Range of motion at the MTP is limited. Forefoot valgus, rigid pes cavus, and multipartite sesamoids have been associated with sesamoiditis. Radiographs of the sesamoids include a lateral, axial sesamoid, and medial oblique view. Radiographic interpretation can be challenging because up to 25% of the population has bipartite sesamoids. This finding is frequently bilateral and is more common in the tibial sesamoid (Figure 13.24). Bipartite fragments typically have smooth sclerotic margins. Irregular fragment margins may be visible with either acute fractures or stress fractures. Treatment of sesamoiditis involves relative rest and immobilization if necessary. A J-shaped pad may help to deweight the painful sesamoid. A stiff last can help by limiting motion at the MTP. The diagnosis of a sesamoid stress fracture should be considered in patients with continued pain. Bone scan or MRI may assist with this diagnosis. For patients with refractory symptoms, excision, partial excision, or bone grafting is performed, depending on the findings at surgery.

Reflex Sympathetic Dystrophy

Complex regional pain syndrome (CRPS), or reflex sympathetic dystrophy (RSD), is a medical condition involving chronic musculoskeletal pain, often with accompanying autonomic dysfunction. It is more common in females and the

FIGURE 13.24. Normal bipartite tibial
sesamoids.

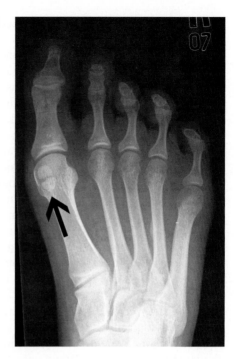

majority of cases involve the lower extremity, including the legs, ankles, or feet
(10). It typically follows a minor injury such as an ankle sprain or overuse syndrome. The pain is clearly out of proportion to the injury, and is often difficult to
localize. The child or adolescent appears tender "everywhere" around the
affected extremity. The individual may complain of "burning," "stinging," or
"tingling." The skin may show color changes, temperature differences, or abnormal sensation compared with the opposite side. The injury responds poorly to
typical treatment modalities. Social issues or psychological stressors may be
present. The evaluation must be exhaustive to rule out significant underlying
pathology or injury. A basic laboratory evaluation helps to exclude an inflammatory or infectious process. Treatment includes aggressive physical therapy, cognitive behavior therapy, and, occasionally, medications such as antidepressants.
Immobilization and inactivity make the condition worse. Antiinflammatory
medications may be used initially as one would prescribe for the initial injury.
The child is encouraged to participate fully in expected school activities. Children
typically recover from the condition, but recurrence may occur.

Developmental and Related Conditions

Osteochondroses

Osteochondroses are disorders unique to the maturing skeleton. These
conditions are thought to be caused by repetitive stress and disruption to
the vascular supply of the bone (51).

Kohler's disease of the tarsal navicular is more common in males and affects children between 4–6 yr of age (42,51). The child presents with the insidious onset of midfoot pain. Tenderness is localized to the medial aspect of the foot and most pronounced over the navicular bone. Gait is often antalgic and toe raises are painful. Basic radiographs demonstrate the sclerotic, narrowed, and sometimes fragmented navicular bone (Figure 13.25) (17,42). Treatment involves a 4–12-wk period of immobilization in either a walking boot or short leg cast. Weight bearing is allowed. The condition is self-limiting, and the goal of treatment is symptom resolution (50,51). Radiographic healing can take 6–12 mo or longer.

Freiberg's infarction most commonly involves the second metatarsal head. Typically, the condition affects adolescent females in the second decade of life (17,25,42,51). Tenderness is localized over the metatarsal head involved. Swelling is present, and range of motion at the MTP joint limited. Early in the condition, the radiographic findings may be subtle and only show some flattening of the metatarsal head (Figure 13.26) or slight sclerosis in the bone. Later, there is further sclerosis, fragmentation, and narrowing of the MTP joint. Prompt diagnosis is important to try to preserve the structure of the metatarsal head and the MTP joint function (42). Initial treatment involves a walking boot or short leg cast with a toe plate to reduce pain. Weight bearing is allowed, but activities must stay below the level of discomfort. Patients are transitioned to a stiff last orthosis to limit motion of the metatarsal head. Surgery is reserved for those with persistent symptoms or presenting late in the disease course (25,42,50).

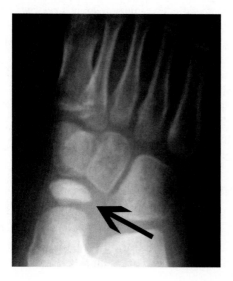

FIGURE 13.25. Kohler's disease of the navicular.

FIGURE 13.26. Freiberg's infarction of the 2nd metatarsal head.

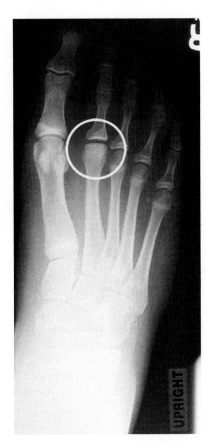

Flat Feet

Flat feet (pes planus) are common in young athletes. The arch of the foot is primarily formed and stabilized by the bones and ligaments (42,51). A "flat" foot refers to a loss of the normal longitudinal arch of the foot (Figure 13.27). The condition is universal in children under the age of three yr and relates to ligamentous laxity through the foot and interposition of fat in the arch (42,51). Children can "develop" an arch up through the age of 6 yr (52,53). The condition is more common in individuals with ligamentous laxity. Expensive shoes and orthotics will not influence the development of an arch (51,52). Flat feet have been associated with conditions such as medial tibial stress syndrome, lower leg stress fractures, and knee pain. The critical aspect of the examination is to determine if the foot is flexible or rigid. A flexible flat foot forms an arch when non–weight bearing and when completing a toe raise (Figure 13.28). Gross inspection of the patient weight

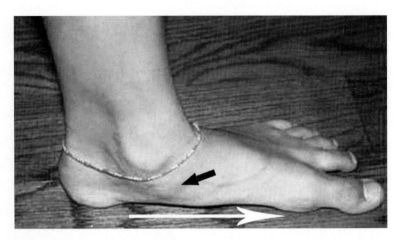

FIGURE 13.27. Moderate relaxed flat foot deformity with no arch (white arrow) and talar head sag (black arrow).

bearing can determine the severity of the flat foot. A valgus deformity of the hind foot in combination with a flat foot is termed a "planovalgus" foot. With toe raise, the hind foot should move into neutral or varus (Figure 13.28). The medial border of the foot is observed for the degree of talar head sag (Figure 13.27). As the medial border of the foot becomes more

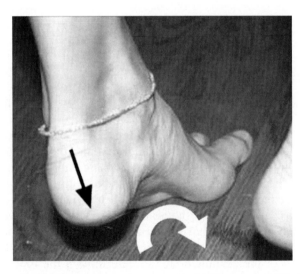

FIGURE 13.28. Normal foot motion with toe raise–hindfoot varus (black arrow) and arch formation (white arrow).

prominent with severe deformities, the lateral border of the foot will appear more concave in contour. Subtalar and midfoot motion should be assessed to rule out a tarsal coalition. Standard radiographs are obtained in patients with painful or rigid flat feet. Weight bearing films demonstrate the true functional and anatomic relationship.

The patient with a painless, flexible flat foot does not need any treatment. Supportive shoes are encouraged, with the hope of preventing any foot pain in the future. Flexibility in the calf and plantar fascia may be helpful. Intervention is warranted for the athlete with painful, flexible, flat feet. An over-the-counter mid- or full-length semirigid foot orthosis can be helpful, and is an inexpensive first-tier treatment. Associated weakness, tendonitis, and poor flexibility must be addressed. Severe flat foot with pain or a rigid flat foot requires surgical referral. Surgery for severe flexible flat foot is rarely considered for individuals before skeletal maturity (51,52).

Tarsal Coalition

Tarsal coalition is a condition in which two or more of the tarsal bones develop together or fail to separate. This connection can be cartilage, fibrous tissue, or bone. The condition is bilateral in approximately 50% of patients (17,42,51). Most coalitions involve the calcaneus and the navicular (calcaneonavicular) and the talus and calcaneus (talocalcaneal) (12,13,51). The etiology of the coalition is unknown. A failed differentiation of mesenchymal tissue has been proposed (51,54). The coalition limits the normal subtalar motion. Pain often develops in the second decade of life, corresponding with sport-related demands, increased body weight, and the period when the coalition typically ossifies (42,54). Participation in sports involving running, jumping, and cutting place a tremendous stress on the subtalar complex. Tarsal coalition should be considered with recurrent ankle sprains or foot/ankle pain seen with flat feet; it is often associated with rigid or stiff flat feet. Thus, motion in the hind foot and subtalar joint is limited. The arch will not be present with toe raise, and the athlete is unable to walk on the lateral border of the foot. Pain is typically nonspecific and diffuse through the hind and midfoot. Peroneal and calf muscle tightness may be present. Standard three-view radiographs demonstrate the calcaneal-navicular coalition best on the oblique projection (Figure 13.29). The lateral view may demonstrate the elongation of the talar head, the so-called "anteater" sign (Figure 13.30) (51). The talocalcaneal coalition is more difficult to appreciate on standard radiographs, except for early degenerative changes throughout the foot related to the abnormal biomechanics. When radiographs fail to demonstrate the coalition, further investigation is warranted. Both CT and MRI have advantages (17,42,51). CT can best detect bony coalitions, particularly talocalcaneal bridges (Figure 13.31), but MRI is superior in detecting fibrous or cartilaginous connections.

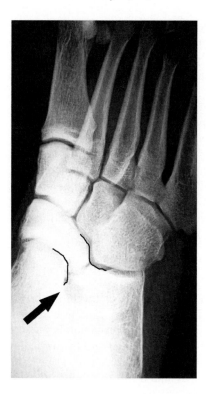

FIGURE 13.29. Oblique projection of the foot demonstrating a calcanealnavicular bar.

Nonoperative measures should be attempted to reduce pain and allow sports participation. Immobilization in a short-leg cast or walking boot can be utilized to reduce pain. Physical therapy can address associated muscle tightness or weakness. A custom foot orthosis and ankle support orthotic can be used to support the ankle and subtalar complex. Referral is war-

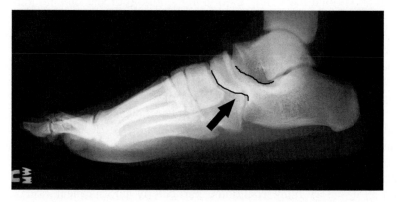

FIGURE 13.30. Lateral projection of the foot demonstrating a calcanealnavicular bar (the anteater sign).

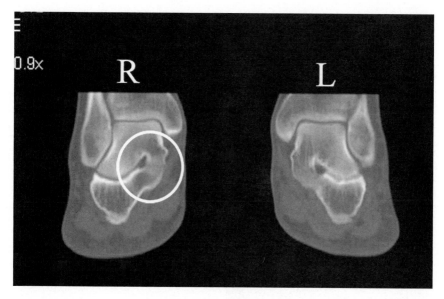

FIGURE 13.31. CT of the foot demonstrating a bilateral talocalcaneal bar (right circled).

ranted for athletes with continued symptoms. Surgery typically involves bar resection and fat or other soft tissue interposition (42).

Accessory Bones of the Foot

Young athletes with a symptomatic accessory navicular bone present with pain along the medial aspect of the foot. Pain is often gradual in onset with no known preceding trauma. Weight gain, arch collapse, sports participation, injuries, or narrow shoe wear may all aggravate the condition. Accessory navicular bones are frequently bilateral, which can help if there is trauma and question of a fracture. A tender prominence is noted in the proximal medial arch. Swelling and redness may be present. Resisted inversion and a single-leg toe raise are often painful because of posterior tibialis inflammation. Radiographs are diagnostic, and the accessory bone is best appreciated on the AP or oblique view (Figure 13.32). Nonoperative treatment includes relative rest, ice, and antiinflammatory medications. Shoe wear or orthotics with a supportive medial wedge may help. Restrictive or tight shoes are discouraged. A brief period of immobilization in a cast or walking boot may be required to settle down the pain and inflammation. Adults with the condition rarely have symptoms (51). Surgery is reserved

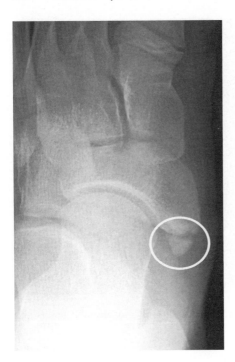

FIGURE 13.32. Accessory navicular bone.

for patients with continued symptoms. Removal of the accessory bone and, in some cases, advancement of the posterior tibialis tendon to the remaining navicular bone is the standard surgical management (51).

The os trigonum is the most common accessory bone in the foot. This ossicle forms at the posterior aspect of the talus and ossifies early in the second decade of life. These bones can become symptomatic in athletes who participate in sports involving repetitive ankle plantarflexion or inversion (i.e., ballet, gymnastics, dance, and soccer). The pain often is a result of overuse-related mechanical posterior ankle impingement. This impingement can be bony or soft tissue related. The diagnosis is difficult because many structures can cause pain in the posterior ankle (i.e., peroneal tendons, flexor hallucis longus, Achilles tendon, retrocalcaneal bursa, etc.) and because the unfused os trigonum can be seen in up to 10% of the general population. The athlete presents with posterior ankle pain that is worse with maximal ankle plantarflexion. Direct or medial/lateral compression tenderness may be elicited. Drawer testing may show instability creating the specific symptoms. The lateral radiograph will demonstrate the bony ossicle posterior to the talus (Figure 13.18). A lateral view with the ankle in maximal plantarflexion may demonstrate impingement. Treatment involves avoidance of pain-producing positions, cryotherapy, and an anti-inflammatory. Immobilization may be necessary initially in a walking boot or ankle-stabilizing orthotic. The athlete may not be able to return to optimal participation without surgical resection of the bony fragment.

Adolescent Bunion

Adolescent bunion (also known as juvenile hallux valgus) primarily affects adolescent females. The term "adolescent" bunion infers the growth centers of the foot are still open (51). In some cases, there is a familial pattern to the disorder. The adolescent may present because of pain, difficulty with shoe wear, or simply cosmetic concerns. Young athletes with a problematic bunion are often involved in sports that require narrow and firm shoe wear or repetitive foot movements, such as soccer, cheerleading, and dance. For young ballet dancers going on point, hallux valgus may be particularly bothersome. The deformity varies in severity. Soft tissue and bursa inflammation develop over the medial prominence. MTP motion is usually full, but rotation causes "pinch" calluses and an abnormal arc of motion. Radiographic evaluation involves weight bearing AP and lateral projections (Figure 13.33). The intermetatarsal (IMT) angle and MTP angle are

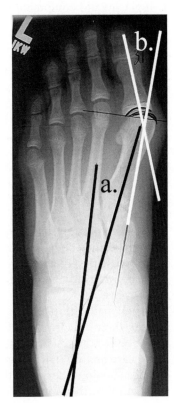

FIGURE 13.33. Adolescent bunion deformity. The IMT angle (a) and metatarsophalangeal angle (b) are labeled.

calculated (51). The IMT angle is normally less than 10 degrees and MTP angle less than 15 degrees. Subluxation of the proximal phalanx on the 1st metatarsal head is a worrisome sign for further progression (51).

Treatment of the condition depends on the severity of the deformity and the age of the child. Milder cases respond to proper shoe wear with medial support and a wide toe box. A stiffer last can help limit motion and pain at the joint. Surgery is reserved for intractable pain, increased deformity, or pain interfering with lifestyle activities in skeletally mature individuals (13). There is an increased recurrence rate compared to adults.

Prevention of Foot and Ankle Injuries

Prevention of foot and ankle injuries can be divided into external influences and internal influences. External influences include:

1. a quality pre-participation exam,
2. having individuals "walk the field" before practices or games to note uneven playing surfaces or debris on playing fields,
3. proper protection and shoe wear (i.e., shin guards),
4. replacing old equipment (i.e., running shoes every 300–500 miles),
5. athletic taping and supportive brace wear,
6. and avoiding dangerous recreation equipment (i.e., trampolines).

Of note, most studies have failed to demonstrate a protective benefit of ankle taping or bracing unless a prior injury has occurred (55). Also, high-top shoes versus low-top shoes have not been found to reduce ankle injuries (25). Intervention strategies to decrease ankle injuries have been reported in the literature with some success (3,56–60). These programs have focused on various braces or taping, as well as tasks such as a structured warm-up, balance training, and practicing cutting, jumping, and landing to improve strength, flexibility, and neuromuscular control.

Internal influences include items such as:

1. overall fitness level and body weight. Elevated BMI (presumed elevated fat mass) has been linked to prolonged ankle morbidity after an injury and musculoskeletal surgical complications (61,62).
2. proper nutrition and healthy lifestyle behaviors.

The challenge with preventive strategies is standardizing these efforts and proving their effectiveness. Education plays a huge role in injury prevention. Young athletes, parents, and coaches should learn topics such as basic injury care and when it is important to seek medical attention. Parents and coaches should understand that if the athlete cannot complete the return to sport tasks, they may worsen the injury if allowed to participate.

Return to Play

Return to sports participation after an injury can be complicated. With acute injuries, the treating physician should be comfortable that the injury has healed sufficiently to begin weight bearing. Certain activities, such as batting or shooting baskets, may even be possible while in a walking boot or cast. When the athlete is ready, a removable splint or foot orthosis will allow physical therapy to improve range of motion and strength, and reduce edema. With certain injuries the athlete will need to work on proprioception as well. When the athlete is walking comfortably with routines of daily living, a prescribed functional return to sport protocol can commence. This is best detailed under the direct supervision of a certified athletic trainer, physical therapist, or physician. The athlete should not feel any "sharp" pain while advancing to more difficult tasks. A prototype progression is shown in Table 13.2. Typically, the athlete should advance as tolerated every 1–2 encounters. The athlete can perform non–sport-specific aerobic activity, such as swimming or stationary biking, before completing the functional task. This will increase blood flow to the extremity and help with cardiovascular endurance when the athlete is ready to return to sport. Directed physical therapy can be continued each day after completing the functional task. Mild discomfort is acceptable. If the symptoms resolve with ice and a night's rest, advancement can continue. If pain is increasing, the athlete should move back to the previous task and allow another 2–3 d before trying to advance again. It is common to have some mild soreness and swelling until the athlete is able to truly take a break from the particular activity. It is also common practice to utilize an ankle-stabilizing orthosis, athletic taping, or foot orthotic, depending on the specific problem for the duration of that particular athletic season to hopefully prevent re-injury. It may be possible for the athlete to advance to a less demanding player position sooner than his or her typical athletic position.

Clinical Pearls

- Remember that fractures to the growth center are more common than ankle "sprains" in young athletes, even with "normal" appearing radiographs.
- With any ankle injury, it is important not to overlook bony tenderness at the base of the fifth metatarsal and the proximal fibula, as associated fractures can be present.
- Ossification centers can be present on the medial malleolus (Figure 13.34), and lateral malleolus and should not be confused with fractures.
- The proximal great toe physis may be bipartite, resembling a Salter–Harris type 3 fracture (Figure 13.35). Clinical correlation is required.

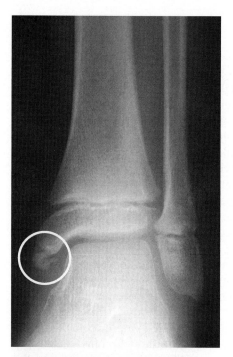

FIGURE 13.34. Medial malleolus ossification center.

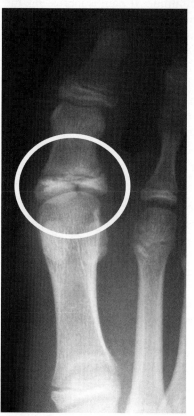

FIGURE 13.35. Bipartite proximal great toe physis.

FIGURE 13.36. Heterotopic ossification in the syndesmosis seen after a "high" sprain.

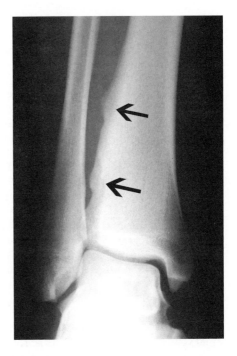

- Nail bed injuries associated with underlying distal phalanx fractures are considered open fractures requiring prophylactic antibiotics and close observation for osteomyelitis.
- The apophysis of the fifth metatarsal runs parallel to the shaft of the bone. Fractures are often oblique or perpendicular to the shaft.
- Flexible, flat feet that are nonpainful require no evaluation or treatment.
- Consider tarsal coalition in the young athlete with recurrent ankle "sprains".
- Consider conditions such as juvenile idiopathic arthritis in the young athlete with an ankle effusion or recurrent midfoot pain.
- The 1st metatarsal physis is proximal. All others are distal (Figure 13.4).
- Deltoid ligament sprains are usually associated with a significant ankle injury and rarely occur in isolation. The examiner should look closely for associated fractures.
- Heterotopic ossification may be present in the syndesmosis after a "high" ankle sprain (Figure 13.36).
- MRI, rather than bone scan, is utilized with localized tenderness in the evaluation of stress fractures.
- Care should be taken when splinting or casting the foot and ankle, especially in the first 1–2 d after the injury. Compartment syndrome is a potential complication of the injury or the cast/splint.

References

1. Hamilton WG. Surgical anatomy of the foot and ankle. 1985. In: Bean KJ, ed. Clinical Symposia. Volume 37, Number 3. Summit, New Jersey; CIBA-GEIGY Corporation; 1985:2–32.
2. Hamilton WG. Biomechanics of the foot and ankle. In: Lutter LD, Mizel MS, Pfeffer GB, eds. Orthopaedic Knowledge Update: Foot and Ankle. Rosemont, Il.: American Academy of Orthopaedic Surgeons; 1994:1–13.
3. DiGiovanni BF, Partal G, Baumhauer JF. Acute ankle injury and chronic lateral instability in the athlete. Clin Sports Med 2004;23:1–19.
4. Vander Griend RA, Savoie FH, Hughes JL. Soft Tissue Injuries of the Foot and Ankle. In: Lutter LD, Mizel MS, Pfeffer GB, eds. Orthopaedic Knowledge Update: Foot and Ankle. Rosemont, Il.: American Academy of Orthopaedic Surgeons; 1994:241–247.
5. Moore KL. The lower limb. In: Satterfield TS, ed. Clinically Oriented Anatomy. 3rd ed. Baltimore: Williams and Wilkins; 1992:432–495.
6. Rubin A. Ankle and foot anatomy. In: Sallis R, Massimino F, eds. ACSM's Essentials of Sports Medicine. St. Louis: Mosby; 1997:446–452.
7. Jahss, Melvin H. Examination of the foot and ankle. In: Jahss MH, ed. Disorders of the Foot and Ankle, Vol. 1. 2nd ed. Philadelphia: WB Saunders; 1991:35–48.
8. Crawford AH, Al-Sayyad MJ. Deformities of the first ray. In: Lutter LD, Mizel MS, Pfeffer GB, eds. Orthopaedic Knowledge Update: Foot and Ankle. Rosemont, Il.: American Academy of Orthopaedic Surgeons; 1994:141–162.
9. Jaffe WL, Gannon PJ, Laitman JT. Paleontology, embryology, and anatomy of the foot. In: Jahss MH, ed. Disorders of the Foot and Ankle, Vol. 1. 2nd ed. Philadelphia, PA: WB Saunders; 1991:11–34.
10. Crawford AH, Al-Sayyad MJ. Fractures and dislocations of the foot and ankle. In: Greene NE, Swiontkowski MF, eds. Skeletal Trauma in Children. 3rd ed. Philadelphia: Saunders; 2003:516–586.
11. McBryde AM. Ankle fractures in athletes. In: Sallis R, Massimino F, eds. ACSM's Essentials of Sports Medicine. St. Louis: Mosby; 1997:453–457.
13. Marsh JS, Daigneault JP. Ankle injuries in the pediatric population. Curr Opin Pediatr 2000;12:52–60.
13. Chambers HG. Ankle and foot disorders in skeletally immature athletes. Orthop Clin North Am 2003;34:445–459.
14. Kay RM, Tang CW. Pediatric foot fractures: evaluation and treatment. J Am Acad Orthop Surg 2001;9:308–319.
15. Heckman JD. Fractures and dislocations of the foot. In: Rockwood CA, Green DP, Bucholz RW, eds. Rockwood and Green's Fractures in Adults. 3rd ed. Philadelphia: JB Lippencott Co.; 1991:2041–2082.
16. Richardson EG. Foot and ankle: an overview. In: Greene W, ed. Essentials of Musculoskeletal Care. 2nd ed. Rosemont, Il.: American Academy of Orthopaedic Surgeons; 2001:408–486.
17. Pommering TL, Kluchursky L, Hall SL. Ankle and foot injuries in pediatric and adult athletes. Primary Care: Clinics in Office Practice. 2005;32:133–161.
18. Stiell IG, McKnight RD, Greenberg GH, et al. Implementation of the Ottawa ankle rules. JAMA 1994;271(11):827–832.

19. Leddy JJ, Smolinski RJ, Lawrence J, Snyder JL, Priore RL. Prospective Evaluation of the Ottawa Ankle Rules in a University Sports Medicine Center. Am J Sports Med 1998;26:158–165.
20. Plint AC, Bullock B, Osmond MH, et al. Validation of the Ottawa ankle rules in children with ankle injuries. Acad Emerg Med 1999;6(10):1005–1009.
21. Simons S. Rehabilitation of ankle injuries. In: Sallis R, Massimino F, eds. ACSM's Essentials of Sports Medicine. St. Louis: Mosby; 1997:458–462.
22. Vander Griend RA, Savoie FH, Hughes JL. Fractures of the ankle. In: Rockwood CA, Green DP, Bucholz RW, eds. Rockwood and Green's Fractures in Adults. 3rd ed. Philadelphia: JB Lippencott Co.; 1991:1983–2040.
23. Nussbaum E, Hosea TM, Gatt CD. Managing "high" ankle sprains. J Musculoskelet Med 2004:621–630.
24. Uys HD, Riijke AM. Clinical Association of Acute Lateral Ankle Sprain with Syndesmotic Involvement: A stress radiography and magnetic resonance imaging study. Am J Sports Med 2002;30(6):816–822.
25. Richardson GE. Leg, foot, and ankle. In: Miller MD, Cooper DP, Warner JJP, eds. Review of Sports Medicine and Arthroscopy. 2nd ed. Philadelphia: WB Saunders Co.; 2002:78–113.
26. Chambers HG. Fractures of the ankle. In: Lutter LD, Mizel MS, Pfeffer GB, eds. Orthopaedic Knowledge Update: Foot and Ankle. Rosemont, Il.: American Academy of Orthopaedic Surgeons; 1994:193–197.
27. DiGiovanni BF, Partal G, Baumhauer JF. Injuries to the Midfoot and Forefoot. In: Lutter LD, Mizel MS, Pfeffer GB, eds. Orthopaedic Knowledge Update: Foot and Ankle. Rosemont, Il.: American Academy of Orthopaedic Surgeons; 1994:259–262.
28. Mologne TS, Lundeen JM, Clapper MF, O'Brien TJ. Early screw fixation versus casting in the treatment of acute Jones fractures. Am J Sports Med 2005; 33(7):970–975.
29. Reese K, Litsky A, Kaeding C, Pedroaza A, Shah N. Cannulated screw fixation of Jones fractures: a clinical and biomechanical study. Am J Sports Med 2004;32(7):1736–1742.
30. Wright RW, Fischer DA, Shively RA, Heidt RS, Jr., Nuber GW. Refracture of proximal fifth metatarsal (Jones) fracture after intramedullary screw fixation in athletes. Am J Sports Med 2000;28(5):732–736.
31. Mantas JP, Burks RT. Lisfranc injuries in the athlete. Clin Sports Med 1994;13(4):719–730.
32. Nunley JA, Vertullo CJ. Classification, investigation, and management of midfoot sprains: Lisfranc injuries in the athlete. Am J Sports Med 2002;30(6): 871–878.
33. Mullen JE, O'Malley MJ. Sprains: Residual Instability of subtalar, lisfranc joints, and turf toe. Clin Sports Med 2004;23:97–121.
34. Thompson MC, Matthew MA. Injury to the tarsometatarsal joint complex. J Am Acad Orthop Surg 2003;11:260–267.
35. Thompson MC, Mormino MA. Foot and ankle injuries. In: Garrick JG, Webb DR, eds. Sports Injuries: Diagnosis and Management. 2nd ed. Philadelphia: WB Saunders Co.; 1999:358–403.
36. Strauss JE, Lippert FG. Chronic lateral ankle instability: incidence of associated conditions and rational for treatment. Presented at the American Academy of Orthopaedic Surgeons 72nd Annual Meeting. 2005. Feb 23–27. Washington, DC.

37. Lebrun CT, Krause JO. Variations in mortise anatomy. Am J Sports Med 2005;33(6):852–855.
38. Schachter AK, Chen AL, Reddy PD, Tejwani NC. Osteochondral Lesions of the Talus. J Am Acad Orthop Surg 2005;13:152–158.
39. Vincent KA. Arthroscopy. In: Lutter LD, Mizel MS, Pfeffer GB, eds. Orthopaedic Knowledge Update: Foot and Ankle. Rosemont, Il.: American Academy of Orthopaedic Surgeons; 1994:65–67.
40. Berndt AL, Harty M. Transchondral fractures (osteochondritis dissecans) of the talus. J Bone Joint Surg Am 1959;41:988–1020.
41. Mintz DN, Tashjian GS, Connell DA, Deland JT, O'Malley M, Potter HG. Osteochondral lesions of the talus: a new magnetic resonance grading system with arthroscopic correlation. Arthroscopy 2003;19(4):353–359.
42. Tachdjian MO. The foot and ankle. In: Greenfield S, ed. Clinical Pediatric Orthopaedics: The Art of Diagnosis and Principles of Management. Stamford, CT: Appleton & Lange; 1997:1–85.
43. Philbin, TM, Lee, TH, Berlet, GC. Arthroscopy for Athletic Foot and Ankle Injuries. Clin Sports Med. 2004;23:35–53.
44. Tuan K, Wu S, Sennett B. Stress Fractures in Athletes: Risk Factors, Diagnosis, and Management. Orthopaedics. 2004;27:583.
45. Korpelainen R. Risk Factors for Recurrent Stress Fractures in Athletes. Am J Sports Med 2001;29(3):304–310.
46. Kelly AW, Hame SL. Managing stress fractures in athletes: The goal of diagnosis and treatment is speedy return to play. J Musculoskelet Med 2005; 22:463–472.
47. Harmon KG. Lower extremity stress fractures. Clin J Sports Med 2003; 13(6):358–364.
48. Dabners LE, Mullis BH. Effects of nonsteroidal anti-inflammatory drugs on bone formation and soft-tissue healing. J Am Acad Orthop Surg 2004;12:139–143.
49. Ogden JA. Sever's injury: a stress fracture of the immature calcaneal metaphysis. J Pediatr Orthop 2004;24(5):488–492.
50. Omey M, Micheli LJ. Foot and ankle problems in the young athlete. Med Sci Sports Exer 1999;S470–S486.
51. Sullivan JA. The child's foot. In: Morrissy RT, Weinstein SL, eds. Lovell and Winter's Pediatric Orthopaedics. 4th ed. Philadelphia: Lippincott-Raven Publishers; 1996:1077–1135.
52. Sullivan JA. Pediatric flatfoot: evaluation and management. J Am Acad Orthop Surg 1999;7:44–53.
53. Staheli LT, Chew DE, Corbett M. The longitudinal arch: a survey of eight hundred and eighty-two feet in normal children and adults. J Bone Joint Surg Am. 1987;69A:426–428.
54. Vincent KA. Tarsal coalition and painful flatfoot. J Am Acad Orthop Surg 1998;6:274–281.
55. Arnold BL, Docherty CL. Bracing and rehabilitation: what's new? Clin Sports Med 2004;23:83–95.
56. Ubell ML. The effect of ankle braces on the prevention of dynamic forced ankle inversion. Am J Sports Med 2003;31(6):935–940.
57. Verhagen E, Van der Beek A, Twist J, Bouter L, Bahr R, Van Mechelen W. The effect of a proprioceptive balance board training program for the prevention of ankle sprains: a prospective controlled trial. Am J Sports Med 2004; 32(6):1385–1393.

58. Olsen OE, Myklebust G, Engebretsen L, Holme I, Bahr R. Exercises to prevent lower limb injuries in youth sports: cluster randomized controlled trial. Br J Med 2005;330(7489):449.
59. Emery CA, Cassidy JD, Klassen TP, Rosychuk RJ, Rowe BH. Effectiveness of a home-based balance training program in reducing sports related injuries among healthy adolescents: a cluster randomized controlled trial. Can Med Assoc J 2005;172(6).
60. McGuine TA. The effect of a balance training program on prevention of ankle sprains in high school athletes: a prospective randomized controlled intervention study. Presented at the American Orthopaedic Society for Sports Medicine Annual Meeting. 2005. July 14–17. Keystone, CO.
61. Timm NL. Chronic ankle morbidity in obese children following an acute ankle injury. Arch Pediatr Adolesc Medi 2005;159:33–36.
62. Leet AL, Pichard CP, Ain MC. Surgical treatment of femoral fractures in obese children: does excessive body weight increase the rate of complications? J Bone Joint Surg Am 2005;87-A:2609–2613.

Appendices

Appendices

Appendix 1
Sports and Children: Consensus Statement on Organized Sports for Children

FIMS/WHO Ad Hoc Committee on Sports and Children

For children, regular physical activity and sport, together with a balanced diet, are essential to promote optimal growth and maturation and to develop sufficient physical fitness and mental vigour. The psychological and social benefits of regular physical activity help in coping with stress and anxiety, counterbalance the burden and symptoms of quiet sitting and mental concentration, and have a favourable influence on self-image and social relations. Participation in a variety of sports and exercises at a young age is important also for acquiring the necessary skills and experience to maintain regular exercise throughout life.

While children have participated in spontaneous sport and games since the dawn of recorded history, the organization by adults of competitive sports for children and adolescents is relatively recent. This development, however, has now spread worldwide and encompasses both developed and developing countries.

Although the overall goal of the International Federation of Sports Medicine (FIMS) and World Health Organization (WHO) is to encourage all children and young people, including the disabled, to become involved in regular physical activity, the present statement focuses on the benefits and risks of organized sport for children, as one element of physical activity. Its specific purpose is to encourage sports governing bodies, health professionals, parents, coaches, and trainers to take opportune action to ensure the health and well-being of child athletes.

This statement focuses exclusively on competitive sports for children and adolescents within organized sports settings (clubs/associations), including schools.

Benefits of Organized Sports for Children

In the organized sports setting it is possible to manage the amount of exercise taken by children and adolescents as well as the circumstances under which the exercise is administered. Sports-associated illness or injury can thus be minimized. Properly structured, organized sports for children can offer an opportunity for enjoyment and safe participation by all healthy children regardless of age, sex or level of economic development, as well as those with disabilities or chronic diseases.

The potential benefits of organized sport for children and adolescents include improvement of health, enhancement of normal physical and social growth and maturation, as well as improvement of their motor skills and physical fitness, both health-related fitness and sports-specific fitness, particularly for those who are physically and mentally challenged. In addition, organized sports competitions for children: and adolescents can, if properly structured, play an important role in socialization, self-esteem, and self-perception, as well as improving psychological well-being. Organized sports can also establish the basis for a healthy lifestyle and lifelong commitment to physical activity.

Risks of Organized Sports for Children

The potential risks of organized sports include increased occurrence of illness or injury. At present, there is no clear evidence that the risk of acute traumatic injuries is greater in the organized sports setting than in similar exposures in free play activities. On the other hand, the potential for overuse injuries resulting from repetitive microtrauma appears to be specific to children participating in organized sports activities. Overuse injuries are very rare in children who participate in free play or uncontrolled sports activities.

There is also a potential for special catastrophic injuries among children who participate in organized sports, e.g. cardiac arrest following chest wall impact, as well as head and neck injuries. Organization of children's sports activity by adults does have the potential for abuses to occur if those who set the amount of sports participation and the training regimen are inexperienced and use adult models. Concerns have been raised about the potential for excessive amounts of training and/or abnormal nutritional habits or unhealthy dietetic manipulation in the organized sports setting to interfere with normal growth and maturation of children and also to foster development of osteoporosis. There is also the potential for risk of interference with overall health-related fitness by excessive emphasis on sport-specific training. Similarly, examples of pathological socialization or psychopathology, such as excessive anxiety or excessive stress, have been noted among children and adolescents who participate in organized sports. Also, there is growing evidence that excessive, violent, and intensive training may increase the rate of overuse and of catastrophic injuries Fortunately, the organized sports setting can decrease the rate or severity of such injuries by providing the opportunity for monitoring their risk factors and reducing them through rule changes, protective equipment, and alterations in technique or duration of play.

Recommendations

Although organized sports for children are of increasing importance, the growth of organized sports should not be at the expense of physical education or general fitness activities, particularly those in which the family can be involved. Children worldwide must be given equal opportunities to participate in sports, regardless of age, sex, level of skill or economic status.

The specific recommendations shown below were made.

Sports Governing Bodies

- The following obligations apply to sports governing bodies:
  - they should be directly responsible for the safety and training of young athletes engaged in their particular sports;
  - they should institute systems to monitor the level of intensity and categories of competition in their sports;
  - they should be responsible for preparing and maintaining statistics of illness and injury for children and adolescents participating in their sports;
  - they should be responsible for certifying the credentials of coaches for this age level (including direct participation in coaching education, certification, and a reasonable assessment of the ethical and moral character of their coaches);
  - they should have the responsibility to determine standards for protective equipment, playing fields, and duration of competition appropriate for children; and
  - they should formulate the appropriate legislation related to organized sports for children.

Youth Sports Coaches

- Coaches should:
  - participate in special education programmes; and
  - have credentials that encompass the techniques and skills of youth sports; the specific safety risks of children's sports; the psychology and sociology of children and adolescents; and the physiology of growth and development related to physical activity during childhood and adolescence, as well as common medical related issues.

Health Professionals

- Health professionals should take steps to improve their knowledge and understanding of the organized sports environment as well as the risk factors and safety factors inherent to this type of sports participation.

- Physicians should monitor the health and safety of children involved in organized sports whenever possible, in particular those involved in elite sports training.

Sports Training

- Sports training for children and adolescents encompasses the age range from 5–18 years. In the early stages of training, every emphasis should be placed on broad-based participation opportunities to enhance general motor development.
- Sports specialization should be avoided before the age of 10 years.
- During specialized training, there should be careful monitoring of the nutritional status of young athletes. In particular, care should be taken to ensure that child athletes are given adequate diets for the high-energy demands of sports. In addition, every effort should be made to avoid marginal dietary practices, in particular caloric deprivation to delay maturation of physical development during sports training. Such dietetic manipulations must be viewed as a form of child abuse.
- Special attention should be paid to the volume and intensity of sports training of children and adolescents.

Parents

- The Ad Hoc Committee stresses the importance and responsibility of parental participation in the education process concerning the benefits and risks of sports training in childhood.
- Parents must increase their knowledge and awareness of the benefits and risks of competitive sport.
- Parents must be active participants in the process of coaching and training of their children in sports.

Research

- More research is needed to identify the specific benefits and risks of organized sport for children. This information is essential to maximize the benefits, while minimizing the risks that children may incur in organized sports.

Members of the Ad Hoc Committee

Professor Lyle J. Micheli, Chair, Education Commission, International Federation of Sports Medicine, Division of Sports Medicine, Children's Hospital, 300 Longwood Ave, Boston MA 02115, USA

Professor Neil Armstrong, Children's Health and Exercise Research Centre, University of Exeter, UK

Professor Oded Bar-Or, Children's Exercise and Nutrition Centre, McMaster University, Canada

Professor Colin Boreham, Department of Sport and Leisure Studies, University of Ulster, UK

Professor Chan Kai-ming, Department of Orthopaedics and Traumatology, Chinese University of Hong Kong

Dr Roger Eston, School of Sport, Health and Physical Education Sciences, University of Wales, UK

Dr Andrew P Hills, School of Human Movement Studies, Queensland University of Technology, Australia

Dr Nicola Maffulli, Department of Orthopaedic Surgery, University of Aberdeen, UK

Professor Robert M Malina, Institute for the Study of Youth Sports, Michigan State University, USA

Dr Alan Nevill, Centre for Sport and Exercise Sciences, John Moores University, UK

Dr Thomas Rowland, Baystate Medical Center, USA

Professor Craig Sharp, School of Physical Education and Sport, Brunei University College, UK

Professor William D. Stanish, Division of Orthopedic Surgery, Canada

Dr Suzanne Tanner, Division of Orthopaedics, University of Alabama, USA

Appendix 2
Position Statement on Girls and Women in Sport

IOC Medical Commission, Working Group Women in Sport
Chair Dr. Patricia Sangenis

This statement was produced during the Congress "Women and Sport", Lleida, Spain, April 18–20, 2002. Directors of the Scientific Program: Dr. Francisco Biosca and Dr. Patricia Sangenis.

Authors:

Dr. Lyle Micheli: Director, Division of Sports Medicine, Boston Children's Hospital.

Associate Clinical Professor of Orthopaedic Surgery, Harvard Medical School. Vice President of the Fédération International de Médecine Sportive (FIMS). Past President (1990 -91) American College of Sports Medicine.

Dr. Angela Smith: Clinical Associate Professor of Orthopaedic Surgery, University of Pennsylvania Attending Faculty, The Sports Medicine and Performance Children's Hospital Philadelphia.

Chair of the Education Commission FIMS 2002–2005
Past President (2001–02) American College of Sports Medicine

Dr. Francisco Biosca:
Professor of Anatomy in the INEFC of Lleida
President of the Spanish Society of Sports Traumatology
Vice president of the European Society of Sports Traumatology

Dr. Patricia Sangenis; Director of the Institute Deporte y Salud Buenos Aires
Member of the Medical Commission of the IOC
Chair of the Working Group "Women in Sport" International Olympic Committee (IOC) Medical Commission
Member elected of the Executive Committee of FIMS 1998–2002
Fellow of the American College of Sports Medicine
With the collaboration of Mark Jenkins
Opportunities for girls and women to participate in sport have increased dramatically over the last quarter century. A generation ago, women competed in "ladylike" or "graceful" athletic endeavors such as tennis, diving, figure-skating, and gymnastics. Today they also engage in a wide variety of

sports once considered the preserve of boys and men. Rugby and weightlifting are just two of the traditionally male sports in which women now compete ardently for world titles.

It is the position of the IOC Medical Commission that sport is for everyone. Girls and women should not be excluded from participation in athletic activity because of their gender. As with sports participation for all populations, the benefits for girls and women far outweigh any possible risks. The IOC Medical Commission encourages efforts to understand any possible special concerns of female athletes in order to develop and implement measures to reduce these athletes' injuries and enhance the quality of their participation.

Benefits of Sports Participation

The benefits of vigorous physical activity are well-understood, and have important implications for female participants. These benefits include physical and psychosocial components.

Physical Benefits

- Reduced risk of illnesses such as heart disease, hypertension, diabetes, and endometrial and breast cancer
- Improved muscle-to-fat ratio/body composition
- Stronger immune system with moderate physical activity
- Less menstrual discomfort
- Stronger bones and reduced risk of developing osteoporosis later in life

Psvchosocial Benefits

- Improved self-esteem, self-confidence, and perception of competence; better performance in academic settings
- Decreased risk of unwanted pregnancy
- Decreased risk of drug and alcohol abuse

Risks of Sports Participation

As with any competitive activity requiring strength, endurance, and daring, sport carries with it the risk of physical harm. It bears repeating, however, that the benefits of sport outweigh the risks. Put another way—given the perils of a sedentary lifestyle, which include a variety of chronic illnesses, the consequences of physical *inactivity* outweigh possible hazards involved in sports participation.

The two most common questions asked about the participation of girls and women in sports are:

- Are girls/women at greater risk of certain types of injuries?
- Do girls/women get injured more often?

"Female" Injuries?

Gender-specific injuries are rare, and concerns about female participation in sports are outdated and erroneous.

The female reproductive organs are better protected from serious athletic injury than the male organs. Serious sports injuries to the uterus or ovaries are extremely rare. Breast injuries, a commonly heard argument against girls' participation in vigorous sports, are among the rarest of all sports injuries, even when women play a full-contact sport such as rugby.

More Injuries?

Acute injuries are caused by sudden trauma such as impact or a twist. Common acute sports injuries include bone fractures, ligament sprains, and muscle strains and contusions. Girls and women are not generally at greater risk of sustaining "acute" injuries compared to their male athlete counterparts. One exception may be anterior cruciate ligament (ACL) injuries.

Studies show that adolescent and college-aged female athletes—especially soccer and basketball players—are three to four times more likely to sustain an ACL injury than their male counterparts. The reasons for this are not fully understood, but are thought to encompass a complex combination of intrinsic and extrinsic risk factors, possibly including anatomical, hormonal, and conditioning differences. Some measures to reduce the number of ACL injuries in female athletes include: 1) strengthening the leg muscles that stabilize the knee, especially the hamstrings; 2) improving aerobic conditioning to prevent fatigue-related missteps; 3) modifying the usual "cutting," or "side-stepping," maneuver from a two-step to a three-step motion so the knee is never fully extended; 4) performing sports that involve running and pivoting with the weight forward on the balls of the feet, emphasizing soft jump landings; and 5) educating coaches about the increased risk of ACL injuries in female athletes and enhancing the ability of coaches to evaluate female athletes' skills, conditioning, and readiness to participate.

Overuse injuries are caused by repetitive microtrauma to tissue. Common overuse injuries include stress fractures, tendonitis, and bursitis. Female athletes may be more susceptible to overuse sports injuries. Two apparent reasons for this are a lack of long-term preparation for vigorous sports training and not beginning sports training until the height of the growth spurt (typically between eleven and thirteen), a time when musculoskeletal injury incidence is generally greater for all children. The wider female pelvis and greater angulation of the female knee are related to increased incidence of kneecap problems, compared with boys/men. A rapid increase in training volume is the most frequent cause of overuse injuries, so it is important for girls and women beginning a sports or exercise program to only gradually increase the frequency, intensity, and/or duration of their activity regimen, especially if they have not been particularly active since early childhood.

Female athletes may be at a higher risk of stress fractures. The term "Female Athlete Triad" was coined to describe the most common chain of events leading to this type of injury:

1) Intense training plus disordered eating contribute to **menstrual abnormalities**, particularly when nutritional intake is insufficient to meet the energy needed for the training
2) menstrual abnormalities are associated with decrease of the estrogen needed to build bones, which, coupled with a poor diet may lead to osteoporosis or decreased bone mineral content; and,
3) weaker bones are vulnerable to stress **fractures** related to the athlete's training schedule.

The Female Athlete Triad is most frequently seen in endurance runners and those who participate in activities such as gymnastics, figure-skating, and dance—sports where leanness is considered a virtue and therefore where, regrettably, disordered eating is endemic. Treatment of the Female Athlete Triad should be multidisciplinary, as the athlete with this condition will benefit from the input of a sports psychologist and sports nutritionist familiar with the disorders as well as a sports medicine orthopedist and physiotherapist/athletic trainer.

The disproportionate incidence of overload injuries seen in female athletes may partly be a product of sociological factors that make girls' conditioning levels lower than boys'. As social attitudes change and girls begin to participate in sports and fitness activities regularly from a younger age, improved fitness levels should reduce this incidence. Additional gender-related risk factors include: "extrinsic" factors such as lack of knowledge on the part of coaches on appropriate training for girls and women, and "intrinsic" risk factors such as hormonal and tissue differences from boys/men, including but not limited to smaller bone architecture and different upper to lower body proportions in length and strength that appear throughout all populations and are not changed by training. Research into improved training methods for girls and women will continue to ameliorate discrepancies in injuries rates between the genders, though until then these discrepancies should not prevent or discourage female sports participation.

Recommendations to Minimize Injury Risk and Enhance Participation

Sport is becoming increasingly important in the lives of girls and women. The increasing number of competitive and recreational female athletes should be viewed positively. To perpetuate and accentuate the progress that has been made in this area in so many countries—and to inspire progress in countries where none has been made—the IOC Medical Commission makes the following recommendations:

Sports Governing Bodies

- should, in keeping with Rule 2, Paragraph 5 of the Olympic Charter, promote women in sport at all levels and in all structures, particularly in their executive bodies (including medical committees)
- should encourage the participation of girls and women in their particular sport
- should maintain injury and illness statistics pertaining to girls and women in their particular sport

Physical Educators, Coaches, and Other
Exercise and Health Professionals

- should take measures to improve their understanding of the special considerations of the female athlete
- should focus on helping young female athletes (5–18) develop a broad range of skills through exposure to a variety of sports; sports specialization before age 10 is not desirable
- should ensure that increases in training volume are not so great that they cause overuse Injury

Parents

- should encourage daughters to participate in sports and physical activity from a young age
- should increase their understanding of the benefits and risks of sports for girls and women
- should regularly remind themselves that the most important reason children play sports is for *fun*

Research

- should focus on gathering epidemiological data on injury rates in order to develop effective injury prevention strategies

Sources

FIMS/WHO Ad Hoc Committee on Sports and Children—Micheli LJ (Chair), Armstrong N, Bar-Or O, Boreham C, Chan K, Eston R, Hills AP, Maffulli N, Malina RM, Nair NVK, Nevill A, Rowland T, Sharp C, Stanish WD, Tanner S. Sports and children:
   Consensus statement on organized sports for children. Bulletin of the World Health Organization. 1998; 76(5):445–447.
   Clinics in Sports Medicine (The Young Athlete) Vol 19, No.4, 2000.
   U.S. Department of Health and Human Services. The Surgeon General's call to action to prevent and decrease overweight and obesity. (2001) Rockville, MD: U.S. Department of Health and Human Services, Public

Health Service, Office of the Surgeon General; Available from: US GPO, Washington.

The President's Council on Physical Fitness and Sports Report—Physical Activity & Sport in the Lives of Young Girls: Physical & Mental Health Dimensions from an Interdisciplinary Approach .. (1997). Washington DC: President's Council on Physical Fitness and Sports.

Wein D, Micheli LJ. Nutrition, Eating Disorders, & The Female Athlete Triad. In: Mostofsky DL, Zaichkowsky LD, eds. Medical and Psychological Aspects of Sport and Exercise. Morgantown, WV: Fitness Information Technology, Inc. 2002: 91–102.

Tofler IR, Stryer BK, Micheli LJ, Herman LR. Physical and emotional problems of elite female gymnasts. New Engl J Med. 1996; 335(4):281–283.

Omey ML, Micheli LJ, Gerbino PG 2nd. Idiopathic scoliosis and spondylolysis in the female athlete. Tips for treatment. Clin Orthop. 2000; (372):74–84.

Micheli LJ, Metzl JD, Di Canzio J, Zurakowski D. Anterior cruciate ligament reconstruction surgery in adolescent soccer and basketball players. Clin J Sport Med. 1999; 9(3):138–41.

The Encyclopaedia of Sports Medicine VIII Volume: Women in Sport. Edited by Barbara L. Drinkwater. An IOC Medical Commission Publication in collaboration with the International Federation of Sports Medicine.

Appendix 3
IOC Consensus Statement on Training the Elite Child Athlete

Protecting the health of the athlete is the primary goal of the International Olympic Committee's (IOC) Medical Commission. One of its main objectives is the promotion of safe practices in the training of the elite child athlete. The elite child athlete is one who has superior athletic talent undergoes specialised training, receives expert coaching and is exposed to early competition. Sport provides a positive environment that may enhance the physical growth and psychological development of children. This unique athlete population has distinct social, emotional and physical needs which vary depending on the athlete's particular stage of maturation. The elite child athlete requires appropriate training, coaching and competition that ensure a safe and healthy athletic career and promote future well-being. This document reviews the scientific basis of sports training in the child, the special challenges and unique features of training elite children and provides recommendations to parents, coaches, health care providers, sports governing bodies and significant other parties.

Scientific Basis of Training the Elite Child Athlete

Aerobic and anaerobic fitness and muscle strength increase with age, growth and maturation. Improvement in these variables is asynchronous. Children experience more marked improvements in anaerobic and strength performance than in aerobic performance during pubescence. Boys' aerobic and anaerobic fitness and muscle strength are higher than those of girls in late pre-pubescence, and the gender difference becomes more pronounced with advancing maturity. Evidence shows that muscle strength and aerobic and anaerobic fitness can be further enhanced with appropriately prescribed training. Regardless of the level of maturity, the relative responses of boys and girls are similar after adjusting for initial fitness.

An effective and safe strength training programme incorporates exercises for the major muscle groups with a balance between agonists and antagonists. The prescription includes a minimum of two to three sessions per week with three sets, at an intensity of between 50 to 85% of the one maximal repetition (1RM).

An optimal aerobic training programme incorporates continuous and interval exercises involving large muscle groups. The prescription recommends three to four, 40 to 60 minute sessions per week at an intensity of 85 to 90% of maximum heart rate (HRM).

An appropriate anaerobic training programme incorporates high intensity interval training of short duration. The prescription includes exercise at an intensity above 90% HRM and of less than 30 seconds duration to take into account children's relatively faster recovery following high intensity exercise.

A comprehensive psychological programme includes the training of psychological skills such as motivation, self-confidence, emotional control and concentration. The prescription applies strategies in goal-setting, emotional, cognitive and behavioural control fostering a positive self-concept in a healthy motivational climate.

Nutrition provided by a balanced, varied and sustainable diet makes a positive difference in an elite young athlete's ability to train and compete, and will contribute to optimal lifetime health. Adequate hydration is essential. Nutrition requirements vary as a function of age, gender, pubertal status, event, training regime, and the time of the competitive season. The nutrition prescription includes adequate hydration and individualises total energy, macro- and micro-nutrient needs and balance.

With advancing levels of maturity and competitiveness, physiological and psychological training and nutrition should be sport-specific with reference to competitive cycles. Confidential, periodic and sensitive evaluation of training and nutritional status should include anthropometric measures, sport-specific analyses and clinical assessment.

Special Issues in the Elite Child Athlete

Physical activity, of which sport is an important component, is essential for healthy growth and development.

The disparity in the rate of growth between bone and soft tissue places the child athlete at an enhanced risk of overuse injuries particularly at the apophyses, the articular cartilage and the physes (growth plates). Prolonged, focal pain may signal damage and must always be evaluated in a child.

Overtraining or "burnout" is the result of excessive training loads, psychological stress, poor periodisation or inadequate recovery. It may occur in the elite child athlete when the limits of optimal adaptation and performance are exceeded. Clearly, excessive pain should not be a component of the training regimen.

In girls, the pressure to meet unrealistic weight goals often lead s to the spectrum of disordered eating, including anorexia and/or bulimia nervosa. These disorders may affect the growth process, influence hormonal function, cause amenorrhoea, low bone mineral density and other serious illnesses which can be life-threatening.

There are differences in maturation in pubertal children of the same chronological age that may have unhealthy consequences in sport due to mismatching.

Elite child athletes deserve to train and compete in a suitable environment supported by a variety of age-appropriate technical and tactical training methods, rules, equipment, facilities and competitive formats.

Elite child athletes deserve to train and compete in a pleasurable environment, free from drug misuse and negative adult influences, including harassment and inappropriate pressure from parents, peers, health care providers, coaches, media, agents and significant other parties.

Recommendations for Training the Elite Child Athlete

The recommendations are that

- more scientific research be done to better identify the parameters of training the elite child athlete, which must be communicated effectively to the coach, athlete, parents, sport governing bodies and the scientific community
- the International Federations and National Sports Governing Bodies should:
  - develop illness and injury surveillance programmes
  - monitor the volume and intensity of training and competition regimens
  - ensure the quality of coaching and adult leadership
  - comply with the World Anti-Doping Code
- parents/guardians develop a strong support system to ensure a balanced lifestyle including proper nutrition, adequate sleep, academic development, psychological well-being and opportunities for socialisation
- coaches, parents, sports administrators, the media and other significant parties should limit the amount of training and competitive stress on the elite child athlete.

The entire sports process for the elite child athlete should be pleasurable and fulfilling.

Patrick Schamasch IOC Medical & Scientific Director
Susan Greinig IOC Medical Programs Director
Margo Mountjoy Chair
Lyle Micheli Program Consultant

Participants:
Neil Armstrong
Lucio Bizzini
Joe Blimkie
Janet Evans
David Gerrard
Jan Hangen
Serge Herman
Karin Knoll
Willem van Mechelen
Patricia Sangenis

Index